Child Neurology and
Developmental Disabilities

Child Neurology and Developmental Disabilities

Selected Proceedings of the Fourth International Child Neurology Congress

Senior Editors:

Joseph H. French, M.D.
Developmental Disabilities Center
State University of New York
Health Science Center at Brooklyn/
New York State Office of Mental Retardation
and Developmental Disabilities
Institute for Basic Research in Developmental Disabilities
New York

Shaul Harel, M.D.
Pediatric Neurology Unit and Child
Development Assessment Center
Tel Aviv Medical Center
Sackler Faculty of Medicine
Tel Aviv University
Tel Aviv

Paul Casaer, M.D., Ph.D.
University of Leuven
University Hospital Gasthuisberg
Leuven

Associate Editors:

Marvin I. Gottlieb, M.D., Ph.D.
Institute for Child Development
Hackensack Medical Center
University of Medicine and Dentistry of New Jersey
Hackensack

Isabelle Rapin, M.D.
Albert Einstein College of Medicine
Yeshiva University
New York

Darryl C. De Vivo, M.D.
Presbyterian Hospital
College of Physicians & Surgeons
Columbia University
New York

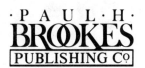

·P·A·U·L·H·
BROOKES
PUBLISHING Co

Baltimore · London · Sydney · Toronto

Paul H. Brookes Publishing Co.
Post Office Box 10624
Baltimore, Maryland 21285-0624

Typeset by the Composing Room, Grand Rapids, Michigan.
Manufactured in the United States of America by
The Maple Press Company, York, Pennsylvania.

Library of Congress Cataloging-in-Publication Data
International Child Neurology Congress (4th : 1986 : Jerusalem)
    Child neurology and developmental disabilities.

    Congress was held in Jerusalem, Mar. 16–20, 1986.
    Includes bibliographies and index.
    1. Pediatric neurology—Congresses.   2. Developmental disabilities—
Congresses. 3. Nervous system—Diseases—Pathophysiology—Congresses.   I.
French, Joseph.   II. Harel, Shaul.   III. Casaer, Paul Jules Maria.   IV. Title.
[DNLM: 1. Child Development Disorders—congresses.   2. Nervous System
Diseases—in infancy & childhood—congresses. W3 IN525 4th 1986c / WS 340 I58
1986c]
RJ486.I525 1986   618.92'8   88-9498
ISBN 1-55766-001-8

Contents

Contributors

Toshiaki Abe, M.D.
Department of Pediatrics
Teikyo University School of Medicine
2-11-1 Kaga
Itabashi-ku
Tokyo 173
Japan

Oded Abramsky, M.D., Ph.D.
Department of Neurology
Hadassah University Hospital
Hebrew University Hadassah Medical School
Jerusalem 91120
Israel

Doris A. Allen, Ed.D.
Associate Professor in Child Psychiatry
Director
Therapeutic Nursery
Nurses' Residence, 3N17
Albert Einstein College of Medicine
1300 Morris Park Avenue,
Bronx, NY 10461

Janette Atkinson, Ph.D.
Visual Development Unit
University of Cambridge
22 Trumpington Street
Cambridge CB2 1QA
Great Britain

Peter G. Barth, M.D., Ph.D.
Department of Pediatric Neurology
Academic Medical Center
Meibergdreef 9
1105 AZ Amsterdam
The Netherlands

Itschak Binderman, M.D.
Hard Tissues Unit
Ichilov Tel Aviv Medical Center
6 Weizmann Street
Tel Aviv 64239
Israel

W. Ted Brown, M.D., Ph.D.
New York State Office of Mental Retardation and
    Developmental Disabilities
Institute for Basic Research in Developmental
    Disabilities
1050 Forest Hill Road
Staten Island, NY 10314

Wolfgang Brück, M.D.
Division of Neuropathology
University of Mainz
Mainz
West Germany

Paul Casaer, M.D., Ph.D.
Professor of Paediatrics, Paediatric Neurology and
    Neurophysiology
University of Leuven
Department of Paediatrics and Neonatal Medicine
University Hospital Gasthuisberg
B-1300 Leuven
Belgium

William J. Cashore, M.D.
Associate Professor of Pediatrics
Brown University
Women and Infants Hospital
Providence, RI 02902

Hanan Costeff, M.D.
Department of Pediatric Rehabilitation
Lewenstein Hospital, Raanana
Sackler Faculty of Medicine
Tel Aviv University
Israel

Philippe de Saint-Georges, M.D.
Research Fellow in Pediatric Neurology
Instructor in Neuroanatomy
University of Louvain Medical School at Brussels
Avenue Hippocrate 10/1303
B-1200 Bruxelles
Belgium

Darryl C. De Vivo, M.D.
Sidney Carter Professor of Neurology
Professor of Pediatrics
Director of Pediatric Neurology
Neurological Institute
Columbia-Presbyterian Medical Center
710 West 168th Street
New York, NY 10032

**Victor Dubowitz, B.Sc., M.D., Ph.D.,
    F.R.C.P., D.C.H.**
Department of Paediatrics and Neonatal Medicine
Royal Postgraduate Medical School
Du Cane Road
London W12 OHS
Great Britain

Yehoshua Earon, M.D.
Division of Pediatrics
Tel Aviv Medical Center
University of Tel Aviv
Child Development Assessment Center
14 Balfour Street
Tel Aviv 65211
Israel

viii   Contributors

Philippe Evrard, M.D.
Professor of Pediatric Neurology and
  Neuroanatomy
University of Louvain Medical School at Brussels
Avenue Hippocrate 10/1303
B-1200 Bruxelles
Belgium

Joseph H. French, M.D.
Deputy Director, Developmental Disabilities Ctr
Clinical Professor of Neurology and Pediatrics
SUNY Health Science Center at Brooklyn
New York State Office of MR/DD
Institute for Basic Research in
  Developmental Disabilities
Box 75, 450 Clarkson Avenue
Brooklyn, NY 11203

Ryochi Fujii, M.D.
Department of Pediatrics
Teikyo University School of Medicine
2-11-1 Kaga
Itabashi-ku
Tokyo 173
Japan

Fons J.M. Gabreëls, M.D., Ph.D.
Center for Child Neurology
University Hospital Nijmegen
P.O. Box 9101
6500 HB Nijmegen
The Netherlands

Jean-François Gadisseux, M.D.
Postdoctoral Research Fellow in Pediatric
  Neurology and
Instructor in Neuroanatomy
University of Louvain Medical School at Brussels
Avenue Hippocrate 10/1303
B-1200 Bruxelles
Belgium

Natan Gadoth, M.D.
Professor of Neurology
Department of Neurology
Beilinson Medical Center, Petah Tiqvah
Sackler Faculty of Medicine
Tel Aviv University
Israel

Hans H. Goebel, M.D.
Professor of Neuropathology
Abteilung für Neuropathologie
Pathologisches Institut der
Johannes Gutenberg-Universität
Langenbeckstr. 1
D-6500 Mainz/
West Germany

Sophie Goldblum, Ph.D.
Department of Biology
University of California-Los Angeles
Los Angeles, CA 90024-1606

Gerald S. Golden, M.D.
Director, Child Development Center
Shainberg Professor of Pediatrics
Professor and Acting Chairman, Department of
  Neurology
University of Tennessee, Memphis
711 Jefferson Avenue
Memphis, TN 38105

Marvin I. Gottlieb, M.D., Ph.D.
Director
Institute for Child Development
Professor of Pediatrics, University of Medicine
  and Dentistry of New Jersey
Hackensack Medical Center
30 Prospect Avenue
Hackensack, NJ 07601

Gorm Greisen, M.D.
Department of Neonatology
Rigshospitalet, DK-2100
Copenhagen
Denmark

Debra A. Gusnard, M.D.
Division of Pediatric Radiology
University of Chicago Hospitals
5841 S. Maryland
Chicago, IL 60637

Shaul Harel, M.D.
Pediatric Neurology Unit and
Child Development Assessment Center
Division of Pediatrics
Tel Aviv Medical Center
Sackler Faculty of Medicine
Tel Aviv University
14 Balfour Street
Tel Aviv 65211
Israel

Hugo S.A. Heymans, M.D., Ph.D.
Department of Pediatrics
University Hospital Groningen
The Netherlands

Mikio Hiraiwa, M.D.
Department of Pediatrics
Teikyo University School of Medicine
2-11-1 Kaga
Itabashi-ku
Tokyo 173
Japan

Takashi Igarashi, M.D.
Department of Pediatrics
Faculty of Medicine
The University of Tokyo
Bunkyo-ku
Tokyo 113
Japan

Masaaki Iio, M.D.
Department of Radiology
Nakano National Chest Hospital
Tokyo 164
Japan

Edmund C. Jenkins, Ph.D.
New York State Office of Mental Retardation and
  Developmental Disabilities
Institute for Basic Research in Developmental
  Disabilities
1050 Forest Hill Road
Staten Island, NY 10314

William G. Johnson, M.D.
Associate Professor of Clinical Neurology
Columbia University
College of Physicians and Surgeons 4-448
630 West 168th Street
New York, NY 10032

Hazim J. Kadhim, M.D.
Postdoctoral Research Fellow in Neuroanatomy
  and Pediatric Neurology
University of Louvain Medical School at Brussels
Avenue Hippocrate 10/1303
B-1200 Bruxelles
Belgium

Ram Kairam, M.D.
Department of Pediatrics
G.H. Sergievsky Center
Columbia University
630 West 168th Street
New York, NY 10032

Murray M. Kappelman, M.D.
Professor, Pediatrics
Director, Division of Behavior and Developmental
  Pediatrics
University of Maryland School of Medicine
Room 5-678 WPCC
Baltimore, MD 21201

Richard J. Kascsak, Ph.D.
New York State Office of Mental Retardation and
  Developmental Disabilities
Institute for Basic Research in Developmental
  Disabilities
1050 Forest Hill Road
Staten Island, NY 10314

Ulf Käsgen, M.D.
Division of Neuropathology
University of Mainz
Mainz
West Germany

Goro Kato, Ph.D.
Department of Biochemistry
Yamanashi Medical College
Yamanashi 409-38
Japan

Alvin M. Kaye, Ph.D.
Department of Hormone Research
Weizmann Institute
Rehovoj
Israel

John H. Kennell, M.D.
Professor of Pediatrics
Case Western Reserve University School of
  Medicine
Chief, Division of Child Development
Rainbow Babies and Children's Hospital
2074 Abington Road
Cleveland, OH 44106

Marcel Kinsbourne, M.D.
Director
Behavioral Neurology
Eunice Kennedy Shriver Center
200 Trapelo Road
Waltham, MA 02254

Mårten Kyllerman, M.D.
Department of Pediatrics II
University of Göteborg
Östra Sjukhuset
S-416 85 Göteborg
Sweden

Perez Lavie, Ph.D.
Unit of Behavioral Biology
Tischniun, Haifa
Israel

Hans C. Lou, M.D., Ph.D.
Chief Physician
Department of Neuropaediatrics
John F. Kennedy Instituttet
GL Landevej 7-9
DK-2600 Glostrup
Denmark

Lois Mendelson, Ph.D.
Therapeutic Nursery
Nurses' Residence, 3N17
Albert Einstein College of Medicine
1300 Morris Park Avenue
Bronx, NY 10461

John H. Menkes, M.D.
Departments of Neurology and Pediatrics
University of California-Los Angeles
Los Angeles, CA 90024-1769

Charles M. Miezejeski, Ph.D.
New York State Office of Mental Retardation and
  Developmental Disabilities
Institute for Basic Research in Developmental
  Disabilities
1050 Forest Hill Road
Staten Island, NY 10314

Wilhelm Mortier, M.D.
Professor
Director of the Kinderklinik Wuppertal
Teaching Hospital of the University of Dusseldorf
Heusnerstr. 40
D-5600 Wuppertal 2
West Germany

Thomas P. Naidich, M.D.
Director of Neuroradiology
Department of Neuroradiology
Baptist Hospital of Miami
8900 North Kendall Drive
Miami, FL 33176-2197

Eiji Nanba, M.D.
Division of Child Neurology
Institute of Neurological Sciences
Tottori University
Yonago 683
Japan

Eike Noack, M.D.
Professor of the Pharmacological Institute of the
  University of Dusseldorf
Moorenstr. 5
D-4000 Dusseldorf
West Germany

Chizuru Nonaka, M.D.
Department of Pediatrics
Teikyo University School of Medicine
2-11-1 Kaga
Itabashi-ku
Tokyo 173
Japan

Kiyoshi Omura, M.D.
National Institute of Neuroscience, NCNP
4-1-1 Ogawahigashi, Kodaira
Tokyo 187
Japan

Michael J. Painter, M.D.
Division of Child Neurology
University of Pittsburgh
Children's Hospital of Pittsburgh
3705 Fifth Avenue at DeSoto Street
Pittsburgh, PA 15213-3417

Nigel Paneth, M.D., M.P.H.
Department of Pediatrics
G.H. Sergievsky Center
Columbia University
630 West 168th Street
New York, NY 10032

Jennifer Pinto, Ph.D.
G.H. Sergievsky Center
Columbia University
630 West 168th Street
New York, NY 10032

Galya Rabinovitz, M.A.
Child Development Assessment Center
Division of Pediatrics
Tel Aviv Medical Center
Sackler Faculty of Medicine
Tel Aviv University
14 Balfour Street
Tel Aviv 65211
Israel

Isabelle Rapin, M.D.
Professor, Neurology and Pediatrics
Albert Einstein College of Medicine
Yeshiva University
1300 Morris Park Avenue
Bronx, NY 10461

N. Paul Rosman, M.D.
Professor of Pediatrics and Neurology
Tufts University School of Medicine
Chief, Division of Pediatric Neurology
Floating Hospital for Infants and Children
New England Medical Center Hospitals
750 Washington Street
Boston, MA 02111

Raoul Rudelli, M.D.
New York State Office of Mental Retardation and
  Developmental Disabilities
Institute for Basic Research in Developmental
  Disabilities
1050 Forest Hill Road
Staten Island, NY 10314

Hitoshi Sakuraba, M.D.
Department of Clinical Genetics
The Tokyo Metropolitan Institute of Medical
  Science
Bunkyo-ku
Tokyo 113
Japan

Hans-Rudolf Scholte, Ph.D.
Professor in Biochemistry
Biochemical Department I of the Erasmus
  University
POB 1738, DR 3000
Rotterdam
The Netherlands

Ruud B.H. Schutgens, Ph.D.
Department of Pediatrics
Academic Medical Center
Meibergdreef 9
1105 AZ Amsterdam
The Netherlands

Caroline A. Sewry, B.Sc., Ph.D.
Department of Paediatrics and Neonatal Medicine
Royal Postgraduate Medical School
Du Cane Road
London W12 OHS
Great Britain

O. Carter Snead, III, M.D.
Professor, Pediatrics and Neurology
Room 654-CHT
1600 7th Avenue, South
Birmingham, AL 35233

Haim Sohmer, Ph.D.
Department of Physiology
Hebrew University-Hadassah Medical School
P.O.B. 1172
Jerusalem 91010
Israel

Dalia Somjen, Ph.D.
Hard Tissues Unit
Ichilov Tel Aviv Medical Center
6 Weizmann Street
Tel Aviv 64239
Israel

Israel Steiner, M.D.
Department of Neurology
Hadassah University Hospital
Hebrew University Hadassah Medical School
Jerusalem 91120
Israel

Leo Stern, M.D.
Professor and Chairman of Pediatrics
Brown University
Rhode Island Hospital
Providence, RI 02902

Yoshiyuki Suzuki, M.D.
Director
Division of Inherited Metabolic Disease
National Institute of Neuroscience, NCNP
4-1-1 Ogawahigashi, Kodaira
Tokyo 187
Japan

Abraham Tomer, M.D.
Pediatric Neurology Unit and
Child Development Assessment Center
Division of Pediatrics
Tel Aviv Medical Center
Sackler Faculty of Medicine
Tel Aviv University
14 Balfour Street
Tel Aviv 65211
Israel

Akihiko Tsuji, Ph.D.
National Institute of Neuroscience, NCNP
4-1-1 Ogawahigashi, Kodaira
Tokyo 187
Japan

Arnold Tweed, M.D.
Professor
Department of Anaesthesia
University Hospital
P.O. Box 5339
London, Ontario N6A 5A5
Canada

Stefan Walter, M.D.
Division of Neuropathology
University of Mainz
Mainz
West Germany

Ronald J. Wanders, Ph.D.
Department of Pediatrics
Academic Medical Center
Meibergdreef 9
1105 AZ Amsterdam
The Netherlands

Yosef Weisman, M.D.
Pediatric Neurology Unit
Hard Tissues Unit
Ichilov Tel Aviv Medical Center
6 Weizmann Street
Tel Aviv 64239
Israel

Gabrielle Weiss, M.D.
Department of Psychiatry
The Montreal Children's Hospital
2300 Tupper Street
Montreal H3H 1P3
Canada

John E. Williams, M.D.
Associate Director
Institute for Child Development
Clinical Assistant Professor of Pediatrics,
University of Medicine and Dentistry of New
 Jersey
Hackensack Medical Center
30 Prospect Avenue
Hackensack, NJ 07601

Henryk M. Wisniewski, M.D., Ph.D.
Director
New York State Office of Mental Retardation and
 Developmental Disabilities
Institute for Basic Research in Developmental
 Disabilities
1050 Forest Hill Road
Staten Island, NY 10314

Krystyna E. Wisniewski, M.D., Ph.D.
Associate Director, Clinical Diagnostic Services
Pediatric Neurologist
New York State Office of Mental Retardation and
    Developmental Disabilities
Institute for Basic Research in Developmental
    Disabilities
1050 Forest Hill Road
Staten Island, NY 10314

Rei-Cheng Yang, M.D.
National Institute of Neuroscience, NCNP
4-1-1 Ogawahigashi, Kodaira
Tokyo 187
Japan

David K. Yousefzadeh, M.D.
Section Chief
Division of Pediatric Radiology
University of Chicago Hospitals
5841 S. Maryland
Chicago, IL 60637

Preface

THE TOPICS THAT ARE INCLUDED IN THIS BOOK WERE CHOSEN ARBITRARILY BY THE EDITORS FROM PAPERS THAT were delivered at the *Fourth International Child Neurology Congress* and the Satellite Symposium, *Child Neurology and Developmental Pediatrics—Sharing Issues of Mutual Concern.* These meetings were held in Jerusalem, Israel, March 16–20, 1986. Authors of the selected papers subsequently were given an opportunity to update their contributions.

Chapters 1 through 12 discuss recent information concerning the etiology, diagnostic categorization, and pathogenesis of some nervous system diseases that occur during the pediatric-age years. Data that assign a hormone-signaling property, for central nervous system maturation, to a vitamin D metabolite are offered in Chapter 13. Chapters 14, 15, and 16 examine possible improvident influences of recurring seizures on the developing nervous system, a potential pathogenetic role of some neuropeptides in the epileptic process, and the recognition and treatment of neonatal seizures.

Epidemiologic data about chronic neurologic diseases of children in a postindustrial society are discussed in Chapter 17. The reported studies, completed prior to the recent recognition of the impact of acquired immune deficiency syndrome's influence on reproductive efficiency, indicate that preterm birth of small-for-gestational-age infants, rather than perinatal birth injury, is a major determinant of the static encephalopathies that are expressed later in life as developmental disabilities. A recorded increase in the prevalence of infantile hydrocephalus may share this cause. An exciting finding is the net gain of healthy infants who currently survive preterm birth. In Chapter 18, some of the biologic and psychologic concomitants associated with this auspicious consequence of contemporary neonatal intensive care unit practices are reviewed.

Chapters 19 through 23 discuss *in utero* pathology, ultrasound neuroimaging (USNI), and potential pathogenesis and pathophysiologic sequel of some nonprogressive encephalopathies that commence pre- and perinatally. Chapter 21 also analyzes the diagnostic efficacy of neonatal USNI when it is validated neuropathologically.

Vascular flow and metabolic study of the neonatal brain are discussed in Chapter 22. Chapter 23 addresses positron emission tomography of intracerebral hemorrhage in infancy. Chapter 24 discusses a clinical model for assessment and treatment of high-risk infants. Methods for primary care pediatricians to initate the early identification of preschool-age children who subsequently may evidence learning disabilities are discussed in Chapter 25. The clinical characteristics of some learning disorders that have a neurological basis are reviewed in Chapter 26. Chapter 27 reviews methods for screening and objectively assessing infants or young children for the presence of visual dysfunction. The use of brain stem auditory–evoked responses as a method for assessing, as well as localizing, auditory dysfunction in infants and young children, is reviewed in Chapter 28. A clinically applicable nosology for developmental language disabilities (DLDs) is presented in Chapter 29. The recommended subtyping is proposed as a basis for design of rational programs of remediation for DLDs during the preschool-age years. Chapter 30 critically analyzes recent findings concerning the therapeutic specificity, optimum dose, delineation of responsive symptoms, and iatrogenic effects of methylphenidate or dextroamphetamine treatment for children with attention deficit disorder (ADD). "Controversial" therapies for children with ADD and learning disabilities are reviewed in Chapter 31.

Chapter 32 discusses difficulties that thwart researchers who attempt to measure early intervention's therapeutic efficacy for some, many, or all developmental disabilities when they use standard study designs. The use of longitudinal—rather than many, more traditional—designs is recommended as a rational response to the inherent problems associated with investigating immature subjects. Long-term follow-up data on cohorts who were found to have ADD during childhood are reviewed critically in Chapter 33. Detailed knowledge of the natural history of ADD, and of other developmental disabilities, is an obvious basic requirement for measuring therapeutic efficacy via longitudinal studies. Designing effective remediation strategies, whose therapeutic efficacies merit measurement, requires an understanding of the pathogenetic mechanism(s) that are expressed clinically as specific developmental disabilities. The final chapter examines this issue apropos neurologically based hypotheses concerning the pathogenesis of developmental reading disorders. A deficiency of selective cerebral hemisphere activation is favored as a likely generative mechanism. Substantiation of this hypothesis would support designing means to enhance selective hemispheral activation in order to treat this group of developmental disorders.

The editors hope that this book will be useful to those readers who aspire to understand rationally nervous system diseases in infants and children. Assuredly, increasingly basic knowledge concerning these diseases will permit clinicians to better serve afflicted children, and will assist scientists in providing clinicians with more efficacious treatments.

Support by the New York State Office of Mental Retardation and Developmental Disabilities aided in the compilation of this volume and is gratefully acknowledged. The editors also are indebted to Peggy Clark and Evelyn Nesbitt for secretarial service, and to Lawrence Black for bibliographic assistance.

JOSEPH H. FRENCH, M.D.
SHAUL HAREL, M.D.
PAUL CASAER, M.D.

This book is dedicated
in memory of
Marilyn Doss French
December 25, 1929–February 18, 1987

Child Neurology and
Developmental Disabilities

Chapter 1

The Biochemical
and Molecular Genetic Bases
of Inherited Neurological Diseases

William G. Johnson

MOLECULAR GENETICS IS RAPIDLY changing the approach to genetic diseases (Johnson, 1979; Old & Primrose, 1986; Rosenberg, 1986). The clinician will not simply be a spectator but also a participant in the process of bringing this technology to the patient. Understanding the principles of molecular genetics will assist clinicians in accomplishing this responsbility.

This discussion focuses first on neurogenetic disorders with unknown gene product and subsequently on disorders whose gene product is known. The chapter will close with an examination of other DNA sequences of potential interest; this will be followed by concluding remarks.

GENE MAPPING AND CLONING
IN DISORDERS WITH
UNKNOWN GENE PRODUCT

Gene Mapping by Restriction Fragment Length Polymorphisms (RFLPs)

The use of restriction fragment length polymorphisms has revolutionized human gene mapping in recent years (Gusella et al., 1983), yet in principle, the technique is little different from gene mapping using earlier markers. The two features that account for the difference are: first, the greatly increased number of informative polymorphic markers that are becoming

available for human gene mapping; and second, the fact that mapping with all of these markers is done with essentially the same methods, the same equipment, and in the same laboratory.

Restriction Fragment Length Polymorphisms Restriction endonucleases are bacterial enzymes that cut DNA in a sequence-specific way (Old & Primrose, 1986). These enzymes, about 300 in number to date, have nothing to do with human DNA, but seem to be involved with the survival of one bacterial strain versus another. However, these enzymes are able to cut human DNA like other kinds of DNA, and they do this by recognizing a particular DNA sequence which they then cut. These enzymes recognize and localize specific DNA sequences that are usually 4–8 base pairs in length.

Restriction fragments are the pieces that result after a restriction endonuclease has cut a length of DNA. The DNA which was cut may have been a small DNA fragment, a phage DNA, a human chromosome, or the entire human genome. Whatever the starting material, the result is a mixture of DNA fragments of a wide variety of lengths.

Restriction fragment lengths can be determined and restriction fragments of different sizes can be separated by means of agarose gel electrophoresis. Specific DNA sequences can be found on such a gel if the complementary sequence (the probe) is available and is radiolabeled. The gel is blotted to transfer the restriction fragments out of the gel and onto the flat surface of a nitrocellulose or nylon filter. Then the filter is soaked under specific conditions (hybridized) with a solution containing radiolabeled probe. The location of the probe radioactivity is determined by autoradiography. The location of the probe on the filter gives its location on the original gel and therefore the length of the original DNA fragment, since distance of migration on the agarose gel is related to the size of DNA.

Restriction fragment length polymorphisms are simply polymorphic variants of restriction fragment lengths. A polymorphism is a common genetic variant that is present in some members of a population but not in others. A polymorphism may be a phenotypic variant, a variant in activity or electrophoretic mobility of an enzyme, a variant in DNA sequence, or another kind of genetic variant. A genetic variant is considered common if it is present in 1% of genes; since each individual has two copies of each autosomal gene, a variant present in 1% of genes will be present in 2% of individuals. Thus, a polymorphism is a genetic variant present in at least 2% of individuals. However, a useful polymorphism should have a higher frequency, 10%–40%, of individuals carrying the minor allele. Individuals carrying the polymorphic variant will have the normal phenotype in nearly all cases. The reason for this is that harmful alleles will rapidly be eliminated from the population by natural selection and will be brought down to frequencies of well below 1%.

A restriction fragment length polymorphism results when a polymorphic variant in a specific DNA base sequence eliminates or adds a restriction endonuclease site. If the variant sequence is in the region recognized by a known probe, then the number or position of bands recognized by the probe will be different in the variant sequence from that in the normal sequence. By convention, the "variant" sequence is the one with the smaller population frequency.

Use of RFLP's for Gene Mapping   The

process of gene mapping using RFLPs is, in principle, little different from gene mapping using other kinds of markers. The basic procedure is: 1) to collect a kindred affected with the particular disorder, 2) to determine by clinical examination whether each individual carries the disease, 3) to determine by DNA blotting whether each individual carries two normal alleles, two variant alleles, or one of each, and 4) to compare the distribution in the pedigree of the clinical disorder and the DNA markers to see if linkage is present.

Each time an individual produces progeny, the two copies of each gene are separated at the first meiotic division of gametogenesis and then go into different cells; only one copy of each parental gene can be transmitted to each child. Genes on different chromosomes assort randomly during meiosis. Because of crossing over at the first meiotic division, genes that are far apart on the same chromosome also assort randomly. Genes that are close together on the same chromosome do not assort randomly, that is, they show linkage (see Figure 1).

Before this transmission process can be followed, the parent's two copies of the genes being tested for linkage must be "marked" so that they can be distinguished from each other in order to follow the transmission of each copy from parent to child. The "informative" individual is informative precisely because each of

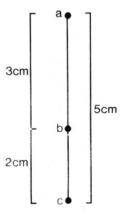

Figure 1.   Three gene loci, a, b, and c, are located close to each other on the same chromosome and are linked. Loci a and b are 3 centimorgans apart; b and c are 2 centimorgans apart; a and c are 5 centimorgans apart.

the two alleles of the two genes being tested for linkage (the disease gene and the RFLP) has been marked because the individual is heterozygous at each of the two loci.

An informative individual is one whose two alleles can be distinguished for the genes being considered. An affected individual, a heterozygote in the usual situation where the gene for a dominant disease gene is being mapped, has one abnormal allele (causing the disease) and one normal allele, and is therefore informative for the disease gene. To be informative for the RFLP being tested for linkage, the individual must be heterozygous at this locus also, with one copy of the normal RFLP allele and one copy of the variant RFLP allele.

A final requirement is that the phase must be established for that individual. Specifically, if the disease gene and the marker RFLP are linked, it is necessary to determine if the variant RFLP allele is on the chromosome that carries the *abnormal* allele of the disease gene or on the chromosome that carries the *normal* allele of the disease gene. Knowing the phase makes possible the construction of haplotypes (a shorthand statement of which alleles of the genes under consideration sit on the same chromosome of a chromosome pair) for the individual; in general, however, this is usually established only by examining the pedigree as a whole.

After the clinical state (affected or not) and the genotype with respect to the RFLP being tested for linkage have been determined for each member of the kindred, the frequency of recombination between the disease gene locus and the RFLP gene locus is determined. Fifty percent recombination is expected if the two gene loci are on different chromosomes or are far apart on the same chromosome; zero percent recombination suggests very tight linkage between the two loci, especially if the pedigree is so large that there were many opportunities for recombination to occur.

In practice, what is done is to use tables or a computer program to calculate lod at different postulated recombination frequencies from the pedigree data. Lod is the logarithm of the odds ratio: odds for linkage/odds against linkage.

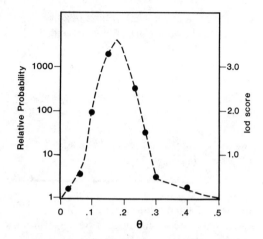

Figure 2.   A graphic representation of the outcome of linkage testing between a disease locus and a restriction fragment length polymorphism (RFLP). The abscissa is θ, the recombination fraction; the ordinate, expressed on the left as relative probability and on the right as lod score, is the relative probability of linkage between the two loci. Note that log (relative probability) = lod. When theta is given different values between 0.0 and 0.5, the lod scores define a curve which in this case has a peak lod > 3 at a θ of 0.19. Therefore, the two loci are linked because lod > 3. The most probable distance between the two loci is 19 centimorgans.

Recombination fraction θ is successively assumed to be 0%, 5%, 10%, and so on, for example, and lod is calculated at each θ. The result is a plot whose abscissa is recombination frequency and whose ordinate is lod. A plot where linkage is present gives a curve with a peak at some value of θ. The height of the peak gives lod at the most likely recombination frequency (see Figure 2). For example, a curve with a peak of 2 at θ = 0.1 is evidence for linkage of the two loci tested at a recombination frequency of 10%; at that recombination frequency, the odds ratio is 100 to 1 in favor of linkage. This sounds impressive: there seems little likelihood that the result is mere coincidence. Nonetheless, an lod score of 3, odds ratio of 1000 : 1 in favor of linkage, is the minimum requirement for general acceptance of a linkage claim.

Since gene loci that are farther apart have a higher recombination frequency, the distance between two gene loci can be measured using recombination frequency: gene loci that have a 1% recombination frequency are 1 centimorgan apart. The distance in centimorgans is approximately linear with recombination frequency for small distances, but not with larger distances. This is due to the increasing frequency of double crossovers with larger distances. The distance in centimorgans does not show linear correlation with chromosomal length measured morphologically with banded chromosome preparations; this is because crossovers are more frequent near the ends of chromosomes than near the centromere.

Having completed linkage testing for a disease locus and an RFLP, it is important to remember that any linkage established is between the two loci and not between any of the specific alleles at these two loci. Association between specific alleles is a different phenomenon called linkage disequilibrium.

If linkage was established, testing can be done with new RFLPs known to be linked to the first RFLP for more accurate mapping. If linkage was not established because the peak of the lod curve was less than 3, then new families can be studied with the same RFLP. Since the lod scores at different values of theta from the new families and from the old families are all in the form of logarithms, old data and new data can simply be added to give new lod scores. When the peak of the lod curve passes 3, linkage has been established. Of course, the new families studied must all have the same disease; if some of the families appear to have the same disease but in fact have a disease not caused by the same gene, the situation will become more confused rather than more clear with the addition of new families.

If, however, linkage was not established because there was no peak, then new RFLPs need to be tested for linkage.

Importance of Large Kindreds   In general, it is easier to do gene mapping with one very large family (Gusella et al., 1983) than with several large families, and easier with several large families than with many small families. Therefore, the clinician should be alert for large families. Since large kindreds are relatively uncommon, they are a valuable resource for research in that disorder. When such a large family is ascertained, a laboratory interested in gene mapping should be contacted so that the

family may have a chance to participate in research that will be of direct benefit to them.

Gene Mapping by Chromosomal Abnormalities

Chromosome abnormalities can give the location of a disease-causing gene (Franke et al., 1985; Labidi & Cassidy, 1986; Ledbetter et al., 1982; Monaco et al., 1986; Worton et al., 1984).

Types of Chromosome Abnormalities Useful for Gene Mapping   Patients with genetic disorders have one or more damaged copies of a particular gene. The damage can come about in a number of ways. One way is that a DNA point mutation in a gene's coding region can lead to an amino acid substitution in the protein gene product. Another way is that a small deletion can remove part or all of a gene's DNA sequence. A larger deletion may remove all of the DNA sequence of the gene in question plus that of one or more neighboring genes. Such a deletion may be large enough to be visible on a banded chromosome preparation. Another possibility is that the gene may be damaged when one breakpoint of a chromosome translocation cuts through the gene's DNA sequence. Such a translocation is likely to be visible on a banded chromosome preparation.

It is likely that a subgroup of patients with nearly every genetic disease has that disease because of chromosome damage significant enough to be visible in banded chromosome preparations. Although this group is not large, it is extremely important to find because the site of chromosome damage gives the chromosomal location of the disease gene directly. Moreover, there are strategies for using the abnormal chromosomes from patients to clone the gene for the disease even though the gene product is unknown. Therefore, it is important to study patients with genetic diseases for chromosome morphology, especially when there is something atypical about their disease.

Gene Mapping with Translocations   In the usual balanced reciprocal chromosome translocations seen in humans, breakage has occurred in two different chromosomes with reassortment of the pieces. For example, breakage may occur in chromosome 21 resulting in two pieces: one piece contains the centromere, the other piece does not contain the centromere. In the same way, breakage may occur in the X chromosome resulting in two pieces: one piece contains the centromere, the other piece does not contain the centromere. In a balanced translocation, the pieces recombine. That is, the centromere-containing piece of the X chromosome joins at its broken end to the broken end of the chromosome 21 piece which does not contain the centromere: this new chromosome is called a derivative X. Also, the centromere-containing piece of chromosome 21 joins at its broken end to the broken end of the X chromosome piece which does not contain the centromere: this new chromosome is called a derivative 21. Since this is a balanced translocation, no DNA has been lost (at least not very much); the existing DNA has simply been recombined. However, the genes located at the two breakpoints may have been cut in two and may no longer function, even though their DNA is still present.

Some girls with Duchenne muscular dystrophy have translocations between the X chromosome and another chromosome (X auto-some translocations) as the cause of their disease (Worton et al., 1984). Duchenne muscular dystrophy is an X-linked recessive disorder that normally occurs in boys. Girls with X autosome translocations can become affected with Duchenne dystrophy in the following way. One Duchenne gene is damaged because it is cut by the translocation event. The other Duchenne gene on the other (uncut) X chromosome is normal. However, the derivative X is now unable to undergo lyonization (Lyon inactivation). Therefore, during development, lyonization is non-random: only the normal uncut X chromosome is inactivated; only the derivative X chromosome remains active. Therefore, such a girl has no functioning copy of the Duchenne gene and develops Duchenne muscular dystrophy.

After examination of several girls with Duchenne muscular dystrophy, it was noticed that the X chromosome breakpoints were always in the Xp21 band (that is, band 2.1 on the short arm of the X chromosome). The conclusion was that this was the location of the Duchenne gene.

A strategy to clone the Duchenne gene was developed making use of an X;21 translocation (see Figure 3) found in a girl with Duchenne

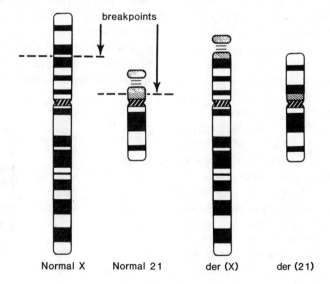

Normal X   Normal 21   der (X)   der (21)

Figure 3. A schematic representation of a balanced translocation between a normal X chromosome and a normal chromosome 21 giving a derivative (der) X chromosome and a derivative (der) chromosome 21. The breakpoints shown cut through the Duchenne locus on the X chromosome and the rRNA locus on chromosome 21. Each derivative chromosome contains a part of the Duchenne locus immediately adjacent to a part of the rRNA locus.

muscular dystrophy. This was chosen because the breakpoint in chromosome 21 was in the middle of a large area of repeated DNA sequences coding for ribosomal RNA (rRNA) and because a DNA probe was available for rRNA (Worton et al., 1984). Cells from the patient were grown in culture, and the two abnormal derivative chromosomes were separated by flow sorting. Next, libraries were made (as discussed later) of these two abnormal chromosomes and clones were sought which contained *both* DNA sequences for rRNA and DNA sequences found on the X chromosome. Such clones could only represent sequences from the breakpoint which was right in the middle of (or at least very close to the middle of) the Duchenne gene.

Study of Duchenne patients with translocations led not only to direct chromosomal localization of the disease gene but also to a direct strategy for cloning it.

Gene Mapping with Deletions In chromosome deletions, two breakpoints occur in the same chromosome, thus giving rise to three pieces. The two end pieces join, and the middle piece is lost or deleted. Often, the deleted piece is so small that the chromosome looks normal under the microscope even with the best banded studies. Sometimes, however, the deletion is large enough to be visible under the microscope. Such deletions can be useful for both mapping and cloning of disease genes.

An example is found again in Duchenne muscular dystrophy. One unusual boy, BB, was found (Franke et al., 1985) who had three X-linked diseases (Duchenne muscular dystrophy, chronic granulomatous disease, and retinitis pigmentosa) as well as the McLeod phenotype, an X-linked blood group abnormality. He also had a small deletion of the X chromosome visible under the microscope by banded chromosome studies in the Xp21 region. This finding was direct evidence that the genes for all three diseases were located in this region. It also provided another strategy for cloning these genes. Using a technique called subtractive hybridization, BB's deleted X chromosome was used to strip away from the normal X chromosome all those DNA sequences not present

in the deletion. The remaining DNA sequences were those which *were* present in the deleted material, that is, the genes for Duchenne muscular dystrophy (Monaco et al., 1986), chronic granulomatous disease, and retinitis pigmentosa.

Another example is Prader-Willi syndrome. This is inherited as a dominant lethal disorder. Dominant lethal disorders are those disorders in which an affected individual does not reproduce. The disorder is not necessarily lethal to the patient. However, because the patients do not reproduce, the disease cannot be transmitted from parent to child. Therefore, nearly all cases are sporadic and result from the new mutation of a parental germ cell. Since the disorder is dominant, only a single copy of the abnormal gene is sufficient to cause the disease. In about 40% of patients with Prader-Willi syndrome, some abnormality (deletion or translocation) is found (Labidi & Cassidy, 1986; Ledbetter et al., 1982) involving a small area of chromosome 15 (15q11–q12, that is, bands 1.1 to 1.2 on the long arm of chromosome 15). This consistent finding gives the location of the gene causing Prader-Willi syndrome (see Figure 4). It is likely that those patients without abnormal appearing chromosomes 15 have either deletions too small to be seen under the microscope or point mutations. It is possible, however, that these patients have genetic damage elsewhere, and that abnormality of a different gene can also cause the clinical appearance of Prader-Willi syndrome. The de-

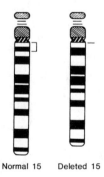

Normal 15   Deleted 15

Figure 4. A normal and deleted chromosome 15 with their banding patterns. The deleted region, 15q1–2, is shown by the bracket on the normal chromosome. The point of deletion is marked by a horizontal line.

leted chromosomes from Prader-Willi boys can also be used for cloning the Prader-Willi gene as just described for Duchenne muscular dystrophy resulting from deletion.

GENE CLONING IN DISORDERS WITH KNOWN GENE PRODUCT

For diseases with a known gene product (usually an enzyme), the gene can usually be readily cloned by screening a cDNA library (Old & Primrose, 1986). A library is simply a collection of DNA sequences that have been inserted into vectors so that they can be more easily manipulated. A cDNA library is chosen because cDNAs usually consist mostly of coding sequence for a protein without the long introns or flanking sequences that are present in genomic DNA. This is because cDNAs are constructed from mRNA, which consists mostly of the coding sequence.

Making cDNA Libraries

cDNA (complementary DNA) is really a DNA made from messenger RNA by reverse transcriptase; the synthesis of the second cDNA strand is usually achieved by allowing the first strand to form a self-priming hairpin loop. The loop is then cleaved by S1 nuclease (which cleaves single-stranded or unpaired DNA) to give a double-stranded cDNA. In this way, the sequence information of unstabile mRNA is converted into stabile DNA, cDNA.

A cDNA library can be prepared by adding linker arms to the ends of the double-stranded cDNA. Each linker arm is designed so that it contains one recognition site for a restriction endonuclease such as EcoR1; that is, each linker arm can be cut by EcoR1. Any internal EcoR1 sites in the cDNA are blocked so that the only place that EcoR1 will cut is on the two linker arms flanking the cDNA. Next, an appropriate vector, usually a self-replicating virus such as the bacteriophage lambda gt10 or lambda gt11, is chosen into which the cDNA with its linker arms (the "insert") will be inserted. Now, both the vector and the insert are cut with the same restriction endonuclease, in this case EcoR1. The vector and the insert are

mixed together, allowed to anneal (bind together at their "sticky ends" produced by the EcoR1 cut), and covalently linked with the enzyme ligase. This DNA is now packaged *in vitro* with bacteriophage capsular proteins and allowed to grow in a suitable host, usually a strain of E. coli. Those pieces of DNA in which one insert has been correctly placed into one vector will replicate and form infective viruses consisting of the insert stably incorporated into the vector. The identical products of one such successful insertion event constitute a single clone. Once inside a vector, the cDNA can be manipulated in useful ways, radiolabeled, or produced in large quantity.

If the original mRNA for preparing the library was obtained from a tissue, such as brain, then each copy of mRNA in the piece of tissue will be represented by a cDNA insert in a vector and will give rise to one clone. In practice, not every mRNA will give rise to a clone in the library. This means that some genes will not be found at all in a cDNA library, especially if their mRNA is an uncommon one in the tissue used to prepare the library. Also, mRNAs that are common in the tissue will be represented in the library by many clones.

Cloning from a cDNA Library

The purpose of making the cDNA library in the first place was to get out from it, that is clone from it, a DNA sequence of interest. There are many cloning strategies, some of them very ingenious or specialized. Two strategies, of general applicability, have proven especially useful for neurological diseases. The specificity required resides either in amino acid sequence for all or part of the protein of interest, or in antibodies raised against the protein of interest. That is, clones containing the gene of interest can usually be pulled out of a cDNA library if either antibodies to the gene product or the sequence of some of its peptide fragments can be obtained. Of course, the sequence has to be in the library in the first place.

In both strategies, the first step is to grow up the library at clonal density. The mixture of insert-containing vectors is diluted and grown with a large excess (a "lawn") of the bacterial host (usually E. coli) on a solid agarose gel plate. Each individual insert-containing bacteriophage will give rise to a single plaque which can be seen as a clear area against the hazy bacterial lawn. A single large plate may have 20,000 tiny plaques spread out over its surface. Next, replicas are made by laying a piece of nitrocellulose paper (a nitrocellulose filter) over the plate: the filter picks up DNA and protein from each plaque in exactly the same spatial pattern as that of the original plate. The problem now is: 1) to identify which of the plaques on the nitrocellulose filter contain the cDNA of interest, 2) to retrieve the plaques of interest from the original plate, and 3) to culture from these plaques the phage whose insert is the cDNA of interest.

If some amino acid sequence for the gene product is known, using the genetic code, a small piece of DNA (an oligonucleotide) can be chemically synthesized that will code for that aminoacid sequence. Since this oligonucleotide is a small piece of the coding sequence of the gene being sought, it should hybridize to one strand of the cDNA insert representing the gene of interest in the library. All that is necessary is to make this oligonucleotide (the "probe") radioactive, to allow it to hybridize in solution with the nitrocellulose filter replica (where it will bind only to the few plaques containing the insert of interest), wash off nonspecific binding, and detect the plaques of interest by autoradiography. In practice, because of the degeneracy of the genetic code, more than one DNA sequence will code for the aminoacid sequence used to make the oligonucleotide probe. All of these sequences must now be synthesized, usually several dozen oligonucleotides, and the mixture used to probe the nitrocellulose filters. In addition, once a clone is found, it must be carefully checked to make sure that it really does contain a sequence complementary to that of one of the probes, before the clone is restriction mapped and sequenced.

If a specific antibody against the gene product is available, then an expressing library is used. Lambda gt11 can be used to make an expressing library. Such expressing vectors will produce in small amounts the protein coded for by the insert which they carry. Thus, the specific antibody, in conjunction with a staining procedure such as immunoperoxidase, can be used to detect the few plaques on the nitrocellulose filter that carry the gene of interest as an insert. The success of this method depends on the specificity and strength of the antibody used.

Genes Cloned by These Methods   Genes for both recessive and dominant diseases have been cloned by the methods mentioned above. Recently cloned genes of particular interest for neurologists are those for beta-glucuronidase (mucopolysaccharidosis type VII, Sly syndrome) (Guise et al., 1985), fucosidosis (alpha-L-fucosidase) (Fukushima, deWet, & O'Brien, 1985), Gaucher disease (beta-glucosidase) (Ginns et al., 1984), Tay-Sachs disease (hexosaminidase alpha-subunit) (Korneluk et al., 1986; Myerowitz, Piekarz, Neufeld, Shows, & Suzuki, 1985), Sandhoff's disease (hexosaminidase beta-subunit) (Korneluk et al., 1986; O'Dowd et al., 1986), alpha-galactosidase (Fabry's disease) (Bishop et al., 1986), all recessive diseases, and those for a form of amyloidosis (Dwulet & Benson, 1984; Mita, Maeda, Shimada, & Araki, 1984; Nakazato et al., 1984; Saraiva, Birken, Costa, & Goodman, 1984; Sasaki et al., 1984), an autosomal dominant disease.

OTHER DNA SEQUENCES OF POTENTIAL INTEREST FOR THE STUDY OF HUMAN DISEASE

An exciting class of genes found in Drosophila melanogaster that may have relevance for human disease research is the homeotic (or homoeotic) gene class (Gehring, 1984; Gehring, 1985; Ruddle, Hart, & McGinnis, 1985; Scott, 1985; Wolgemuth et al., 1986). Molecular genetic studies of homeotic genes in Drosophila, for example, may soon make a contribution to apparently nongenetic human congenital malformations. The term homeosis (also homoeosis) refers to the replacement of one structure of the body by a homologous structure from another body segment. Why should fruit fly diseases interest child neurologists? Because parts of these genes are found in vertebrates, for example: in frogs, mice, and in humans. The fact that these important developmental genes have been evolutionarily conserved in such different organisms suggests that they are doing something important.

One group of these genes, the bithorax complex, specifies the thoracic and abdominal segments (e.g., wings or legs). The other group, the antennapedia complex, controls the development of the head and anterior thoracic segments. Damage to genes in these groups causes congenital malformations in Drosophila melanogaster.

Interestingly, several of these homeotic genes contain the same 180 base pair (bp) sequence; this is called the homeo box. It is this fragment that is conserved in fruit flies, frogs, mice, and humans. There is a suggestion that this homeo box sequence codes for a protein domain that binds to DNA.

Are there certain broadly similar developmental mechanisms in these different species? Will the cloned human homeo box sequences (there are now several) lead to a better understanding of human development? What diseases, if any, result from damage to these developmental gene sequences? These are questions for the future.

CONCLUSIONS

Molecular genetic research will not solve all of the pediatric neurologist's problems, but it will surely make important contributions toward solving them. Child neurologists are now urged to:

1. Look for large families whose members are affected with genetic neurological disorders. These families will make possible the rapid localization and mapping of the genes responsible.
2. Obtain banded chromosome studies looking for deletions, translocation, or other chromosome damage in patients with typical and atypical cases of genetic disorders as well as in patients with selected, apparently nongenetic, disorders. Finding a consistent location for chromosome damage in even a few of these patients will make possible rapid localization and cloning of the gene responsible. Further, it will permit the documentation of the genetic origin of disorders not previously known to be genetic.
3. Identify families with two cases of apparently nongenetic disorders.
4. Arrange for blood collection or skin biopsy from patients with rare or rapidly fatal genetic disorders in order to establish cell lines for further studies.

REFERENCES

Bishop, D.F., Calhoun, D.H., Bernstein, H.S., Hantzopoulos, P., Quinn, M., & Desnick, R.J. (1986). Human alpha-galactosidase A: Nucleotide sequence of a cDNA clone encoding the mature enzyme. *Proceedings of the National Academy of Sciences of the United States of America, 83,* 4859–4863.
Dwulet, F.E., & Benson, M.D. (1984). Primary structure of an amyloid prealbumin and its plasma precursor in a heredo-familial polyneuropathy of Swedish origin. *Proceedings of the National Academy of Sciences of the United States of America, 81,* 694–698.
Franke, U., Ochs, H.D., de Martinville, B., Giacalone, J., Lindgren, V., Disteche, C., Pagon, R.A., Hofker, M.H., van Ommen, G.-J.B., Pearson, P.L., & Wedgewood, R.J. (1985). Minor Xp21 chromosome deletion in a male associated with expression of Duchenne muscular dystrophy, chronic granulomatous disease, retinitis pigmentosa and McLeod syndrome. *American Journal of Human Genetics, 37,* 250–267.

Fukushima, H., de Wet, J.R., & O'Brien, J.S. (1985). Molecular cloning of cDNA for human alpha-L-fucosidase. *Proceedings of the National Academy of Sciences of the United States of America, 82,* 1262–1265.
Gehring, W.J. (1984). Homeotic genes and the control of cell determination. In: E.H. Davidson & R.A. Firtel (Eds.), *Molecular biology of development* (pp. 3–22). New York: A.R. Liss.
Gehring, W.J. (1985). The homeo box: A key to the understanding of development? *Cell, 40,* 3–5.
Ginns, E.I., Choudary, P.V., Martin, B.M., Winfield, S., Subblefield, B., Mayor, J., Merkle-Lehman, D., Murray, G.J., Bowers, L.A., & Barranger, J.A. (1984). Isolation of cDNA clones for human beta-glucocerebrosidase using the lambda-gt11 expression system. *Biochemical and Biophysical Research Communications, 123,* 574–580.
Guise, N.S., Korneluk, R.G., Waye, J., Lamhonwah, A.M., Quan, F., Palmer, R., Ganshow, R.E., Sly,

W.S., & Gravel, R.A. (1985). Isolation and expression in Escherichia coli of a cDNA clone encoding human beta-glucuronidase. *Gene, 34,* 105–110.

Gusella, J.F., Wexler, N.S., Conneally, P.M., Naylor, S.L., Anderson, M.A., Tanzi, R.E., Watkins, P.C., Ottina, K., Wallace, M.R., Sakaguchi, A.Y., Young, A.B., Shoulson, I., Bonilla, E., & Martin, J.B. (1983). A polymorphic DNA marker genetically linked to Huntington's disease. *Nature, 306,* 234–238.

Johnson, W.G. (1979). Principles of genetics in neuromuscular disease. In V.C. Kelley (Ed.), *Practice of pediatrics* (Vol 4). New York: Harper & Row.

Korneluk, R.G., Mahuran, D.J., Neote, K., Klavins, M.H., O'Dowd, B.F., Tropak, M., Willard, H.F., Anderson, M.J., Lowden, J.A., & Gravel, R.A. (1986). Isolation of cDNA clones coding for the alpha-subunit of human beta-hexosaminidase. *Journal of Biological Chemistry, 261,* 8407–8413.

Labidi, E., & Cassidy, S.B. (1986). A blind prometaphase study of Prader-Willi syndrome: Frequency and consistency in interpretation of del 15q. *American Journal of Human Genetics, 39,* 452–460.

Ledbetter, D.H., Mascarello, J.T., Riccardi, V.M., Harper, V.D., Airhart, S.D., & Strobel, R.J. (1982). Chromosome 15 abnormalities and the Prader-Willi syndrome: A follow-up report of 40 cases. *American Journal of Human Genetics, 34,* 278–285.

Mita, S., Maeda, S., Shimada, K., & Araki, A. (1984). Cloning and sequence analysis of cDNA for human prealbumin. *Biochemical and Biophysical Research Communications, 124,* 558–564.

Monaco, A.P., Neve, R.L., Colletti-Feener, C., Bertelson, C.J., Kurnit, D.M., & Kunkel, L.M. (1986). Isolation of candidate cDNAs for portions of the Duchenne muscular dystrophy gene. *Nature, 323,* 646–650.

Myerowitz, R., Piekarz, R., Neufeld, E.F., Shows, T. B., & Suzuki, K. (1985). Human beta-hexosaminidase alpha chain: Coding sequence and homology with the beta chain. *Proceedings of the National Academy of Sciences of the United States of America, 82,* 7830–7834.

Nakazato, M., Kangawa, K., Minamino, N., Tawara, S., Matsuo, H., & Araki, S. (1984). Identification of a prealbumin variant in the serum of a Japanese patient with familial amyloidotic polyneuropathy. *Biochemical and Biophysical Research Communications, 122,* 712–718.

O'Dowd, B.F., Klavins, M.H., Willard, H.E., Gravel, R., Lowden, J.A., & Mahuran, D.J. (1986). Molecular heterogeneity in the infantile and juvenile forms of Sandhoff disease (O-variant G_{M2}-gangliosidosis). *Journal of Biological Chemistry, 261,* 12680–12685.

Old, R.W., & Primrose, S.B. (1986). *Principles of gene manipulation. An introduction to genetic engineering* (2nd ed.). Berkeley: University of California Press.

Rosenberg, R.N. (1986). *Neurogenetics: Principles and practice.* New York: Raven Press.

Ruddle, F.H., Hart, C.P., & McGinnis, W. (1985). Structural and functional aspects of the mammalian homeobox sequences. *Trends in Genetics, 1,* 48–51.

Saraiva, M.J.M., Birken, S., Costa, P.P., & Goodman, D.S. (1984). Amyloid fibril protein in familial amyloidotic polyneuropathy, Portuguese type. *Journal of Clinical Investigation, 74,* 104–119.

Sasaki, H., Sasaki, Y., Matsuo, H., Goto, I., Kuroiwa, Y., Sahashi, I., Takahashi, A., Shinoda, T., Isobe, T., & Tahagi, Y. (1984). Diagnosis of familial amyloidotic polyneuropathy by recombinant DNA techniques. *Biochemical and Biophysical Research Communications, 125,* 636–642.

Scott, M.P. (1985). Molecules and puzzles from the antennapedia homoeotic gene complex of Drosophila. *Trends in Genetics, 1,* 74–80.

Wolgemuth, D.J., Engelmyer, E., Duggal, R.N., Gizang-Ginsberg, E., Mutter, G.L., Ponzetto, C., Viviano, C., & Zakeri, Z.F. (1986). Isolation of a mouse cDNA coding for a developmentally regulated, testis-specific transcript containing homeo box homology. *The EMBO Journal, 5,* 1229–1235.

Worton, R.G., Duff, C., Sylvester, J.E., Schmickel, R.D., & Willard, H.F. (1984). Duchenne muscular dystrophy involving translocation of the dmd gene next to ribosomal RNA genes. *Science, 224,* 1447–1449.

Chapter 2

The Fragile X Syndrome and Developmental Disabilities

*Krystyna E. Wisniewski, Joseph H. French,
W. Ted Brown, Edmund C. Jenkins, and Charles M. Miezejeski*

DISCOVERY OF THE FRAGILE X [FRA(X)] syndrome is a significant advance in the identification of causes of developmental disabilities. Males with a marker on the X chromosome at position q27.3, illustrated in Figure 1, and referred to as the fra(X) chromosome, have a distinct form of inherited mental retardation (MR) called the fra(X) syndrome. Over the last several years, it has been demonstrated that this X-linked syndrome is the most common hereditary form of MR (Brown, Jenkins, Gross, et al., 1987; Lubs, 1969, 1983; Turner, Optiz, Brown, et al., 1986).

The prevalence of affected, live-born males with the fra(X) syndrome is about 1/1350 (Optiz, 1986; Webb, Bundy, Thake, et al., 1986). Approximately twice as many females are carriers; about one-third of these are affected and manifest some degree of cognitive dysfunction, that is, learning disabilities or mild MR. Prevalence surveys suggest that 5%–10% of all MR in males is associated with the presence of the fra(X) chromosome abnormality (Brown, Jenkins, Cohen, et al., 1986; Herbst, 1980). Also, unaffected male carriers have been identified; about one out of every five males who inherit the mutation are unaffected, cytogenetically negative, transmitting males (Sherman, Jacobs, Morton, et al., 1985; Sherman, Morton, Jacobs, et al., 1984). However, approximately one-half of obligate female carriers and 90% of clinically affected females *are* cytogenetically positive. Thus, families of affected persons can be tested cytogenetically, and females who are identified as carriers of the

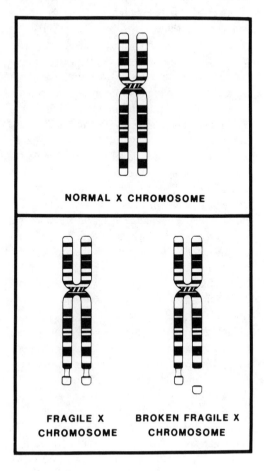

Figure 1. Normal X chromosome and fragile X chromosomes.

fra(X) chromosome abnormality can be counseled regarding their risk of bearing a child with the fra(X) syndrome (Jenkins & Brown, 1986; Jenkins, Brown, Brooks, et al., 1984; Jenkins, Brown, Duncan, et al., 1982; Sherman et al., 1984, 1985).

We previously reported the developmental disabilities and neurological abnormalities associated with 27 cases of the fra(X) chromosome abnormality (Wisniewski, French, Fernando, et al., 1985). This chapter extends these studies to a larger number of fra(X) positive subjects who have developmental disabilities.

MATERIALS AND METHODS

Sixty-two subjects who were fra(X) chromosome positive (55 males, mean age = 23.1 yrs. ± 14.3 SD with a range of 0.6–70, and 7 females, mean age = 15.7 yrs. ± 3.5 SD with a range of 11–20) and who had developmental disabilities were studied. A detailed history, physical examination, and pedigree were obtained for each patient. Appropriate informants were questioned in detail in order to detect potential encephalopathic events during the gestational and perinatal periods. The presence or absence of aberrant development was determined clinically by standard methods (Gesell & Amatruda, 1956). Interpretation of the stability or progress of neurodevelopmental aberrations, that is, mental retardation or dementia, was made by using customary standards (Rapin, 1977). Testicular volumes were measured, and a normal value of 18.2 ml, ± 4.75 SD, was chosen for adult males (Brown, Mezzacappa, & Jenkins, 1981; Turner, Eastman, Casey, et al., 1975). Testicular volumes greater than 25 ml were considered to indicate the presence of macroorchidism. Developmental and neurological examinations were performed on all subjects (Touwen, 1979; Touwen & Prechtl, 1970). Seizures were classified according to accepted conventions (International League Against Epilepsy, 1981; Kirman, 1974). A diagnosis of infantile autism was made according to criteria described in the *Diagnostic and Statistical Manual of Mental*

Disorders [DSM III] (American Psychiatric Association, 1980) (Brown, Jenkins, Friedman, et al., 1982; Cohen, Fisch, Wolf-Schein, et al., 1985). Learning disabilities, when suspected, were diagnosed via the use of accepted standards (Rapin, 1982). Cognitive function was quantified by neuropsychological testing (Anastasia, 1976; Benton, 1975) and the degree of mental retardation was categorized according to standards codified in the DSM III (American Psychiatric Association, 1980). Cytogenetic analysis was performed as previously described (Jenkins, Brown, Brooks, et al., 1984; Jenkins, Brown, Wilson, et al., 1986); at least 50 cells were examined routinely in negative instances.

RESULTS

All 62 cases (55 males and 7 females) with developmental disabilities were fra(X) chromosome positive. Twelve of the 25 mothers who were tested also had the fra(X) chromosome abnormality. The frequency of fra(X) positive cells ranged from 4%–50%; the number of cells examined per tested individual varied from 16 to 100.

Thirty-nine of the 62 cases occurred in 15 pedigrees that evidenced at least a developmentally disabled sibling or first cousin. Twenty-three cases were apparently sporadic and had no known biologic relatives who were developmentally disabled.

Fifty-two of the 55 males (94%) who were fra(X) positive had MR; the MR was mild in 8 (15%), moderate in 25 (48%), severe in 14 (27%), and profound in 5 (10%) of these 52 patients. Cognitive function could not be assessed precisely in an 8-month-old male infant. Males were usually more cognitively impaired than females, for example, there were 19/55 males with severe or profound MR versus 0/7 females. One of the seven females had mild MR and one was moderately retarded. Severity of the MR was not consistent within individual families with more than one developmentally disabled person; severity varied between families. Five of the seven females (70%) and 2/55 males (4%) were learning disabled. Autistic stigmata were present in 10/62 (16%) of the patients.

A past history of hypotonia in infancy was common. Delayed attainment of motor milestones was stated to have occurred in only 15/62 (24%) patients. Delayed language development occurred in all 62 subjects. The eldest subject, a 70-year-old male with severe MR, had exhibited episodes of increasingly disruptive behavior for several years prior to our evaluation. No progressive neurologic dysfunction was delineated as the cause of his behavioral symptoms. None of the remaining patients, 61/62, had any potential clinical stigmata of progressive neurologic dysfunction.

Seizures occurred in 14/62 (22%) patients. Both partial as well as generalized seizures occurred; patients promptly responded to appropriate anticonvulsant medications. There were no corroborated instances of infantile spasms. EEGs were obtained in 10/14 (71%) cases with seizures and in 5/48 cases of individuals who had not experienced seizures. No diagnostically specific pattern was found in the latter group. One patient with seizures had a normal EEG. Seven of ten EEGs in the patients with seizures were characterized by the findings of pharmacologically induced sleep only. Epileptiform activity was restricted to the temporal areas in 2/10 patients with seizures. None of the EEGs evidenced slow spike and wave complexes. No association was found between the occurrence of seizures and the degree of MR.

All of the 62 patients had normal (97th percentile; 3rd percentile), heights and weights; cranial circumferences (CC) were normal in 55/62 (89%). Four patients (6%) had macrocrania (CC > 97th percentile) and three (5%) had microcrania (CC < 3rd percentile). A narrow midface, reduced inner canthal span, prominent forehead, prominent ears, excessively vaulted palate, and mild facial asymmetry were present in 31/62 (50%) patients. All adult males had macroorchidism. No symptoms of cardiovascular dysfunction were present in any of the 62 patients. One young adult male had the general physical examination findings of mitral valve prolapse. Distal joint hyperextensibility, without arthropathy, was present in most adults. No somatic musculature abnormalities were detected.

A lateralized, focal neurologic deficit was present in only 1/62 patients, a late middle-age adult male with severe MR. His pyramidal release signs and an extremital growth arrest were attributed to a contralateral cerebral arteriovenous malformation (AVM) that had been ligated and irradiated during his preschool-age years. Soft neurologic signs were present in 61/62 (98%) cases. These consisted of the persistence of pinch synkinesia, Prechtl's movements, and gait maladroitness beyond their expected ages of disappearance. All older juvenile, adolescent, and adult patients evidenced impaired fine motor coordination: they experienced difficulty in tandem walking, hopping, performing skilled finger movements, and whistling. An 8-month-old, hypotonic, normal-reflexic male with delayed language development could not be tested for the presence or absence of these nonfocal deficits. Twelve of the 62 (19%) patients had generalized hyperreflexia as an isolated finding. In one family, three juvenile patients had unsustained ankle clonus as an isolated finding. None of the 62 patients had extrapyramidal, cerebellar, lower motor neuron or segmental sensory deficit findings. Blindness, secondary to adult-onset glaucoma, was present in a single adult male. Congenital nystagmus was found in 5/62 (8%) patients, and was associated with myopia in 2 of these 5. Auditory function was clinically normal in 61/62 (98%) patients. Brain stem auditory evoked responses (BAER) were normal in 7 of the 12 patients who were tested. Auditory function could not be clinically assessed in 1/62 (2%), (a preschool-age male who had never developed any expressive language). This patient's BAER evidenced ambiguous late waves, especially wave V, that may have prolonged latencies.

Neuroimaging, computerized cranial transaxial tomography (CT scan), was performed on 27/62 (43%) of the patients. Only 8 of these 27 (30%) studies were abnormal. Seven of the 8 abnormal studies evidenced mild ventricular enlargement; the other showed moderate, generalized ventricular dilatation and a left temporal lobe cyst. This patient, as discussed, had a congenital right hemiparesis associated with treatment of an AVM during his preschool-age years. He died, of nonneural causes, at the age of 62. A postmortem examination documented the presence of mild cerebral atrophy, moderate hydrocephalus *ex vacuo,* and a left temporal lobe pseudoporencephaly that was surrounded by a few dural clips. Dendritic spine abnormalities were apparent in Golgi stained sections that were examined via light microscopy. Ultrastructural aberrations of synapses were present in material that was studied by electron microscopy (Rudelli, Brown, Wisniewski, et al., 1985).

The following five fra(X) case summaries illustrate some of the above aggregate data.

Case 1

Case 1 (F43-II-1, DOB: 11/7/81) was a 5-year-old male at the time of our assessment. He was the product of a normal first pregnancy and delivery. Developmental landmarks were normal except for delayed onset of speech (first single words at the age of 2 years). He was evaluated for early-age onset hyperactive behavior and clumsiness.

There were no known occurrences of MR or other developmental disabilities in the family. A 2-year-old sister was normal.

Physical examination noted the presence of large ears and generalized hyperextensibility. The thumbs were easily dislocated.

Neurologic examination documented the presence of impaired fine motor coordination and a short attention span. F43-II-1's speech, spontaneous and responsive, was sparse and agrammatic. He could not name the component parts of common objects. He obeyed three-level verbal commands and appeared to comprehend spoken language at an age-appropriate level.

Lab Investigation The expressive language quotient was 65 (Slosson Intelligence Test) and the Merrill-Palmer Scale IQ was 72. His Peabody Picture Vocabulary Test (Revised) score was 104. The fra(X) chromosome was found in 11/50 (22%) cells.

Diagnosis The diagnosis was attention deficit disorder (ADD) and developmental expressive dysphasia associated with the fra(X) chromosome abnormality.

Case 2

Case 2 (F52-IV-25, DOB: 5/21/77), a boy, was evaluated for disruptive classroom behavior and failure to learn in school when he was 9 1/2 years old. No antenatal abnormalities were known. His delivery was complicated by a prolapsed nuchal cord and breech presentation. The Apgar Score was 3–4 at 1 minute and did not rise to 8 until he was 1 1/2 hours old. Icterus neonatorum occurred; he responded to phototherapy. He sucked poorly while in the newborn nursery. His expressive language development was delayed (first words at the age of 2 ½ years and phrases at 3–4 years). All other developmental landmarks were achieved at normally expected ages. He had evidenced an inability to attend to self-selected, age-appropriate TV programs since late infancy and during his early preschool-age years. He had never completed meals at a single sitting.

Older and younger brothers were normal. One of four maternal aunts had a son who had the fra(X) syndrome; her two other sons were normal. The other maternal aunt's children were not developmentally disabled. A maternal uncle and his son were normal (see Figure 2).

The maternal grandmother had six brothers and sisters. Her eldest sibling, a sister, had 10 progeny; the eldest of these progeny had a first daughter who was learning disabled, and a seventh child, a male, was mentally retarded. Both of these developmentally disabled individuals were fra(X) chromosome positive. The eldest maternal great uncle and his 11 offspring were normal. The youngest maternal great aunt and her 11 progeny were normal. Three other maternal great uncles were normal and had 13

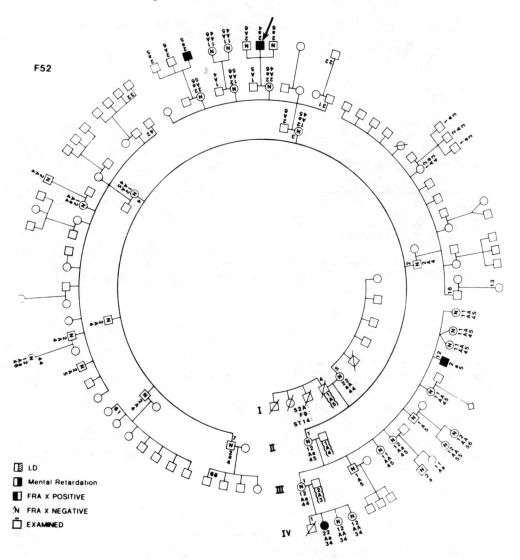

Figure 2. Case two: Pedigree F52.

progeny who did not evidence cognitive abnormalities. F52-IV-25's paternal lineage was entirely normal.

Physical examination noted the presence of a broad forehead, narrow facies, large ears, a gothic-arched palate, and joint hyperextensibility (see Figure 3). Testicular volumes were 10 ml bilaterally.

F52-IV-25 had no focal, lateralized, or space-consuming neurologic deficits. His attention span was brief and he was in constant motion. He evidenced Prechtl's movements,

gait maladroitness, an inability to inhibit the associated movements of ambulation during lateral foot walking, and impaired fine-motor coordination. His mental age was at a 4–6 year-old level.

Lab Investigation   A CT scan was normal. An EEG showed generalized background slowing. The karyotype was fra(X) chromosome positive in 11/50 (22%) cells.

Diagnosis   The diagnosis was fra(X) syndrome (mild MR) and attention deficit disorder (ADD) with hyperkinesia.

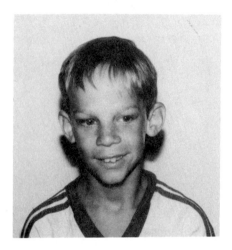

Figure 3. Case two: Physical features.

Case 3

Case 3 (F7-III-3, DOB: 2/28/66), a 21-year-old male who resided with his family, was the product of his mother's first pregnancy and delivery. The past medical history failed to elicit any potential encephalopathic events. Expressive language and ambulatory motor development were delayed (first words at 18 months; walked alone at 24 months). All other developmental milestones were achieved at normally expected ages. He was evaluated because his parents were concerned about the familial occurrence of developmental disabilities.

One sister was learning disabled and a second sister had moderate MR (see Figure 4). Both sisters had fra(X) chromosome abnormalities. The mother's sister had two retarded male children who were fra(X) chromosome positive; one was also autistic.

F7-III-3 had a normal general physical examination, except for the presence of a narrow mid-face, a high-arched palate, and a broad forehead. Testis sizes were 45 ml bilaterally.

Neurologic examination found a mental age at the 4–5 year level and deficient fine motor coordination.

Lab Investigation A CT scan evidenced enlarged sulci over the vertex of the cerebral hemispheres. The EEG and BAER were normal. Karyotype testing detected the presence

of the fra(X) chromosome in 16/50 (32%) cells.

Diagnosis The diagnosis was fra(X) syndrome (moderate MR) with macroorchidism.

Case 4

Case 4 (F59-II-1; DOB: 9/29/53), a male who was evaluated when he was 33 years old, was seen because his behavior had "deteriorated" recently. The reputed worsening began when two workers in his group home had taken other jobs; he was stated to have been "close" to them. F59-II-1 was the product of a normal second pregnancy and delivery. There were no known remote encephalopathic experiences. His mother was unable to supply any details of his early development other than "early brain damage." Unspecified "behavior problems" had commenced in "early" life and he had lived in group residences since the age of 9 years. Current behavioral complaints included diminished participation in, and occasional rejection of, a daily habilitative program. He also refused to enter the group home upon return from the program on "Wednesdays." Efforts to engage F59-II-1 in programmatic activities and to enter his residence were associated with mild self-injury and acting out.

No biologic relatives had developmental disabilities or psychiatric disorders.

Physical examination noted the presence of large ears and a narrow face. A midsystolic

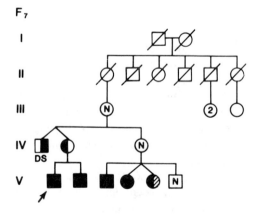

Figure 4. Case three: Pedigree F7.

click and subsequent systolic murmur, both augmented by the Valsalva maneuver, were heard over the apex. No other clinically evident abnormalities of cardiovascular function were found. Testicular volumes were 60 ml bilaterally.

Neurologic examination found a questionable deficit in eye contact. Visual acuity on the left was reduced to finger counting and/or movement. Visual acuity on the right was 20/50. The left eye was severely myopic. A left esotropia and bilateral, horizontal nystagmus were present. F59-II-1's cognitive performance was at a 7–9 year level.

Laboratory Investigation The Vineland IQ score was 50. An EEG and a CT scan were normal. Karyotype study noted the fra(X) chromosome in 23/50 (46%) cells.

Diagnosis The diagnosis was fra(X) syndrome (moderate MR) with probable mitral valve prolapse and macroorchidism, accompanied by adjustment disorder and congenital myopia, o.s., with amblyopia *ex anopsia* and pendular nystagmus.

Case 5

Case 5 (F46-III-1, DOB: 12/27/16), a male, was evaluated at the age of 70 years because of increasingly frequent episodes of negativism, agitation, and refusal to participate in his daily program of habilitative activities. This "change" had occurred over a period of "several" years. He was the product of his mother's first pregnancy; no ante- or perinatal abnormalities were known. Motor and speech development were delayed (first walked alone at 3 years and first spoke single words at 5 years). "Difficult" behavior had commenced in "early" childhood, and F46-III-1 was placed in a congregate-care setting at the age of 20 years. He had been given neuroleptic drugs for many years because of "behavior problems."

Two younger brothers were mentally retarded and fra(X) chromosome positive. A sister was reputed to be "slow" and had two sons who resided in an institution for the "mentally retarded."

F46-III-1 had large ears and a long, narrow face. The right testicular volume was 40 ml and the left was 46 ml.

Neurologic examination noted the presence of marked negativism and episodic agitation; F46-III-1 spat and periodically cursed without apparent provocation. Self-injurious behaviors occurred and included hair pulling as well as face slapping. Pendular nystagmus was present on lateral gaze. Fine motor coordination was impaired, and no cognitive performances beyond a mental age at the 2–3 year level could be elicited.

Lab Investigation An EEG and a CT scan were normal. Sixteen of 50 (32%) cells in the karyotype were fra(X) chromosome positive.

Diagnosis The diagnosis was fra(X) syndrome (severe MR) with episodic agitation, negativism, self-injurious behavior, and macroorchidism.

DISCUSSION

This study found an association between the presence of the fra(X) chromosome abnormality and symptomatic diagnoses of varying degrees of severity of MR, learning disabilities, attention deficit disorder, autism, and seizures. Thus, our findings support the conclusion that the fra(X) chromosome abnormality is a cause of developmental disabilities that have cognitive, behavioral, and/or seizure manifestations.

As previously reported (Wisniewski et al., 1985), fra(X) syndrome patients do not exhibit any alterations of somatic growth. The complete constellation of dysmorphic stigmata that suggest a clinical diagnosis of the fra(X) syndrome were present in only 50% of our cases. Loehr, Synhorst, Wolfe, and Hagerman (1986) have reported that aortic root dilatation and mitral value prolapse occur in patients with the fra(X) syndrome. None of our patients had experienced symptoms that are potentially related to the presence of these cardiovascular disorders, and only one, case 4, had the physical signs of mitral valve dysfunction. All adult males had macroorchidism.

A marked impairment of fine motor coordination in all older patients was the only motor sign that was present in this series. Monoparesis, hemiparesis, and generalized spasticity as well as involuntary movement disorders, potential manifestations of cerebral palsy, have been described in patients with the fra(X) chromosome abnormality by others (Herbst, 1980; Optiz, Kaveggia, Durkin-Stamm, et al., 1978; Optiz, Segal, Klove, et al., 1965; Turner & Optiz, 1980). None of our patients had extrapyramidal, cerebellar, or lower motor neuron deficits. We did identify a congenital hemiparesis that was contralateral to a surgically treated and irradiated AVM, in 1/62 patients. No other patients in this series had clinical, EEG, or neuroradiologic evidence of having an intracranial vascular anomaly. Therefore, a chance association of two unrelated etiologies of nervous system disease cannot be discounted in this patient. We are not aware of any literature reports of an association between the occurrence of intracranial vascular anomalies and the fra(X) chromosome.

Only 24% (15/62) of our patients had a history of delayed motor development. This rate is lower than that reported by Schmidt (1980). There was a similar rate of occurrence of a history of hypotonia in early life, and the only two infants we examined were hypotonic. Both of these infants had normal musculature, muscle strength, and deep tendon reflexes. Hypotonia also was found in fra(X) chromosome positive individuals by Allan and Herndon (1944), Allan, Herndon, and Dudley (1944), Hagerman (1983), and Herbst (1980).

Most patients in this series of fra(X) positive individuals were not felt to be developmentally abnormal until the usual age for commencing the use of single words. This delay in expressive language development could not be attributed to congenital deafness. Strabismus (Herbst, 1980; Schmidt, 1980), pale blue irises (Turner, 1982), and congenital optic atrophy (Herbst, 1980) have been described in fra(X) positive individuals. We have not found strabismus sans an error of refraction in this

group of patients, and cannot state that pale blue irises or congenital optic atrophy are visual system stigmata of the fra(X) chromosome abnormality.

An association between the occurrence of severe myopia and congenital nystagmus is well known (Ford, 1973). Two of our five cases with congenital nystagmus had severe myopia; three of the cases did not have myopia and are pathogenetically unexplained.

Mental retardation is the most frequently occurring developmental disability that was found in the males of this study. The MR was of mild to moderate severity in 60% of the cases, and severe to profound in 35% of the cases. However, two males (5%), Case 1 and a male who was learning disabled, did not have MR. Females more commonly evidenced learning disabilities, 5/7 (72%) cases; mild to moderate MR was present in only 2/7 (28%) of the cases. This has been described by Chudley, Knoll, Gerrard, et al. (1983), Jacobs, Glover, Mayer, et al. (1980), and Brown, Gross, Chan, et al. (1985). Since the severity of cognitive handicap among males in this series varied within and between individual families, the degree of MR in a specific case does not appear to have predictive value in regard to potential, afflicted, biologic relatives (Miezejeski, Jenkins, Hill, et al., 1984).

The prevalence of seizures in our patients is 22%. This is lower than the rate of 42% reported by Herbst (1980). However, both rates fall within the range that is expected in an etiologically heterogenous population with MR. The occurrence of seizures in our patients did not correlate with the severity of MR or with the presence of autism, and an EEG abnormality that correlated with the occurrence of seizures was found only infrequently.

Infantile autism and autistic behavioral manifestations occur in patients who manifest the fra(X) chromosome (Brown, Cohen, Fisch, et al., 1986; Brown, Jenkins, Friedman, et al., 1984; Cohen, Fisch, Wolf-Schein, et al., 1985; Turner, 1982). This observation is also true for 16% (10/62) of the patients in this series.

A disruption of single carbon group transfers is the apparent metabolic basis for making the fra(X) chromosome abnormality apparent in laboratory culture systems (Erbe & Wang, 1984). However, treatment with high doses of folic acid, potentially to augment single carbon group transfers, did not, as previously reported (Brown, Cohen, Fisch, et al., 1986; Brown, Jenkins, Gross, et al., 1987b), significantly change the cognitive performances or behavioral characteristics of the patients that are the subject of this report.

The longitudinal courses of symptomatic patients with the fra(X) chromosome abnormality suggest that they have a nonprogressive and diffuse CNS disorder. Electrophysiologic (EEG & BAER) and neuroimaging (CT scan) studies are not diagnostically specific. An absence of prominent long tract signs and the occurrence of seizures potentially implicate neuronal dysfunction as the pathogenetic basis for their symptoms. A single neuropathologic study (Rudelli et al., 1985) supports this hypothesis.

The fra(X) chromosome abnormality should be sought as the etiologic basis for developmental disabilities in all adult males who have macroorchidism and for younger males who have etiologically uncharacterized mental retardation, learning disabilities, and/or autism that may or may not be associated with easily controlled seizures. The manifestation of etiologically uncharacterized learning disabilities or mild to moderate MR in females, especially if such afflicted persons are related to developmentally disabled males via their maternal lineage, should also lead one to consider obtaining a fra(X) chromosome test. If the fra(X) chromosome abnormality is found to be the etiologic basis for a rather diverse spectrum of developmental disabilities, it is advisable to provide maternal lineage relatives with precise genetic counseling, and preventive and habilitative services. As discussed in Chapter 1, families with this chromosome abnormality may exhibit informative restriction fragment polymorphisms that are associated with the fra(X) locus (Brown, Gross, Chan, et al., 1988; Brown, Jenkins, Gross, et al., 1987b; Oberle, Heilig, Moisan, et al., 1986). The future availability of such DNA probes may significantly augment the clinicians' current use of cytogenetic methods to identify carriers, and may permit them to better understand the molecular biology of this important cause of developmental disabilities.

REFERENCES

Allan, W., & Herndon, C.N. (1944). Retinitis pigmentosa and apparently sex-linked idiocy. *Journal of Heredity, 35,* 41–43.

Allan, W., Herndon, C.N., & Dudley, F.C. (1944). Some examples of the inheritance of mental deficiency: Apparently sex-linked idiocy and microcephaly. *American Journal of Mental Deficiency, 48,* 325–334.

American Psychiatric Association (1980). *Diagnostic and statistical manual of mental disorders* (3rd ed.). Washington, DC: American Psychiatric Association.

Anastasia, A. (1976). *Psychological testing* (4th ed.). New York: Macmillian.

Benton, A. (1975). The clinical neurosciences. In D.B. Tower (Ed.), *The nervous system* (Vol. 2, pp. 67–74). New York: Raven.

Brown, W.T., Cohen, I.L., Fisch, G.S., et al. (1986). High dose folic acid treatment of fragile (X) males. *American Journal of Medical Genetics, 23,* 263–271.

Brown, W.T., Gross, A., Chan, C., et al. (1988). Multilocus analysis of the fragile (X) syndrome. *Human Genetics, 78,* 201–205.

Brown, W.T., Jenkins, E.C., Cohen, I.L., et al. (1986). Fragile X and autism: A multicenter survey. *American Journal of Medical Genetics, 23,* 341–352.

Brown, W.T., Jenkins, E.C., Friedman, E., et al. (1982). Autism is associated with the fragile X syndrome. *Journal of Autism and Developmental Disorders, 12,* 303–308.

Brown, W.T., Jenkins, E.C., Friedman, E., et al. (1984). Folic acid therapy in the fragile X syndrome. *American Journal of Medical Genetics, 17,* 289–297.

Brown, W.T., Jenkins, E.C., & Gross, A. C., et al. (1987a). Genetics and the expression of the fragile X syndrome. *Upsala Journal of Medical Sciences, 44* (Suppl.), 137–154.

Brown, W.T., Jenkins, E.C., Gross, A. C., et al. (1987b). Further evidence for genetic heterogeneity in the fragile X syndrome. *Human Genetics, 75,* 311–321.

Brown, W.T., Mezzacappa, P.M., Jenkins, E.C. (1981). Screening for fragile X syndrome by testicular size measurement. *Lancet, 2,* 1055.

Chudley, A.E., Knoll, J., Gerrard, J.W., et al. (1983). Fragile (X) X-linked mental retardation. I: Relationship between age and intelligence and the frequency of expression of fragile (X) (q28). *American Journal of Human Genetics, 14,* 699–712.

Cohen, I.L., Fisch, G.S., Wolf-Schein, E.G., et al. (1985). Fragile (X) and autism: A preliminary analysis of non-verbal behavioral characteristics. *American Journal of Human Genetics, 37,* A50.

Erbe, R.W., & Wang, J.C. (1984). Folate metabolism in humans. *American Journal of Human Genetics, 17,* 277–288.

Ford, F.R. (Ed.). (1973). Congenital (hereditary) nystagmus. In *Diseases of the nervous system in infancy, childhood and adolescence* (6th ed.). Springfield, IL: Charles C Thomas.

Gesell, A., & Amatruda, C.S. (1956). *Developmental Diagnosis.* New York: Harper & Brothers.

Hagerman, R., & Smith, A.C.M. (1983). The heterozygous female. In R. Hagerman & P.M. McBogg (Eds.), *The fragile X syndrome: Diagnosis, biochemistry and intervention* (pp. 83–94). Dallon, CO: Spectra Publishing Co.

Herbst, D.S. (1980). Non-specific X-linked mental retardation. A review with information from 24 new families. *American Journal of Human Genetics, 7,* 443–460.

International League Against Epilepsy. (1981). Proposal for revised clinical and electroencephalographic classification of epileptic seizures. *Epilepsia, 22,* 489–501.

Jacobs, P.A., Glover, T.W., Mayer, M., et al. (1980). X-linked mental retardation: A study of 7 families. *American Journal of Medical Genetics, 7,* 471–489.

Jenkins, E.C., & Brown, W.T. (1986). The prenatal diagnosis of the fragile X syndrome. In A. Milunsky (Ed.), *Genetic disorders and the fetus: Diagnosis, prevention and treatment* (pp. 185–204). New York: Plenum.

Jenkins, E.C., Brown, W.T., Brooks, J., et al. (1984). Experience with prenatal fragile X detection. *American Journal of Medical Genetics, 17,* 215–239.

Jenkins, E.C., Brown, W.T., Duncan, C.J., et al. (1981). Feasibility of fragile X chromosome prenatal diagnosis demonstrated. *Lancet,* Dec. 5, 1292.

Jenkins, E.C., Brown, W.T., Krawczun, M.S., et al. (1984). Fra (X) (p22) not associated with infantile autism. *Lancet* II, 1397.

Jenkins, E.C., Brown, W.T., Wilson, M.G., et al. (1986). The prenatal detection of the fragile X chromosome: Review of recent experience. *American Journal of Medical Genetics, 23,* 297–311.

Kirman, B.H. (1974). Clinical aspects: Epilepsy. In J. Wortis (Ed.), *Mental retardation and developmental disabilities* (Vol 6, pp. 1–49). New York: Brunner/Mazel.

Loehr, J.P., Synhorst, D.P., Wolfe, R.R., & Hagerman, R.I. (1986).Aortic root dilatation and mitral valve prolapse in the fragile X syndrome. *American Journal of Medical Genetics, 23,* 189–194.

Lubs, H.A. (1969). A marker X chromosome. *American Journal of Human Genetics, 21,* 231–244.

Lubs, H.A. (1983). X-linked mental retardation and the marker X. In E.H. Allan, D. Emery, & D.L. Rimoin (Eds.), *Principals and practices of medical genetics* (Vol 1, pp. 216–223). New York: Churchill Livingston.

Miezejeski, C.M., Jenkins, E.C., Hill, A.L., et al. (1984). Verbal vs. nonverbal ability, fragile X syndrome, and heterozygous carriers. *American Journal of Human Genetics, 36,* 227–229.

Oberle, I., Heilig, R., & Moisan, J.P., et al.(1986). Genetic analysis of the fragile-X mental retardation syndrome

with two flanking polymorphic DNA markers. *Proceedings of the National Academy of Sciences of the United States of America, 83,* 1016–1020.

Optiz, J. M. (1986). On the gates of hell and a most unusual gene [Editorial comment]. *American Journal of Medical Genetics, 23,* 1–10.

Optiz, J.M., Kaveggia, E.G., Durkin-Stamm, M.V., et al. (1978). Diagnostic/genetic studies in severe mental retardation. *Birth defects, 14*(6B), 1–38.

Optiz, J.M., Segal, A.T., Klove, H., et al. (1965). X-linked mental retardation: Study of a large kindred with 20 affected members. *Journal of Pediatrics, 67,* 713–714.

Rapin, I. (1977). Progressive genetic-metabolic diseases of the central nervous system. In A.M. Rudolph (Ed.), *Pediatrics* (16th ed.) (pp. 1892–1939). New York: Appleton-Century-Crofts.

Rapin, I. (1982). *Children with brain dysfunction.* New York: Raven.

Rudelli, R.D., Brown, W.T., Wisniewski, K., et al. (1985). Adult fragile X syndrome. *Acta Neuropathologica, 929,* 1–7.

Schmidt, A. (1980). Fragile site Xq2/ and mental retardation: Clinical and cytogenetic manifestation in heterozygotes and hemizygotes of five kindreds. *Human Genetics, 60,* 322–327.

Sherman, S.L., Jacobs, P.A., Morton, M.E., et al. (1985). Further segregation analysis of the fragile (X) syndrome with special reference to transmitting males. *Human Genetics, 69,* 289–299.

Sherman, S.L., Morton, N.E., Jacobs, P.A., et al. (1984). The marker (X) syndrome: A cytogenetic and genetic analysis. *Annals of Human Genetics, 43,* 21–37.

Touwen, B.C.L. (1979). Examination of the child with minor neurological dysfunction (2nd ed.). (Clinics in Developmental Medicine, Vol. 71). Philadelphia: J.B. Lippincott.

Touwen, B.C.L., & Prechtl, H.F.R. (1970). The neurological examination of the child with minor nervous dysfunction (Clinics in Developmental Medicine, Vol. 28). Philadelphia: J.B. Lippincott.

Turner, G. (1982). Fragile X-linked mental retardation. In B. Borne-Tamir (Ed.), *Human Genetics, Part B: Medical Aspects* (pp. 311–314). New York: Alan R. Liss.

Turner, G., Eastman, C., Casey, J., et al. (1975). X-linked mental retardation associated with macroorchidism. *Journal of Medical Genetics, 12,* 367–371.

Turner, G., & Optiz, J.M. (1980). Editorial comment: X-linked mental retardation. *American Journal of Medical Genetics, 7,* 407–415.

Turner, G., Optiz, J.M., Brown, W.T., et al. (1986). Conference report: Second international workshop on the fragile X and other X-linked mental retardation. *American Journal of Medical Genetics, 23*(1/2), 11–68.

Webb, T.P., Bundey, S.E., Thake, A.L., et al. (1986). Population incidence and segregation ratios in the Martin-Bell syndrome. *American Journal of Medical Genetics, 23*(1/2), 573–580.

Wisniewski, K.E., French, J.H., Fernando, S., et al. (1985). Fragile X syndrome: Associated neurological abnormalities and developmental disabilities. *Annals of Neurology, 18*(6), 665–669.

Chapter 3

Lysosomopathies

Analysis of Intracellular Abnormalities of Functional Proteins and a Survey of New Therapeutic Approaches

Yoshiyuki Suzuki, Kiyoshi Omura, Eiji Nanba, Akihiko Tsuji,
Rei-Cheng Yang, Goro Kato, Hitoshi Sakuraba, and Takashi Igarashi

L YSOSOMES ARE FUNCTIONAL CELLULAR organelles that digest macromolecules such as proteins, carbohydrates, and lipids; these substrates are degraded by lysosomal hydrolytic enzymes in an intraorganelle acidic environment (pH 4–5). If a defect of a specific lysosomal enzyme that catalyzes one or more degradation pathways occurs due to a gene mutation, a substrate accumulates in lysosomes and dysfunction of pertinent cells ensues. Such dysfunction may cause disease with clinical manifestations, such as severe damage in the central nervous system (lysosomal storage diseases or lysosomopathies [Hers & van Hoof, 1973]). At present, lysosomopathies are characterized by the accumulation of lipids (mainly sphingolipids), mucopolysaccharides, glycogen, and glycoprotein oligosaccharides.

Assays of lysosomal enzymes are now widely performed to screen for the presence of lysosomopathies in patients with neurological, as well as somatic, signs and symptoms that commence in infancy and childhood. Cases of rare adult varieties of lysosomopathies have been found, and their enzyme deficiencies also have been identified. Although extensive studies have been performed on various aspects of these diseases, our understanding is not sufficient to explain the pathogenesis of intra-

cellular and intercellular abnormalities that occur in afflicted patients.

In this report, recent results in three different lysosomopathies from our laboratories are presented. These data focus on the correlation between clinical and biochemical phenotypes, on analytical biochemical data on intracellular changes that occur in lysosomal enzyme deficiency diseases, and on the pathogenesis of functional disturbances of pathological lesions, especially in relation to possible therapeutic approaches.

RESULTS OF BIOCHEMICAL SCREENING

We started enzymatic and analytical screening for lysosomopathies using clinically available specimens such as serum or plasma, urine, leukocytes, fibroblasts, and other biopsy samples in 1972 (Suzuki, 1982b). Assays of lysosomal enzymes in leukocytes were performed and almost every type of lysosomopathy has been found (Table 1). The patient's clinical manifestations have been quite variable. The presence of progressive deterioration of neurological function, often associated with convulsive seizures, congenital somatic anomalies, and visceromegaly were the major indica-

This work was supported by grants from the Ministry of Education, Science, and Culture, and from the Ministry of Health and Welfare of Japan.

Table 1. Lysosomal diseases found by biochemical screening (1972–1986)

Tay-Sachs disease	23
Sandhoff disease	4
G_{M1}-gangliosidosis	19
Niemann-Pick disease	7
Gaucher disease	22
Metachromatic leukodystrophy	17
Krabbe disease	17
Fabry disease	18
Farber disease	1
Pompe disease	6
Hurler disease	4
Scheie disease	4
Sanfilippo disease A	2
B	6
C	1
Morquio disease	2
Galactosialidosis	26
Sialidosis	1
I-cell disease	12
Fucosidosis	2
Total	194

tions for biochemical analysis (Suzuki, 1982b). This is not a nationwide survey of metabolic diseases, although clinical samples were sent to us from almost every part of Japan. Thus, the incidence of each lysosomal disease cannot be calculated, but some diseases, like globoid cell leukodystrophy, have been diagnosed almost exclusively in our laboratory. The incidence for this lysosomopathy was roughly calculated on the basis of our diagnostic results (Suzuki & Suzuki, 1983). New genetic diseases and new variants of known diseases have been observed among these patients.

CLINICAL AND BIOCHEMICAL CORRELATION IN GALACTOSIALIDOSIS

Galactosialidosis is a recently recognized metabolic disease that occurs mainly in adults (Suzuki et al., 1985). This disease is characterized by the deficiency of lysosomal β-galactosidase and neuraminidase activity in somatic cells. The activities of these enzymes can be restored by a specific protein that is present in the culture medium of control fibroblasts. The

deficiency of β-galactosidase activity is also restored by thiol protease inhibitors. Deficiency of a 32 kDa protein that is normally associated with β-galactosidase molecules was reported by D'Azzo, Hoogeveen, Reuser, Robinson, & Galjaard (1982); but this has not been confirmed subsequently, except in one report (Suzuki et al., 1985). In that study, the antibody that had been prepared by D'Azzo et al. (1982) for detection of enzyme molecules was used. Our current studies indicate that there is a defect in the biosynthesis and processing of a low molecular weight protein (Nanba, Tsuji, Omura, & Suzuki, 1987) in this disease.

Clinically, the patients with this disease present with almost stereotypic neurosomatic manifestations: loss of vision and/or gait disturbance in the teens followed by action myoclonus, cherry-red spots, convulsive seizures, and angiokeratomata, as well as mild dysmorphism involving face, skin, and bones. The clinical course of this disease has been variable in the 24 cases we collected by the end of 1985 (Figure 1). We have encountered one infantile patient who developed cardiorespiratory as well as neurological signs and symptoms immediately after birth. The infant died of heart failure at 6 months of age.

We have initiated a comparative biochemical study on infantile and adult patients with this disease. Sucrose density gradient centrifugation was performed according to the method described by Hoogeveen, Verheijen, and Galjaard (1983) in order to separate the molecular species of β-galactosidase that are present in fibroblasts (Nanba et al., 1987). Three peaks of β-galactosidase activity were demonstrated in control fibroblasts, a minor fraction of a very large molecular size (peak 1) and two major fractions of smaller molecular sizes (peak 2: 400–500 kDa and peak 3: 100 kDa). These three peaks were detected in galactosialidosis fibroblasts, but exhibited a marked decrease in the enzymatic activities that are associated with the two major peaks, peaks 2 and 3 (Table 2). Early onset cases (the case described above and another reported previously by Kleijer et al., 1979), showed a more

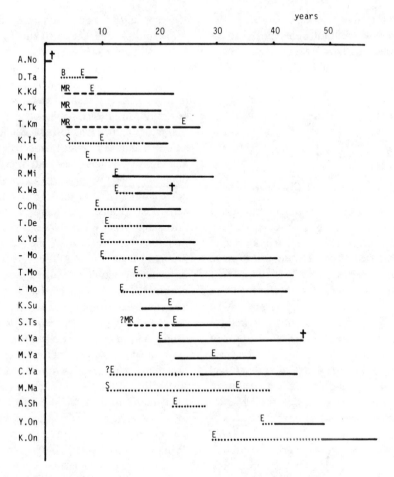

Figure 1. Clinical course in 24 cases of galactosialidosis. (····· = nonneurological manifestations; E = loss of vision and/or cherry-red spots; B = bone deformities; S = angiokeratoma; ----- = mental retardation or deterioration [MR]; _____ = neurological manifestations.)

drastic decrease of peak 2 activity. The two major peaks (2 and 3) were relatively higher in an asymptomatic, that is, a "presymptomatic" adult patient (Suzuki et al., 1985), than in symptomatic adults. The clinical manifestations of these cases correlated well with the degree of biochemical abnormalities. Similar results on the amount of a 52 kDa protein that was separated and detected by electrophoresis

have been reported by Palmeri, Hoogeveen, Verheijen, and Galjaard (1986).

Only peak 3 activity was restored by the addition of thiol protease inhibitors; the protein concentrate of the culture medium of both control and G_{M1}-gangliosidosis fibroblasts effected an almost complete normalization of the pattern of sucrose density gradient centrifugation (Nanba et al., 1987). It can be concluded

Table 2. Distribution of β-galactosidase molecular species fractionated by sucrose density gradient centrifugation

		Peak 1	Peak 2	Peak 3
Infant and fetus	(2)	14.6	0.7	10.6
Adult, symptomatic	(8)	40.5	3.6	13.0
Adult, asymptomatic	(1)	30.4	4.9	23.0

Values are expressed as percent of controls. Number of patients in parentheses.

that the "protective" protein causes an aggregation of monomer molecules (peak 3) of β-galactosidase, and leads to an increase of peak 2, an aggregate form of this enzyme. No significant difference was observed among early and late onset form patients in the degree of molecular size increase in these experiments.

INTRACELLULAR TRANSPORT OF LYSOSOMAL ENZYMES IN I-CELL DISEASE

Extensive studies of intracellular turnover of lysosomal enzymes have been stimulated by the finding that enzyme molecules are abnormally secreted from I-cell disease fibroblasts. These glycoprotein enzymes are recognized by a specific receptor for mannose 6-phosphate in oligosaccharide moieties of enzyme molecules; receptor recognition is apparently required for transport to and incorporation into lysosomes of fibroblasts (Sly & Fischer, 1982). Two receptor types are known, but details of their functional properties are not fully understood. Although most lysosomal enzymes are decreased in activity in I-cell disease, a few enzymes such as β-glucosidase, α-glucosidase, and acid-phosphatase are protected from abnormal secretion, and their intracellular activities are normal in I-cell disease fibroblasts. Furthermore, a question is raised by the fact that nonfibroblastic cells and some tissues from patients with this disease only exhibit a decrease of β-galactosidase activity; other lysosomal enzyme activities are apparently normal (Table 3). Thus, an alternative pathway for these enzymes to be transported to and incorporated into lysosomes must exist.

Because of these problems, we prepared membrane-bound enzymes from human liver and evaluated the effects of environmental

(solvent) changes on enzyme molecules (Kato & Suzuki, 1985). After treatment of human liver cell material by exhaustive washing and solubilization with detergents, a final membrane fraction was dissociated at pH 4.0 in order to recover free and solubilized lysosomal enzyme activities. The acid-soluble enzyme that was obtained was tested for binding to purified mannose 6-phosphate receptor. The amount of binding was extremely variable; 80% in β-glucuronidase, 50% in N-acetyl-β-hexosaminidase, and only 2% in α-glucosidase activities. β-glucuronidase and N-acetyl-β-hexosaminidase in this "acid-soluble" fraction from the liver of a patient with I-cell disease did not bind to the receptor, although intracellular activities of these enzymes were normal. It was concluded that there are alternate mechanisms for the transport of lysosomal enzymes in tissues other than fibroblasts in this disease (Kato & Suzuki, 1985).

Some mammalian lectins (sugar-binding proteins) act as receptors for the processing and sorting of carbohydrate chains in glycoprotein molecules. Liver membrane fractions containing enzyme activity were treated with various sugars, and the results are summarized in Table 4. In the control liver, 10 mM mannose 6-phosphate dissociated the largest amount of N-acetyl-β-hexosaminidase activity and the dissociation was lower with other sugars. On the contrary, there was little dissociation from the membrane preparation of the I-cell disease liver with mannose 6-phosphate; fucose, mannose, and N-acetylglucosamine caused significant dissociation. Due to technical limitations, only N-acetyl-β-hexosaminidase was tested in this experiment. This lysosomal enzyme is bound mainly to the phosphomannosyl receptor under the physiological conditions that are present in control human liver. In I-cell dis-

Table 3.   Lysosomal enzyme activities in I-cell disease

	βGal	Others	GGA
Solid tissues	Decreased	Normal	Normal
Fibroblasts	Decreased	Decreased	Normal
Extracellular fluids	Increased	Increased	Normal

βGal: β-galactosidase.
GGA: α-glucosidase, β-glucosidase, acid phosphatase.

Table 4. Dissociation of membrane-bound N–acetyl–β–hexosaminidase from human liver by various sugars

Sugars added	Control	I-cell disease
Mannose 6-phosphate (10mM)	71	3.4
Galactose (10mM)	14	11
Mannose (50mM)	10	40
Fucose (50mM)	7	56
N-Acetylglucosamine (50mM)	Trace	27

Values are expressed as percent released of the total enzyme activity.

ease, N-acetyl-β-hexosaminidase may be sorted and transported, possibly as a glycoprotein with complex type oligosaccharides, by other binding proteins such as fucose-binding protein and/or mannose/N-acetyl-D-glucosamine binding protein. Such alternative sorting and transport would compensate for a defective phosphomannosyl pathway. Further investigations are currently in progress.

PREVENTION OF VASCULAR LESIONS IN FABRY'S DISEASE

Fabry's disease is a genetic lipid storage disease caused by deficiency of α-galactosidase activity that is transmitted by an X-linked gene (Desnick & Sweeley, 1983). Major clinical manifestations of this disease are caused by accumulation of ceramide trihexoside in the vascular endothelium and in other varieties of cells. This accumulation leads to ischemia, infarction, and thrombosis in the central nervous system, heart, and kidneys, usually in male patients after middle age. We have evaluated hemizygous males and heterozygous females with thromboembolism. These cases have been followed from the relatively early stages of the disease (Sakuraba et al., 1986). Recently, a trial has been started for preventing vascular complications of this disease by the administration of antiplatelet drugs.

Platelet aggregation and plasma β-thromboglobulin levels, indicators of platelet function, were increased in both hemizygotes and heterozygotes. The plasma content of 6-keto-prostaglandin $F_{1\alpha}$, an indicator of vascular endothelial antiplatelet function, was somewhat decreased in most patients (Igarashi, Sakuraba, & Suzuki, 1986). Electron microscopic studies

did not detect any remarkable morphological changes in platelets from the patients. It was concluded that a vascular endothelial lesion causes the characteristic enhanced platelet aggregation that is associated with this disease (Sakuraba, Igarashi, Shibata, & Suzuki, 1987).

Platelet hyperfunction can accelerate atherosclerotic as well as thromboembolic vascular damage and can cause a wide variety of vascular complications that determine the overall prognosis of this disease. Consequently, we investigated the effects of vitamin E and ticlopidine administration on platelet aggregation during the course of Fabry's disease. Vitamin E inhibits the release of arachidonic acid from phospholipids in platelets, and inhibits peroxidation of arachidonic acid in vascular endothelium (Pangramala & Cornwell, 1982). Ticlopidine, which is an inhibitor of phospholipase A_2, increases cyclic AMP in platelets and consequently decreases thromboxan A_2 synthesis (Ashida & Abiko, 1978). Preliminary results of administering these drugs to Fabry's patients are summarized in Table 5. A moderate inhibitory effect was observed in vitamin E treatment. Ticlopidine

Table 5. Effects of vitamin E and ticlopidine on platelet aggregation in Fabry's disease

	ADP	Collagen
Vitamin E (2)	100/86	100/90
Ticlopidine (5)	100/35	100/24
Normal range	48–80	58–82

Values are expressed as percent (mean) aggregation with ADP (5μM) or collagen (2 μg/ml) added (numbers of patients in parentheses), before/after the administration of vitamin E (20 mg/kg body weight) or triclopidine (4–5 mg/kg body weight) for 7 days.

therapy showed more drastic changes in the platelet aggregation after 7 days of administration. These results suggest that the intravascular abnormality, which develops at an early stage of the clinical course, may be ameliorated by these drugs; medical treatment of this type promises a more favorable prognosis for this disease (Sakuraba et al., 1987). Further evaluation on a long-term basis is necessary, and a follow-up study has been started in order to establish the ultimate consequences of this treatment in Fabry patients.

CONCLUSION

Major biochemical insights concerning the nature of lysosomopthies have been achieved during the past 2 decades. However, a detailed pathogenesis for many of their clinical manifestations is not sufficiently understood at present. The molecular basis of their respective enzyme deficiencies is not uniform, and elucidation of this knowledge, in order to initiate rational therapeutic trials, is mandatory. Even though gene therapy may be the final target of investigators of genetic metabolic diseases, there are many problems to be surmounted before experimental therapeutic procedures at the cellular level are applied to human patients.

In some diseases, prevention and treatment of the biochemical lesions causing clinical signs and symptoms, especially those of the central nervous system, have been accomplished by diet therapy (amino acid, carbohydrate, and other disorders) and drug therapy (Wilson disease, etc.), as well as other approaches. However, lysosomopathies are more difficult to treat because substrates of the deficient enzymes are accumulated tightly in lysosomes. Also, the clinical manifestations of central nervous system dysfunction associated with these diseases frequently commence in early infancy and childhood, and often have rapidly progressive courses. Enzyme replacement therapy may be possible in the form of bone marrow and other organ transplantation procedures, but the presence of the blood-brain barrier and the delivery of exogenous enzymes to specific target organs are major technical problems that await favorable solutions.

We have investigated a therapeutic possibility that corrects functional abnormalities of platelets and their interaction with vascular endothelium in Fabry's disease; this trial is successful in a few patients at present. Another therapeutic strategy that can be considered in lysosomopathies with rapid turnover of precursor and mature enzyme molecules, specifically, galactosialidosis (Suzuki et al., 1985) and metachromatic leukodystrophy (von Figura, Steckel, & Hasilik, 1983), is to inhibit proteolysis of deficient lysosomal enzymes that have a shortened biologic half-life. Such approaches promise to augment our basic understanding of the pathogenetic mechanisms of disease, and may contribute to the prevention and more rational treatment of some lysosomopathies in the future.

REFERENCES

Ashida, S., & Abiko, Y. (1978). Effect of ticlopidine and acetylsalicylic acid on generation of prostaglandin I₂-like substance in rat arterial tissue. *Thrombosis Research, 13,* 901–908.

D'Azzo, A., Hoogeveen, A., Reuser, A.J.J., Robinson, D., & Galjaard, H. (1982). Molecular defect in combined β-galactosidase and neuraminidase in man. *Proceedings of the National Academy of Sciences of the United States of America, 79,* 4535–4537.

Desnick, R.J., & Sweeley, C.C. (1983). Fabry's disease: α-Galactosidase A deficiency. In J.B. Stanbury, J.B. Wyngaarden, D.S. Fredrickson, J.L. Goldstein, & M.S. Brown (Eds.). *The metabolic basis of inherited disease* (5th ed., pp. 906–944). New York: McGraw-Hill.

Hers, H.G., & van Hoof, F. (Eds.). (1973). *Lysosomes and storage diseases.* New York: Academic Press.

Hoogeveen, A.T., Verheijen, F.W., & Galjaard, H. (1983). The relation between human lysosomal β-galactosidase and its protective protein. *Journal of Biological Chemistry, 258,* 12143–12146.

Igarashi, T., Sakuraba, H., & Suzuki, Y. (1986). Activation of platelet function in Fabry's disease. *American Journal of Hematology, 22,* 63–67.

Kato, G., & Suzuki, Y. (1985). Membrane-bound N-acetyl-β-glucosaminidase: Different binding specificity in control and I-cell disease livers. *FEBS Letters, 193,* 222–226.

Kleijer, W.T., Hoogeveen, A., Verheijen, F.W., Niermeijer, M.F., Galjaard, H., O'Brien, J.S., & Warner,

T.G. (1979). Prenatal diagnosis of sialidosis with combined neuraminidase and β-galactosidase deficiency. *Clinical Genetics, 16*, 60–61.

Motegi, Y., Fujinaga, T., Tamura, H., Kuroume, T., Omura, K., Nanba, E., & Suzuki, Y. (1987). Severe infantile galactosialidosis: A case report. *Nihon Shonika Gakkai Zasshi, 91*, 1459–1464.

Nanba, E., Tsuji, A., Omura, K., & Suzuki, Y. (1987). Galactosialidosis: Studies on residual enzymes in early and late onset clinical phenotypes. *Journal of Clinical Biochemistry and Nutrition, 3*, 149–157.

Palmeri, S., Hoogeveen, A.T., Verheijen, F.W., & Galjaard, H. (1986). Galactosialidosis: Molecular heterogeneity among distinct clinical phenotypes. *American Journal of Human Genetics, 38*, 137–148.

Pangramala, R.V., & Cornwell, D.G. (1982). The effects of vitamin E on arachidonic acid metabolism. *Annals of the New York Academy of Sciences, 393*, 376–391.

Sakuraba, H., Igarashi, T., Shibata, T., & Suzuki, Y. (1987). Effect of vitamin E and ticlopidine on platelet aggregation in Fabry's disease. *Clinical Genetics, 31*, 349–354.

Sakuraba, H., Yanagawa, Y., Igarashi, T., Suzuki, Y., Suzuki, T., Watanabe, K., Ieki, K., Shimoda, K., & Yamanaka, T. (1986). Cardiovascular manifestations in Fabry's disease. A high incidence of mitral valve prolapse in hemizygotes and heterozygotes. *Clinical Genetics, 29*, 276–283.

Sly, W.S., & Fischer, H.D. (1982). The phosphoman-

nosyl recognition system for intracellular and intercellular transport of lysosomal enzymes. *Journal of Cellular Biochemistry, 18*, 67–85.

Suzuki, Y. (1982a). Heredodegenerative diseases of the central nervous system and inborn errors of metabolism. *No to Hattatsu, 14*, 271–275.

Suzuki, Y. (1982b). Enzymatic diagnosis of lysosomal diseases. An experience in a clinical laboratory during the period 1972–1980. *Acta Paediatrica Japonica, 24*, 25–30.

Suzuki, Y., Sakuraba, H., Yamanaka, T., Ko, Y.M., Iimori, Y., Okamura, Y., & Hoogeveen, A.T. (1985). Galactosialidosis: A comparative study of clinical and biochemical data on 22 patients. In M. Arima, Y. Suzuki, & H. Yabuuchi (Eds.), *The developing brain and its disorders* (pp. 161–175). Basel: Karger.

Suzuki, K., & Suzuki, Y. (1983). Galactosylceramide lipidosis: Globoid cell leukodystrophy (Krabbe's disease). In J.B. Stanbury, J.B. Wyngaarden, D.S. Fredrickson, J.L. Goldstein, & M.S. Brown (Eds.), *The metabolic basis of inherited disease* (5th ed., pp. 857–880). New York: McGraw-Hill.

von Figura, K., Steckel, F., & Hasilik, A. (1983). Juvenile and adult metachromatic leukodystrophy: Partial restoration of arylsulfatase A (cerebroside sulfatase) activated by inhibitors of thiol proteinases. *Proceedings of the National Academy of Sciences of the United States of America, 80*, 6066–6070.

Chapter 4

Ultrastructural Pathology of Blood Lymphocytes and Skin in Lysosomal Disorders of Childhood

*Hans H. Goebel, Wolfgang Brück,
Ulf Käsgen, and Stefan Walter*

THE ADVENT OF ELECTRON MICROSCOPY was instrumental in initiating the concept of lysosomal storage disorders (lysosomopathies). In addition, the electron microscope became a major laboratory tool for the diagnosis of neurodegenerative diseases. Ultrastructural investigations of biopsied brain tissue from children afflicted with lysosomopathies, in particular those who had Tay-Sachs disease, provided seminal data on the fine structure of the diseased brain. The subsequent development of biochemical analyses of blood, urine, and skin fibroblasts to demonstrate the presence or absence of lysosomal enzymes in the homozygously affected individual, even prenatally, or a reduction of their activity in heterozygous carriers, rendered brain biopsies for the diagnosis of neurodegenerative diseases—especially those of lysosomal origin—generally inappropriate and obsolete.

Subsequently, it became apparent that many lysosomal diseases, which clinically exhibit a neurodegenerative course, have biochemical and morphological manifestations in extraneural tissues. Hence, the technique of mor-phologically examining blood lymphocytes, skin, and conjunctiva has become a firmly established diagnostic procedure that enables clinicians to:

1. Demonstrate the presence or absence of a lysosomal disease, sometimes by demonstrating the presence of disease-specific residual bodies
2. Establish the diagnosis of lysosomal disorders that cannot be currently diagnosed by biochemical assays
3. Ascertain homozygosity for a lysosomopathy in patients whose biochemically determined enzyme data are at a borderline level between homozygously affected individuals and heterozygotes
4. Detect lysosomal disorders, hitherto undescribed, that require further biochemical characterization

Similar morphologic study of amniocytes has also established the prenatal diagnosis of a lysosomal storage disease which meets the criteria of "1" and "2" *sub verbo* (MacLeod et al., 1985).

Results incorporated in this paper represent parts of the medical theses by W. Brück, U. Käsgen, and S. Walter. Also, we are grateful to Prof. Dr. Anton-Lamprecht, University of Heidelberg, for her helpful advice. Additionally, Mrs. I. Warlo kindly provided the electron microscopic work, Mr. W. Meffert provided the photographic work, and Mrs. M. Messerschmidt and Ms. L. Halbig provided secretarial and editorial assistance.

BLOOD LYMPHOCYTES IN
LYSOSOMAL STORAGE DISEASES

Lysosomal accumulation of glycogen when plasma cell lysosomal acid maltase activity is deficient in patients with type II glycogenosis (Pralle, Schroeder, & Löffler, 1974) signals the involvement of B-lymphocytes in this disease. Morphologic changes of both B- and T-lymphocytes have been found in patients with juvenile neuronal ceroid-lipofuscinosis (NCL) and aspartylglucosaminuria (Aula, Rapola, & Andersson, 1975). Gold (Figure 1a) or peroxidase (Figure 1b) markers, used to discriminate between antisera labeled B-cells (Figure 1a) and T-cells (Figure 1b) indicate that both of these lymphocyte types evidence nonvacuolar as well as vacuolar morphologic alterations in lysosomal diseases.

Ultrastructural abnormalities in blood cells associated with lysosomal diseases are exhibited only by blood lymphocytes and B-lymphocyte derivative plasma cells. Thus, pellets of separated lymphocytes from blood are a better material for diagnostic study than buffy coats, which contain the entire spectrum of circulating nucleated cells, when a lysosomopathy is suspected. Circulating lymphocytes are easily and repeatedly available via phlebotomy. Sedimented lymphocytes may be isolated from uncoagulated blood by use of a Ficoll-Hypaque density gradient (Böyum, 1968). The availability of a micromethod, requiring only 500μl of blood (Kohlschütter, Sieg, Schulte, Hayek, & Goebel, 1982), enables study of lymphocytes from very young children or children with extremely small and fragile veins. Sedimentation-isolated lymphocytes can be used for both the morphologic demonstration of disease-specific lysosomal residual bodies and the biochemical documentation of a suspected enzyme deficiency (Tsuji, Yamada, Tsutsumi, & Miyatake, 1982).

Lymphocytes from patients with lysosomal diseases may be categorized morphologically as: 1) showing lysosomal vacuolation, 2) exhibiting nonvacuolar lysosomal residual bodies, and 3) failing to reveal lysosomal ab-

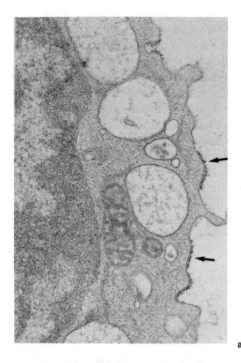
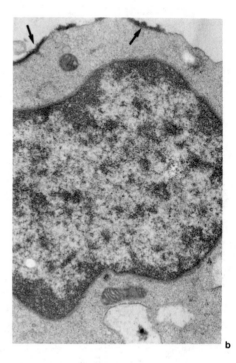

a

b

Figure 1.   Labeling of lymphocytic surfaces with: **a)** gold (arrows), original magnification × 45.000; **b)** peroxidase (arrows), original magnification × 25.300, allows differentiation of B-(a) and T-lymphocytes (b) with B- or I-specific antisera.

normalities (Ikeda, Goebel, Burck, & Kohl-schütter, 1982). Lymphocytes from normal subjects usually reveal minute groups of small membrane-bound granular bodies, apparent lysosomes. Among these lysosomes, a larger lipid-containing inclusion, the Gall body, is frequently seen (Figure 2). Enlarged lysosomes in the lymphocytes from patients with some lysosomal diseases occur in cytoplasmic aggregates, and individual lysosomes are surrounded by an obvious trilaminar unit membrane. Ten percent to over 75% of lymphocytes may display such disease-specific changes in some lysosomal diseases.

The frequency of circulating lymphocytes that contain disease-specific lysosomal residual bodies is determined, at least in part, by the specific lysosomal disease that is present. However, individual patient characteristics such as the duration of the neurodegenerative process at the time of study, the presence or absence of an intercurrent infection, and the preparative technique for morphologic study may also be determinants.

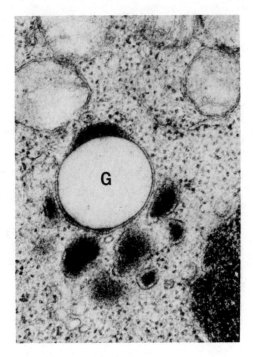

Figure 2.   A Gall (G) body within a normal lymphocyte, original magnification × 189.500.

The longitudinal frequency of intralymphocytic-lysosomal residual bodies and the influence(s) of transient infections on the relative frequency of lysosomal changes have not been determined to date. Lymphocytes appear to be capable of endocytosis-phagocytosis in the presence of bacteria, and may incorporate their own cellular organelles (autophagocytosis), (as with, for example, mitochondria). The methods used to make lymphocyte preparations (i.e., smears), plastic embedded semithin sections, and electron microscopic ultrathin sections, may also be confounding. Spurious vacuolation can be caused by preparative swelling of grouped mitochondria and nuclear membrane enlargement; pseudovacuolation may be the result of the presence of superficial villous processes.

Lysosomal Diseases that Evidence Nonvacuolar Lysosomal Aggregates in Blood Lymphocytes

The number of lysosomal disorders that evidence nonvacuolar lysosomal aggregates in blood lymphocytes is small. However, the ultrastructural findings are often diagnostically specific.

Neuronal Ceroid-Lipofuscinosis (NCL)
The presence of membrane-bound, granular inclusions (Figure 3) is the predominant ultrastructural abnormality that is found in the circulating lymphocytes of patients with infantile NCL. The fine structure of these inclusions resembles that of the granular lysosomes that accumulate in the cells of other tissues from patients with this form of NCL (Ikeda & Goebel, 1979). The presence of curvilinear bodies in circulating lymphocytes (Figure 4) is the hallmark of late infantile NCL; fingerprint profiles within curvilinear bodies are extremely rare in this clinical variety of NCL. Fingerprint profiles *are* present in the avacuolar conglomerates of lipopigments that accumulate in the circulating lymphocytes of patients with early juvenile NCL (Lake & Cavanagh, 1978). In the juvenile form (Spielmeyer-Sjögren) of NCL, fingerprint profile-containing lipopigment aggregates are usually intravacuolar. However, occasional non-

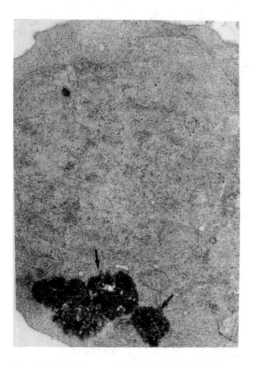

Figure 3.   Infantile neuronal ceroid-lipofuscinosis: two membrane-bound granular lipopigment bodies (arrows), original magnification × 71.500.

course may assist in resolving any controversy concerning the presence or absence of ultrastructural abnormalities in lymphocytes from patients with adult NCL.

Mucolipidosis IV   Lysosomal lamellar bodies that partially resemble membranous cytoplasmic bodies are present in the circulating lymphocytes (Figure 5) from patients with mucolipidosis IV (Goebel, Kohlschütter, & Lenard, 1982). This morphologic finding is consistent with an earlier biochemical report (Bach, Cohen, & Kohn, 1975) that lysosomal gangliosides accumulate in this disorder.

Niemann-Pick Disease   The vacuoles observed by light microscopy in the circulating lymphocytes of patients with Niemann-Pick disease are found to contain membranous material when examined by electron microscopy (Lazarus, Vethamany, Schneck, & Volk, 1967). The occurrence and/or absence of this finding in the individual forms of Niemann-Pick disease remain to be reported.

Miscellaneous   "Tubular arrays" (Figure 6) have been identified occasionally in the cir-

vacuolar lipopigment aggregates may be present in circulating lymphocytes from patients whose clinical courses and skin biopsy findings are compatible with a diagnosis of juvenile NCL (Goebel, 1985). Transitions between these differing ultrastructural patterns of lipopigment accumulation in lymphocytes do not, to the authors' knowledge, occur in these four different varieties of NCL. Admittedly, this statement must be qualified by the previously discussed lack of sequential studies in patients with NCL.

Ultrastructural abnormalities are not usually found in the circulating lymphocytes of patients with the adult form of NCL, even though abnormalities have been reported at least once (Badurska, Fidziańska, & Jedrzejowska, 1981). A precise differentiation between patients with adult NCL and those with juvenile NCL, which evolves in a protracted fashion (Goebel, Pilz, & Gullotta, 1976), is often difficult. Thus, knowledge of the sequential involvement of circulating lymphocytes in those cases of juvenile NCL that evince a protracted

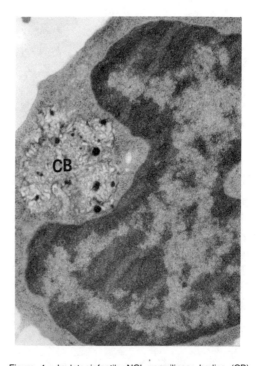

Figure 4.   In late infantile NCL, curvilinear bodies (CB) prevail, original magnification × 160.760.

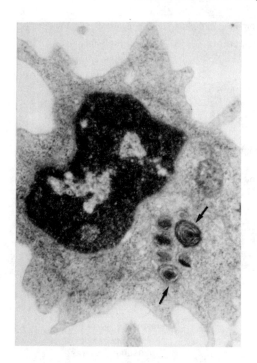

Figure 5. Nonvacuolar lamellar bodies (arrows) mark muco-lipidosis IV, original magnification × 52.500.

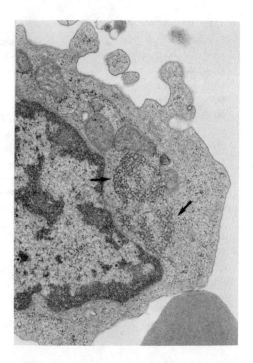

Figure 7. Undulating tubules or tubulo-reticular inclusions (arrows) mark immune-mediated disorders such as dermatomyositis, original magnification × 26.400.

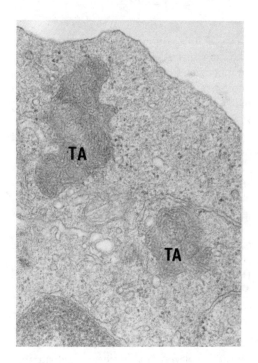

Figure 6. Tubular arrays (TA) are a frequent nonspecific finding in otherwise normal lymphocytes, original magnification × 61.750.

culating lymphocytes of patients affected by lysosomal diseases, as well as in patients with other disease processes. This attests to the non-specificity of this inclusion. "Undulating tubules" or "tubuloreticular inclusions" have been observed in such immune-mediated disorders as lupus erythematosus, scleroderma, dermatomyositis (Figure 7) and AIDS; these findings are a possible result of interferon stimulation. Experimentally administered drugs may also induce the formation of lysosomal storage bodies (Lüllmann-Rauch, 1974).

Lysosomal Diseases that Evidence Abnormal Lysosomal Vacuolation of Blood Lymphocytes

Circulating lymphocytes from patients with the lysosomal diseases listed in Table 1 are characterized by aggregates of membrane-bound vacuoles. These vacuoles contain histochemically demonstrable acid phosphatase: a finding that is compatible with the vacuoles' lysosomal origin. Even though most of the vacuoles are clear, occasional examples of finely amor-

Table 1. Lysosomopathies with vacuolated cytosomes in circulating lymphocytes

Disease	Disease eponym	Enzyme deficiency
MPS, type I-H	Hurler syndrome	α-L-iduronidase
MPS, type II	Hunter syndrome	L-iduronsulfate sulfatase
MPS, type III A	Sanfilippo syndrome A	Heparan-N-sulfatase
MPS, type III B	Sanfilippo syndrome	N-acetylglucosaminidase
MPS, type IV A	Morquio syndrome A	N-acetylagalactosamin-6-sulfatase
MPS, type IV B	Morquio syndrome B	β-galactosidase
MPS, type VI A	Maroteaux-Lamy syndrome A	Arylsulfatase B
MPS, type VI B	Maroteaux-Lamy syndrome B	Arylsulfatase B
MPS, type VII (?)	Sly syndrome	β-glucuronidase
GM$_1$-gangliosidosis, type I	Landing disease	β-galactosidase
GM$_1$-gangliosidosis, type II	Derry disease	β-galactosidase
Mannosidosis	—	α-D-mannosidase
Fucosidosis	—	α-L-fucosidase
Sialidosis	—	α-neuraminidase
Aspartyl-glucosaminuria	—	aspartyl-glucosaminidase
Juvenile neuronal ceroid-lipofuscinosis	Spielmeyer-Sjögren type	unknown
Salla disease	Salla disease	unknown
Mucolipidosis II	I-cell disease	N-acetylglucosaminyl-phosphotransferase
Mucolipidosis III	Pseudo-Hurler polydystrophy	N-acetylglucosaminyl-phosphotransferase
Multiple sulfatase deficiency (?)	—	multiple sulfatases

Modified from Ikeda et al., 1982.

phous granular material have been seen, and sometimes the vacuolar granule content is prominent. Preparative loss of lysosomal contents is the probable explanation for the absence of granular material in most of the lymphocytes from patients with these lysosomal diseases.

Clear vacuoles, whose lysosomal glycogen was washed out, are encountered in the circulating lymphocytes of patients with type II glycogenosis (Figure 8a). However, lymphocytes from patients with both the juvenile and adult forms of this disease may contain solid, nonvacuolar lysosomal inclusions (Figure 8b).

Aggregates of lysosomal vacuoles are a prominent ultrastructural finding in the circulating lymphocytes of patients with the juvenile form of NCL. However, the vacuoles that are seen in this disease frequently contain a granular matrix and fingerprint profiles (Figure 9).

Rarely, fingerprint inclusions are also found in the vacuoles of lymphocytes from patients with mucopolysaccharidoses (MPS) (Goebel,

Ikeda, Schulz, Burck, & Kohlschütter, 1981). The fingerprint inclusions that occur in the lymphocytes from patients with MPS are morphologically similar to, but much less frequent than, those present in juvenile NCL. Thus, lysosomal vacuolation of circulating lymphocytes is associated with a number of lysosomal diseases, including the juvenile variety of NCL. However, only juvenile NCL can be separated from this diagnostic list by morphologically demonstrating a sufficient number of fingerprint profiles in addition to vacuolation.

Lysosomal Diseases that Do Not Evidence Morphologic Abnormalities in Blood Lymphocytes

Histiocytes in the bone marrow, lymphoreticular organs (Figure 10), and skin nodules of patients with Gaucher's and Farber's disease, respectively, exhibit lysosomal storage. However, there is no apparent electron microscopic abnormality in the circulating lympho-

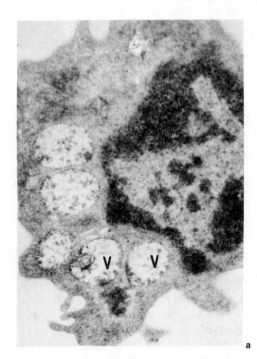

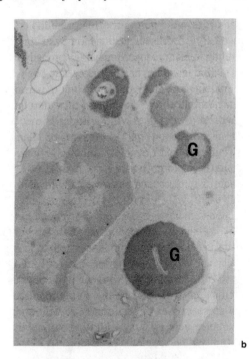

Figure 8.   Adult type II glycogenosis: **a)** glycogen is almost completely washed out, leaving nearly empty vacuoles (V), original magnification × 51.033; **b)** in another specimen, glycogen (G) is densely packed in lysosomes, original magnification × 31.850.

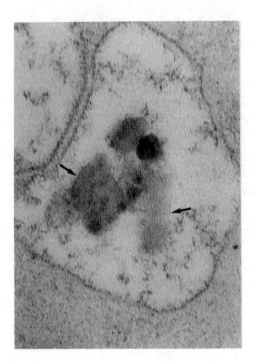

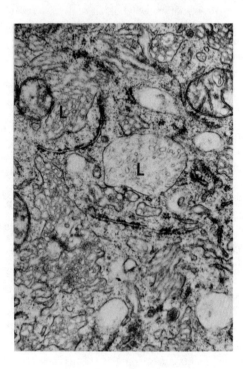

Figure 9.   Juvenile NCL is marked by fingerprint profiles (arrows) within membrane-bound vacuoles, original magnification × 157.500.

Figure 10.   In Gaucher's disease, membrane-bound lysosomes (L) contain hollow profiles, original magnification × 97.600.

cytes from such patients, even though their circulating lymphocytes express a deficiency of either glucocerebrosidase or acid-ceramidase activities, respectively. Therefore, an absence of morphologic abnormalities in circulating lymphocytes does not rule out the presence of a lysosomopathy in a small number of currently identified lysosomal storage diseases.

DERMAL MORPHOLOGIC ABNORMALITIES IN LYSOSOMAL DISORDERS

Even though a morphologic examination of blood for the diagnostic evaluation of a lysosomopathy utilizes lymphocytes only, the diagnostic evaluation of a sufficiently sized and an appropriately executed skin biopsy requires an examination of all of this tissue's structural components. Skin and conjunctiva, in contradistinction to circulating cells, are composed of cell types that have more diverse embryonal origins than blood cells. These cell types and constituents include: mesenchymal (e.g., vascular endothelial, smooth muscle and fibroblastic), cutaneous epithelial (e.g., dermal, glandular, and epidermal), and neuroectodermal (e.g., myelinated and unmyelinated axonal, Schwann cell, and perineural elements). This diversity of cellular origins is the most likely explanation for the presence of cutaneous morphologic abnormalities in nearly all of the currently identified lysosomal storage diseases.

Slight accumulation of lipopigments in cutaneous elements, which are composed of a granular matrix and lipid droplets, occurs in association with normal function and aging. Such accumulations are infrequent in comparison to those associated with both nonlysosomal and lysosomal disease pathologies. Skin biopsies from patients with neurodermatitis, a nonlysosomal disease, may exhibit relatively prominent accumulations of lipopigments in a number of tissue components, including sudoriferous epithelia. Nonspecific lipopigments can be found in the Schwann cells of unmyelinated axons in skin. Nonspecific pi granules, thought to contain sulfatides, occur

normally in Schwann cells of the myelinated axons in intradermal nerve fascicles. The epithelial cells of sweat gland ducts that ascend through the epidermis of normal skin regularly evidence aggregates of membranous bodies (Figure 11).

The morphologic evaluation of a skin biopsy to determine the presence of a lysosomal disease requires the study of vascular endothelial cells, smooth muscle cells, fibroblasts, and glandular and sweat gland ductal cells, as well as any infiltrating cells. As in lymphocytes, the presence of a lysosomal disease is signalled by finding lysosomal vacuoles (Figure 12) and nonvacuolar lysosomal inclusions. The lysosomal vacuoles that are found in skin biopsy specimens from patients with lysosomal diseases are similar ultrastructurally to those that are present in the circulating lymphocytes from these patients. However, those that are present in dermal specimens from patients with the juvenile variety of NCL are an exception to this generalization.

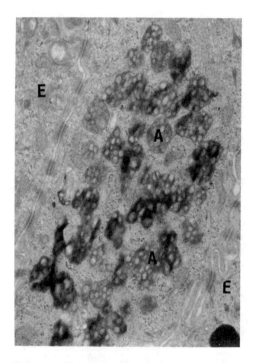

Figure 11. Normal ductal sweat gland epithelia regularly contain lamellar aggregates (A) when traversing the epidermis (E), original magnification × 105.600.

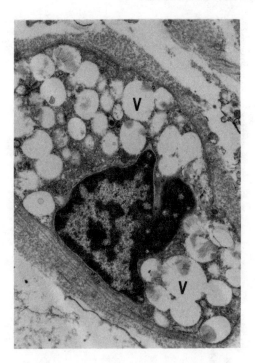

Figure 12.   In mucopolysaccharidosis I, many dermal cells are marked by vacuolar (V) lysosomes, original magnification × 71.820.

Lysosomal Diseases Characterized by Involvement of Epidermal Cells

Skin biopsy specimens may be extremely small in size and may only contain the superficial layers of the integument. Thus, an absence of ultrastructural pathology in epidermal cells does not permit researchers to confidently rule out the diagnostic possibility of a lysosomopathy. However, some lysosomal storage diseases are characterized by such changes.

Sandhoff's disease, Farber's disease, Salla's disease, the MPS, and the mucolipidoses exhibit morphologic features of lysosomal storage in epidermal cells. Lysosomal inclusions within epidermal cells are of two types:

1. Vacuolar, seen in GM_1-gangliosidosis, the mucopolysaccharidoses I, II, and III, and in Salla's disease; in type II glycogenosis, lysosomal glycogen, which is occasionally washed out, may also impart the impression of lysosomal vacuolation.

2. Avacuolar, membranous-lamellar inclu-

sions are seen in Fabry's disease (Figure 13), Farber's disease (Figure 21b), and in mucolipidosis IV, while curvilinear bodies are encountered in late infantile neuronal ceroid-lipofuscinosis (Figure 14).

Both vacuolar and nonvacuolar lysosomal changes are present in specimens from patients with mucolipidosis I and mucolipidosis IV (Goebel et al., 1982). Epidermal cell involvement also has been stated to be present in the infantile and juvenile forms of NCL by some investigators (Ceuterick, Martin, Casaer, & Edgar, 1976; Martin & de Groote, 1974) but most researchers have been unable to confirm this observation.

Lysosomopathies that are Characterized by Changes in Cutaneous Nerve Fibers

The peripheral axons of myelinated and unmyelinated cutaneous nerves rarely exhibit specific features of lysosomal storage. However, their terminal segments do show dystrophic

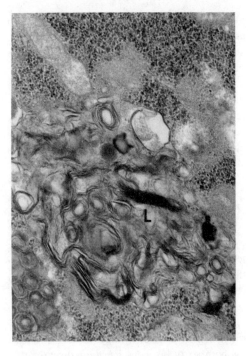

Figure 13.   A large lamellar (L) lysosomal body marks Fabry's disease, even in the carrier state, original magnification × 186.960.

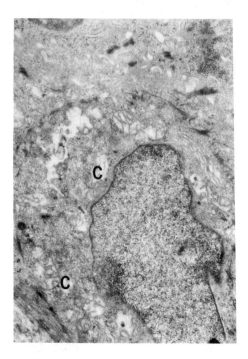

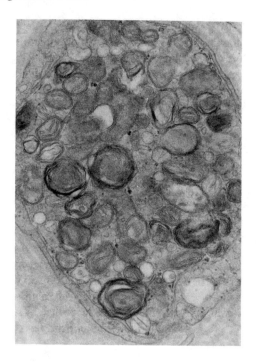

Figure 14. Several curvilinear bodies (C) within a keratinocyte, NCL, original magnification × 6750.

Figure 15. Juvenile NCL: an unmyelinated axon is filled with mitochondria and dense bodies, original magnification × 178.125.

axonal changes (Orfanos & Runne, 1975) such as accumulated mitochondria, dense bodies, and nonspecific lysosomes (Figure 15). Some of the dense bodies are probably derived from degenerating mitochondria. The NCL, MPS, gangliosidoses, and mannosidosis characteristically exhibit such changes. Dense body accumulation in these diseases is probably caused by impaired axonal transport and/or involvement of the parent neuronal perikaryon. Verification of these hypotheses obviously requires study of an axon terminal along with its attached perikaryon. Disease-specific lysosomal inclusions such as the membranous cytoplasmic body are found occasionally in the terminal segments of cutaneous axons of patients with GM_2 − gangliosidosis (Figure 16) (Burck et al., 1980) and mucolipidosis IV.

Thoroughly studying dermal nerve fascicles of patients who have an undiagnosed neurodegenerative disease may greatly increase the number of lysosomal storage diseases that can be identified by skin biopsies (Dolman, 1984). Even though vacuolar lysosomes do not

occur in enlarged cutaneous axon terminals, disease-specific inclusions may be found on occasion, and their presence can be pathognomonic. The search for such inclusions must include unmyelinated axon terminals that are usually located beneath the epidermis (Figure 16); such terminals also occasionally extend into the epidermis (Figure 17).

Disease-specific lysosomal residual bodies are also present in Schwann cells and, less frequently, in intrafascicular mesenchymal cells of myelinated dermal nerve fascicles from patients with metachromatic leukodystrophy (MLD) (Figure 18) and Krabbe's disease (Figure 19). The inclusions have a tufaceous/tuffstone or prismatic/herringbone appearance in MLD, whereas they are needle-like in Krabbe's disease.

Lysosomopathies that Are Characterized by Endothelial Cell Changes

The membrane-bound, lysosomal residual bodies within cutaneous vascular endothelial

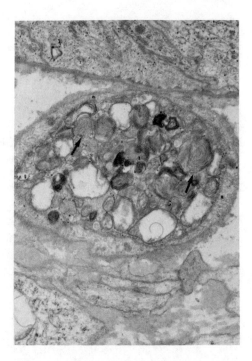

Figure 16. In GM$_2$-gangliosidosis, a subepidermal unmyelinated axonal terminal is filled with numerous disease-specific membranous cytoplasmic bodies (arrows), original magnification × 24.225.

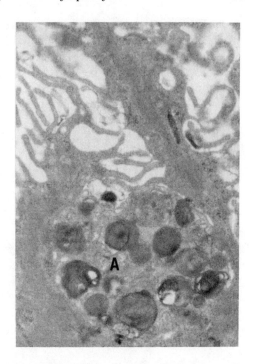

Figure 17. A dystrophic axon (A) is located inside the epidermis, original magnification × 102.000.

cells of patients with lysosomopathies must not be confused with ''undulating tubules'' that are surrounded by membranes of the smooth endoplasmic reticulum. ''Undulating tubules'' are sometimes found in nonlysosomal diseases, for example, dermatomyositis. Pathological lysosomal residual bodies are most frequently perinuclear in location and occur in aggregates. Lysosomal vacuolation may be so marked that endothelial cells become distorted and reduce or obliterate their vascular lumen. The lysosomopathies that evidence such vascular changes are those that show lysosomal vacuolation in other mesenchymal cells such as the mucopolysaccharidoses, mucolipidosis II, GM$_1$-gangliosidosis, mannosidosis, aspartylglucosaminuria, and Salla's disease. Sandhoff's disease (Figure 20), Fabry's disease, Niemann-Pick disease, and fucosidosis mainly have membranous inclusions within endothelial cells.

Lysosomal accretion within endothelial cells may be so massive that peripheral circulation

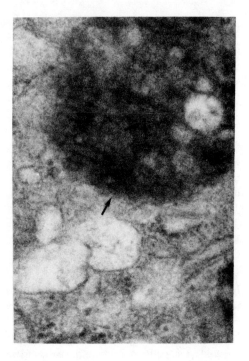

Figure 18. Lysosomes in metachromatic leukodystrophy have a characteristic prismatic (arrows) fine structure, original magnification × 136.000.

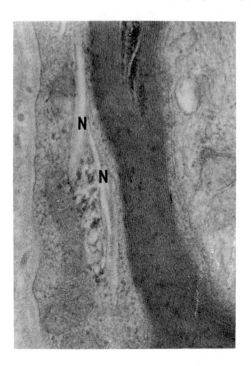

Figure 19.   In Krabbe's globoid cell leukodystrophy, needle-like (N) inclusions are seen in Schwann cells, original magnification × 30.800.

SUMMARY

Light microscopic studies may indicate the presence of lysosomal abnormalities in patients who have lysosomopathies by revealing autofluorescent lipopigments as well as vacuolation in blood smears and semithin plastic embedded sections. However, electron microscopy is required to confirm the presence of a lysosomal storage disease via examination of circulating lymphocytes or biopsied skin from the patient who is suspected to have such a diagnosis.

Reliable and valid electron microscopic examination of circulating lymphocytes and biopsied skin necessitates instant and sufficient fixation in an appropriate fixative. This essential step is usually the responsibility of the clinician collaborating with the neuropathologist who will subsequently postfix, process, and study the specimen.

The cytologic diversity of skin (Martin & Ceuterick, 1978) or conjunctiva (Libert, 1980)

may be compromised. It may result in conspicuous tortuosity of superficial vessels as emphasized by the phenomenon called angiokeratoma diffusum in Fabry's disease and fucosidosis (Kornfeld, Snyder, & Wenger, 1977), or may also be seen in the conjunctiva. Cutaneous vascular compromise can also be seen by light microscopy in some of these lysosomal diseases, as well as by the unaided eye (e.g., angiokeratoma diffusum in Fabry's disease and fucosidosis) (Kornfeld et al., 1977).

Lysosomal Diseases that are Characterized by Changes in Infiltrating Cells

Histiocytes within the characteristic skin nodules of patients with Farber's disease exhibit hollow profiles (Figure 21a) (Burck, Moser, Goebel, Grüttner, & Held, 1985). In addition, the epidermal cells contain membranous inclusions (Figure 21b).

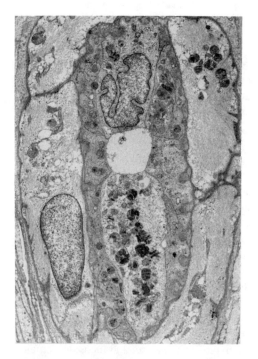

Figure 20.   A cutaneous vessel shows numerous membrane-bound lamellar bodies in several endothelial and smooth muscle cells with only a small lumen in Sandhoff's disease, original magnification × 6500.

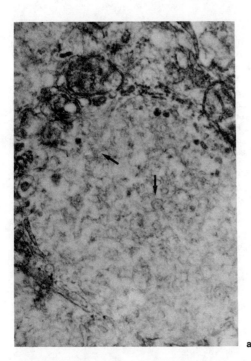 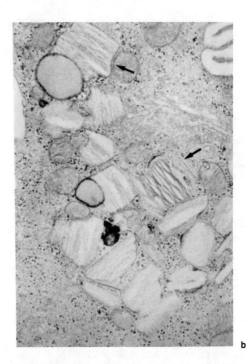

Figure 21. Farber's disease: **a)** curved hollow profiles (arrows) within lysosomes mark histiocytes, original magnification ×
131.760; **b)** lamellar bodies (arrows) are encountered in epidermal cells, original magnification × 71.500.

favors them over circulating lymphocytes as a diagnostic specimen resource when the presence of a lysosomal storage disease is suspected; both skin and blood are available for prenatal diagnosis.

The morphologic changes that are associated with lysosomopathies cannot be evaluated with certainty in cultured cells that are derived from biopsied skin. Lysosomes nonspecifically accumulate as tissue cultures age. Ultrastructural changes in cultured cells must always be compared to any changes that are present in age- + medium-matched controls, as well as to changes that were present in the parent skin biopsy specimen. However, cultured cells from diseased tissue are a resource for studying relationships between *in vitro* substrate feeding, substrate accumulation, and the pathological manifestations of lysosomal storage. Tissue culture techniques also support studies of lymphocyte function in diseased B and T cells that may be stimulated and transformed.

Even though biochemical assays delineate heterozygotes with lysosomopathies that man-

ifest autosomal recessive inheritance, there are, to the best of our knowledge, no ultrastructural manifestations of the carrier state in this category of lysosomal storage diseases. However, Fabry's disease, an X-linked disorder, is characterized by the presence of abnormal lysosomal residual bodies in cells from certain carrier females. Elucidation of similar findings in MPS-type II has not been effected to date.

Ultrastructural investigation of skin biopsies may also be used for the diagnosis of some nonlysosomal neurodegenerative diseases. Lafora's disease (Kamei, Yokota, Ishihara, Kusunose, & Yamada, 1986) and neuroaxonal dystrophy (Martin, Leroy, Libert, van Eygen, & Logghe, 1979) specimens have been found to exhibit characteristic morphologic findings. In the latter instance, conjunctival biopsies may be more easily studied than skin specimens because of their more abundant nerve fiber content. Since some mitochondrial disorders are multisystem diseases, morphologic study of blood cells and skin from patients with these disorders may prove to be profitable.

REFERENCES

Aula, P., Rapola, J., & Andersson, L.C. (1975). Distribution of cytoplasmic vacuoles in blood T and B lymphocytes in two lysosomal disorders. *Virchows Archiv. B. Cell Pathology, 18,* 263–271.

Bach, G., Cohen, M.M., & Kohn, G. (1975). Abnormal ganglioside accumulation in cultured fibroblasts from patients with mucolipidosis IV. *Biochemical and Biophysical Research Communications, 66,* 1483–1490.

Badurska, B., Fidziańska, A., & Jedrzejowska, H. (1981). A dominant form of neuronal ceroid-lipofuscinosis. An ultrastructural study of sural nerve and peripheral lymphocytes. *Journal of Neurology, 226,* 205–212.

Böyum, A. (1968). Separation of leucocytes from blood and bone marrow. *The Scandinavian Journal of Clinical & Laboratory Investigation* (Vol. 21). Supplement *97,* 1–109.

Burck, U., Harzer, K., Goebel, H.H., Elze, K.L., Held, K.R., & Carstens, L. (1980). Ultrastructural pathology of skin biopsy and fibroblast enzyme studies in a case of GM_2-gangliosidosis with deficient hexosaminidase A and thermolabile hexosaminidase B. *Neuropädiatrie, 11,* 161–175.

Burck, U., Moser, H.W., Goebel, H.H., Grüttner, R., & Held, K.R. (1985). A case of lipogranulomatosis Farber: Some clinical and ultrastructural aspects. *European Journal of Pediatrics, 143,* 203–208.

Ceuterick, C., Martin, J.J., Casaer, P., & Edgar, G.W.F. (1976). The diagnosis of infantile generalized ceroid-lipofuscinosis (type Hagberg-Santavuori) using skin biopsy. *Neuropädiatrie, 7,* 250–260.

Dolman, C.L. (1984). Diagnosis of neurometabolic disorders by examination of skin biopsies and lymphocytes. *Seminars in Diagnostic Pathology, 1,* 82–97.

Goebel, H.H. (1985). Fingerprint inclusions in non-vacuolated lymphocytes in juvenile neuronal ceroid-lipofuscinosis. *Clinical Neuropathology, 4,* 210–213.

Goebel, H.H., Ikeda, K., Schulz, F., Burck, U., & Kohlschütter, A. (1981). Fingerprint profiles in lymphocytic vacuoles of mucopolysaccharidoses I-H, III-A, and III-B. *Acta Neuropathologica* (Berlin), *55,* 247–249.

Goebel, H.H., Kohlschütter, A., & Lenard, H.G. (1982). Morphologic and chemical biopsy findings in mucolipidosis IV. *Clinical Neuropathology, 1,* 73–82.

Goebel, H.H., Pilz, H., & Gullotta, F. (1976). The protracted form of juvenile neuronal ceroid-lipofuscinosis. *Acta Neuropathologica* (Berlin), *36,* 393–396.

Ikeda, K., & Goebel, H.H. (1979). Ultrastructural pathology of lymphocytes in neuronal ceroid-lipofuscinoses. *Brain & Development, 1,* 285–292.

Ikeda, K., Goebel, H.H., Burck, U., & Kohlschütter, A. (1982). Ultrastructural pathology of human lymphocytes in lysosomal disorders: A contribution to their morphological diagnosis. *European Journal of Pediatrics, 138,* 179–185.

Kamei, T., Yokota, T., Ishihara, T., Kusunose, Y., & Yamada, M. (1986). Diagnostic significance of skin in

Lafora disease. Abstract 788, International Congress of Neuropathology, Stockholm, September 7–12, p. 390.

Kohlschütter, A., Sieg, K., Schulte, F.J., Hayek, H.W., & Goebel, H.H. (1982). Infantile cardiomyopathy and neuromyopathy with β-galactosidase deficiency. *European Journal of Pediatrics, 139,* 75–81.

Kornfeld, M., Snyder, R.D., & Wenger, D.A. (1977). Fucosidosis with angiokeratoma. *Archives of Pathology and Laboratory Medicine, 101,* 478–485.

Lake, B.D., & Cavanagh, N.P.C. (1978). Early-juvenile Batten's disease—A recognizable sub-group distinct from other forms of Batten's disease. *Journal of the Neurological Sciences* (Amsterdam), *36,* 265–271.

Lazarus, S.S., Vethamany, V.G., Schneck, L., & Volk, B.W. (1967). Fine structure and histochemistry of peripheral blood cells in Niemann-Pick disease. *Laboratory Investigation, 17,* 155–170.

Libert, J. (1980). Diagnosis of lysosomal storage diseases by the ultrastructural study of conjunctival biopsies. In S.C. Sommers & P.P. Rosen (Eds.), *Pathology Annual, Part 1* (Vol. 15, pp. 37–66). New York: Appleton-Century-Crofts.

Lüllmann-Rauch, R. (1974). Lipidosis-like ultrastructural alterations in rat lymph nodes after treatment with tricyclic antidepressants or neuroleptics. *Naunyn-Schmiedeberg's Archives of Pharmacology* (Berlin), *286,* 165–179.

MacLeod, P.M., Dolman, C.L., Nickel, R.E., Chang, E., Nag, S., Zonana, J., & Silvey, K. (1985). Prenatal diagnosis of neuronal ceroid-lipofuscinoses. *American Journal of Medical Genetics, 22,* 781–789.

Martin, J.J., & Ceuterick, C. (1978). Morphological study of skin biopsy specimens: A contribution to the diagnosis of metabolic disorders with involvement of the nervous system. *Journal of Neurology, Neurosurgery, and Psychiatry, 41,* 232–248.

Martin, J.J., & de Groote, C. (1974). Involvement of the skin in late infantile and juvenile amaurotic idiocies (neuronal ceroid-lipo-fuscinoses). *Pathologia Europea, 9,* 263–272.

Martin, J.J., Leroy, J.G., Libert, J., van Eygen, M., & Logghe, N. (1979). Skin and conjunctival biopsies in infantile neuroaxonal dystrophy. *Acta Neuropathologica* (Berlin), *45,* 247–251.

Orfanos, C.E., & Runne, U. (1975). Tumor- and drug-induced cutaneous neuro-phospholipidosis. *Journal of Cutaneous Pathology, 2,* 232–239.

Pralle, H., Schroeder, R., & Löffler, H. (1974). Plasmazelleinschlüsse bei Mangel an saurer Maltase (Glycogenose Typ II). Plasma cell inclusions in acid maltase deficiency (Type II glycogenosis). *Klinische Wochenschrift, 52,* 653–654.

Tsuji, S., Yamada, T., Tsutsumi, A., & Miyatake, T. (1982). Neuraminidase deficiency and accumulation of sialic acid in lymphocytes in adult type sialidosis with partial β-galactosidase deficiency. *Annals of Neurology* (Boston), *11,* 541–543.

Chapter 5

Encephalomyopathies and Defects in Energy Metabolism

Fons J.M. Gabreëls

THE FIRST REPORTS ON BIOCHEMICAL AND morphologic aberrations that exist in human mitochondria initiated a fascinating field of research on a new group of metabolic diseases. In 1966, Price used the term mitochondrial myopathies for these diseases. Cases with mental retardation and other neurological symptoms subsequently made it evident that the nervous system is a prominent target for this group of disorders. In 1977, Shapira coined the term "mitochondrial encephalomyopathies," a clinically heterogeneous group of disorders that can affect multiple systems, but always with nervous system and muscle involvement. In 1981, Walter used the more general term "mitochondriopathy" to designate pathologic states of morphologically and/or functionally abnormal mitochondria. Classification based on clinical or histopathological characteristics of these disorders has proved to be unsatisfactory. However, since the late 1970s, great progress has been made in the identification of specific biochemical defects in some of these disorders. Such information will make a rational classification of these diseases possible.

CLINICAL CONSIDERATIONS

The usefulness of clinical criteria for the identification and classification of mitochondrial encephalomyopathies is limited because there is no consistent clinical phenotype, and because symptoms and signs may be similar in patients with different biochemical defects. The special vulnerability of muscle and brain to mitochondrial dysfunction may be due to the high energy demand of these tissues.

We have observed a diversity of clinical presentations: congenital or late onset, static, progressive, and episodic. Even though the literature concerning these disorders is confusing, some characteristic syndromes have emerged. Representatives of this group are: Kearns-Sayre syndrome, myoclonus epilepsy with ragged-red fibers, lactic acidosis and stroke-like episodes, Alpers syndrome, dysmyelination, Leigh syndrome, and intermittent ataxia. While the syndromes can be distinguished from each other, there are many common symptoms and signs, including exercise intolerance and decompensation during infections.

Laboratory Considerations

Findings on electrocardiography are characteristically abnormal in Kearns-Sayre syndrome.

Electromyography and nerve conduction velocities of patients with mitochondrial encephalomyopathies are usually normal; infrequently, nonspecific or "myopathic" changes or slightly decreased nerve conduction velocities are present in some patients.

Electroencephalography, evoked potentials, and computed tomography usually reveal nonspecific abnormalities. Occasionally, computed tomography reveals the presence of symmetrical focal lucencies and calcification of basal ganglia.

The variability in clinical presentation and the lack of specific laboratory tests frequently make the process of detecting defects of pyruvate metabolism a difficult diagnostic problem in clinical practice. In the screening of encephalomyopathies, assessment of pyruvate and lactate levels of serum under standard conditions after exercise and after glucose loading, play an important role. Assessment of pyruvate and lactate levels of cerebrospinal fluid (CSF), and 24-hour urine lactate excretion, are also helpful. The abnormalities in these levels vary considerably in severity in different patients. Occasionally, all the screening results are normal. In order to find a procedure that would provide direct indication of a disturbance of pyruvate metabolism, we examined the intravenous pyruvate loading test.

In the author's opinion, this test is a specific and sensitive procedure to detect disturbances in pyruvate metabolism, especially if other diagnostic procedures provide insufficient information. It is a useful method for studying patients who are suspected of having mitochondrial encephalomyopathies. Thus, if pyruvate and lactate levels in body fluids are normal, and oral glucose loading and intravenous pyruvate loading yield normal results, pyruvate metabolism must be considered to be undisturbed.

Morphological Considerations

The pathological hallmarks of mitochondrial encephalomyopathies in the central nervous system are the presence of focal and bilaterally symmetrical lesions. These lesions may extend from the cerebral cortex to the spinal cord. Under light microscopy, these lesions show spongy degeneration with neuronal loss, vascular proliferation, astrocytosis, and demyelination. Some electron microscopic studies describe enlarged and disorganized mitochondria in the neuronal perikarya and axons.

Some, but not all, encephalomyopathies are associated with morphological mitochondrial abnormalities in muscle tissue.

Light Microscopy In light microscopic evaluation, application of the modified Gomori trichrome stain and stains for oxidative enzymes may show ragged-red fibers or fibers with abnormally intense oxidative enzyme reactions. Sometimes, excessive accumulation of Sudan black-positive droplets is present.

Electron Microscopy When muscle tissue is examined by electron microscopy, the following structural changes may be observed:

Large aggregates of mitochondria, usually beneath the sarcolemma but also between the myofibrils

Enlarged mitochondria are often present

Cristae may be increased in number and irregularly oriented, or they may form "honeycomb" patterns and/or concentric whorls

A paucity of cristae, giving the mitochondria a vacuolated or empty appearance

Mitochondria that may contain different abnormal inclusions, such as crystalline structures and globular bodies, and there may be enlargement and proliferation of mitochondrial granules

Accumulation of glycogen particles and triglyceride droplets

A classification of encephalomyopathies by morphological criteria is inappropriate for several reasons. First, morphological abnormalities do not distinguish between different encephalomyopathies. We found similar morphological changes in patients with different biochemical errors at varying sites of mitochondrial metabolism. Second, morphological abnormalities of mitochondria are not restricted to mitochondrial encephalomyopathies. Changes of mitochondria have been described in other well known myopathies, as for example, in muscular dystrophy and polymyositis. Third, morphological alterations of mitochondria may be lacking in patients with some biochemically defined errors of mitochondrial metabolism.

Thus, morphological examination of muscle tissue clearly has limitations as a means of detecting and classifying mitochondrial encephalomyopathies.

BIOCHEMICAL CONSIDERATIONS

Enzymatic studies of appropriate tissues must be performed if a patient is suspected of having an encephalomyopathy, especially when studies of body fluids and loading tests reveal elevated levels of lactate and pyruvate.

Mitochondrial encephalomyopathies can be divided biochemically into two groups. The first group consists of those disorders in which there are defects of substrate transport and utilization. The second group comprises disorders in which there are defects of respiratory chain function.

Defects of Substrate Transport and Utilization

The central intermediate substance of oxidative metabolism is acetyl-CoA. Acetyl-CoA can originate from fatty acids, pyruvate, or amino acids. Fatty acids have to be transferred across the mitochondrial membrane in order to be transformed into acetyl-CoA. This process requires a carrier molecule, carnitine, and two enzymes: CPT (carnitine palmitoyl transferase) A and B. Fatty acids are degraded to acetyl-CoA via sequential β-oxidation. Pyruvate undergoes oxidative decarboxylation to acetyl-CoA, catalyzed by PDH-complex. The mitochondrial transaminases can convert amino acids into pyruvate or other keto acids.

To our knowledge, two defects with disturbed substrate transport or disturbed substrate utilization have been identified as the cause of mitochondrial encephalomyopathy: systematic carnitine deficiency and PDH (pyruvate dehydrogenase) complex deficiency. A deficiency of citric acid cycle enzymes has not yet been found, at least not in muscle tissue.

PDH-complex is a multi-enzyme system consisting of three catalytic and two regulatory peptide components. The following encephalomyopathies can be associated with PDH-complex deficiency: Alpers syndrome, dysmyelination, Leigh syndrome, and intermittent ataxia.

Defects of the Respiratory Chain

The respiratory chain is divided into four functional units or complexes, each composed of several proteins. Abnormalities of the complexes have been identified by studies of substrate oxidation, cytochrome spectra, and enzyme assays. A combination of these studies has pinpointed the site of abnormality in many patients, and permitted a classification of the defects.

Some mitochondrial encephalomyopathies have been associated with defects in complex I (diphosphopyridine nucleotide) or NADH-coenzyme Q oxidoreductase in muscle tissue: Kearns-Sayre syndrome, Alpers syndrome, and Leigh syndrome.

Several encephalomyopathies have been associated with complex IV or cytochrome c oxidase deficiency in muscle and brain tissue: Kearns-Sayre syndrome, myoclonus epilepsy with ragged-red fibers, Alpers syndrome, dysmyelination, and Leigh syndrome.

Well-defined pathologic patterns such as those found in Kearns-Sayre syndrome, Alpers syndrome, and Leigh syndrome are associated with various abnormalities in pyruvate metabolism. However, all of these abnormalities in pyruvate metabolism have also been associated with other neurologic disorders. It seems probable that different disorders of the nervous and neuromuscular system can be associated with any kind of biochemical abnormalities in pyruvate metabolism.

The author proposes that mitochondrial encephalomyopathy is a primary or secondary nervous system dysfunction or muscular dysfunction that is caused by a defect in pyruvate metabolism. This dysfunction is sometimes associated with morphologic abnormalities in mitochondria. However, much more scientific work must be done before insight may be obtained in the pathogenesis of mitochondrial encephalomyopathies.

GENETIC CONSIDERATIONS

The mitochondrial encephalomyopathies, inherited as Mendelian traits, may be classified as autosomal recessive, X-linked recessive, and autosomal dominant conditions. However, the hereditary transmission of encephalomyopathies is very complex because the mitochondrion has some nonnuclear DNA.

Most mitochondrial proteins are encoded by nuclear DNA. Nonnuclear mitochondrial DNA codes for at least 13 polypeptides. These include subunits of cytochrome c oxidase, cytochrome b, ATPase, and complex I.

The mitochondrial genome should be transmitted by maternal inheritance in a nonMendelian fashion. An affected mother would pass a mutant disease to all her children, but only her daughters would transmit the trait in subsequent generations.

There are many copies of mitochondrial DNA in each cell, in contrast to the two sets of genes that are present for each nuclear-encoded character. Thus, the phenotypic expression of a mitochondrially coded gene depends on the relative proportion of mutant and wild-type mitochondrial DNA within a cell, and a mutant phenotype is expressed only when the proportion of mutant DNA reaches a threshold.

In conclusion, encephalomyopathies can be transmitted by Mendelian or maternal inheritance; clearly, genetic counseling in these instances is particularly difficult.

Some of the biochemically defined encephalomyopathies are confined to one tissue: for instance, cytochrome c oxidase deficiency may affect brain alone or muscle alone. These data suggest the existence of tissue-specific isoenzymes. The specificity may be the property of one, presumably nuclear-encoded, subunit. Electrophoretic, kinetic, and immunological evidence suggest that one of the subunits differs in different tissues.

These findings suggest that modern techniques of molecular genetics hold great promise for the study of encephalomyopathies.

SUGGESTED READINGS

DiMauro, S., Bonilla, E., Zeviani, M., Nakagawa, M., & DeVivo, D.C. (1985). Mitochondrial myopathies. *Annals of Neurology, 17*, 521–538.

Gabreëls, F.J.M., Prick, M.J.J., Trijbels, J.M.F., Renier, W.O., Jaspar, H.H.J., Janssen, A.J.M., & Slooff, J.L. (1984). Defects in citric acid cycle and the electron transport chain in progressive poliodystrophy. *Acta Neurologica Scandinavica, 70*, 145–154.

Pavlakis, S.G., Phillips, P.C., Di Mauro, S., DeVivo, D.C., & Rowland, L.P. (1984). Mitochondrial myopathy, encephalopathy, lactic acidosis, and strokelike episodes: A distinctive clinical syndrome. *Annals of Neurology, 16*, 481–488.

Petty, R.K.H., Harding, A.E., Moreau-Hughes, J.A. (1986). The clinical features of mitochondrial myopathy. *Brain, 109*, 915–938.

Price, H.M. (1966). Mitochondrial myopathies in man? A review of the evidence. In A.T. Milhorat (Ed.), *Exploratory concepts in muscular dystrophy and related disorders* (pp. 341–350). Amsterdam: Excerpta Medica.

Sengers, R.C.A., Stadhouders, A.M., & Trijbels, J.M.F. (1984). Mitochondral myopathies: Clinical, morphological and biochemical aspects. *European Journal of Pediatrics, 141*, 192–207.

Shapira, Y., Harel, S., Russell, A. (1977). Mitochondrial encephalomyopathies: A group of neuromuscular disorders with defects in oxidative metabolism. *Israel Journal of Medical Sciences, 13*, 161–164.

VanErven, P.M.M., Gabreëls, F.J.M., Wevers, R.A., Doesburg, W.H., Ruitenbeek, W., Renier, W.O., & Lamers, K.J.B. (1987). Intravenous pyruvate loading test in Leigh syndrome. *Journal of Neurological Sciences, 77*, 217–227.

Walter, G.F. (1981). Neuromuskuläre Mitochondriopathie: Ein morphologischer Ausdruck von Störungen des Energiestoffwechsels. In G.F. Walter (Ed.), *Veröffentlichungen aus der Pathologie* (Vol. 117, pp. 1–111). Stuttgart: Gustav Fischer.

Walter, G.F. (1983). Myoencephalopathies with abnormal mitochondria: A review. *Clinical Neuropathology, 2*, 101–113.

Chapter 6

Mitochondrial Dysfunction in Some Neuromuscular Diseases

Wilhelm Mortier, Eike Noack, and Hans-Rudolf Scholte

THE AIM OF THIS CHAPTER IS TO FOCUS ON the clinical problem of diagnosing mitochondriopathies and to present data of selected patients with primary and secondary mitochondrial dysfunctions. The importance of a specific etiologic diagnosis is discussed.

The clinical findings of patients with mitochondrial myopathies and encephalopathies are diverse. Signs and symptoms usually fall into one of four groups (Table 1). From these clinical presentations, only the first very rare circumstance is specific; the others are often similar in patients with different biochemical defects (Di Mauro, Bonilla, Zeviani, Nakagawa, & DeVivo, 1985; Mortier, 1981). The same enzyme defect may manifest itself differently depending on the degree, time of manifestation, and possible protein polymorphism of enzyme subunits (McKay et al., 1986). In addition to obtaining a complete history and physical, as well as a neurological workup, the clinician needs further support by some laboratory investigations (Table 2). Lactate, pyruvate, and ketone body determinations in blood, cerebrospinal fluid, and urine before and after fasting or exercise may indicate—together with carnitine levels in serum and muscle tissue—a defect in substrate utilization. Conducted together with urine investigations of amino or organic acids, such tests may also reveal a defect in mitochondrial dehydro-

Table 1. Mitochondrial myopathies: Symptoms

1. Hypermetabolism (euthyroidism) = Luft's syndrome
2. Feeding/sucking problems, motor retardation, hypotonia, cardiomyopathy, rapid fatigue, weakness, and/or pains after exercise
3. Myopathy and encephalopathy
4. Muscle weakness of unknown etiology

genases in the citric acid cycle, or in the respiratory chain. Loading tests—glucose, pyruvate, or alanine—may be necessary for demonstrating a defect in the metabolism of pyruvate. Ophthalmological investigations, electroencephalograms (EEG), electrocardiograms (ECG), nerve conduction velocity studies, electromyography, and muscle biopsy (including histological, histochemical, and electronmicroscopical techniques) may contribute useful information about the individual patient.

PATIENTS AND METHODS

In the last 3 years, the authors have investigated systematically 11 adults and 37 children with different neuromuscular diseases for primary and secondary mitochondrial dysfunctions (Table 3). Out of special diagnostic procedures (Table 4), we selected the polarographic studies as a screening of oxidative phosphorylation, and obtained valid results by

The authors want to thank Mrs. I.E.M. Luyt-Houwen (Dept. of Biochemistry I, Erasmus University, Rotterdam), Mrs. M.H.M. Vaandrager-Verduin (Dept. of Clinical Genetics, Erasmus University, Rotterdam), and Mrs. C. Wellern (Kinderklinik Wuppertal) for the expert biochemical and histochemical assistance.

Table 2. Routine diagnostic procedures

Determination of	In
Lactate, Pyruvate	Blood (B[a],F[b],L[c],E[d]), Urine (B,F,L), CSF (B)
β-Hydroxybuturate, Acetacetate	Blood (B,F,E), Urine (B,F)
Protein	Blood, CSF
Carnitine	Serum, skeletal muscle
pH, amino, and organo acids	Urine
CK	Serum
Investigation	
Nerve conduction time	Electromyography
Evoked potentials	Muscle biopsy

[a]B = Basal after overnight fast.
[b]F = Fasting test.
[c]L = Loading test (glucose, pyruvate, or alanine).
[d]E = Exercise test.

Table 3.   Investigations

Neuromuscular disease	N
Malignant hyperthermia (at risk)	18
Duchenne muscular dystrophy	6
Myotonic muscular dystrophy	6
Mitochondrial diseases	3
Myopathy nonspecific	4
Myositis	3
Kearns-Sayre syndrome	3
Spinal atrophy (Kugelberg-Welander)	3
Paramyotonia	2
Total number of patients	48
Controls	25

N = 73.

using 150 mg–600 mg wet weight muscle tissue (Barth et al., 1983; Noack & Mortier, 1984). The results of such a polarographic study are available in 1 day, allowing for further and more precise investigations of enzyme activities and cytochrome spectra in frozen samples of about 600 mg–800 mg muscle tissue. In special situations, the workup was complemented by the investigation of mitochondrial calcium uptake kinetics and P[31] MRI spectra.

Table 4.   Special diagnostic procedures

Enzyme activities	Ca^{2+}-transport
Cytochrome spectra	Immunostaining
Oxydative phosphorylation	P[31]-NMR

RESULTS

Out of 48 investigated patients, we found defects in 12 patients (25%); half of the defects were believed to be primary, and the other half of the defects were believed to be secondary (Table 5). Two patients are discussed to underline the difficulties in identifying mitochondrial dysfunctions in the routine workup.

The First Patient

The first patient is a 38-year-old woman (Figure 1) who, since the age of 16, has annually experienced the sudden onset of a high body temperature that reaches up to 40°C within minutes. The high temperature is accompanied by tachycardia, excessive sweating, dyspnea, polydipsia, and polyphagia with 3500 cal. daily and increased irritability. At the age of 37 years, the patient's dramatic episodes increased to four per year. She suffered respiratory arrest twice, was hospitalized, and was successfully intubated and eventually released. The patient still lives at home and is able to perform light housework, but is in communication with an emergency service around the clock. After an episode, she usually recovers fully within 48 hours. She had been in different hospitals and had received extensive workups, but tests for hyperthyroidism had repeatedly been excluded.

Because the patient suffered from unexplained high fever, and because an atypical ma-

Table 5. Primary and secondary mitochondrial defects

Defect	No.	Nature of the defect
Utilization of fatty acids	2	
Carnitine deficiency	1	Secondary ?
Carnitine palmitolytransferase deficiency	1	Primary
Respiratory chain	3	Primary
Oxydation-phosphorylation coupling	7	
Loose coupling with hypermetabolism	1	Primary
Loose coupling without hypermetabolism	6	Secondary

lignant hyperthermia reaction was suspected, she was referred to us for further and special investigation. The patient's history of recurrent symptoms led us to speculate that this patient may suffer from Luft's syndrome (Table 6), a condition which so far has been recognized in only two patients (Haydar et al., 1971; Luft, Ikkos, Palmieri, Ernster, & Afzelius, 1962). Though physically and neurologically normal, the patient's lactate and pyruvate concentrations in the blood after exercise rose pathologically from 0.7 to 4.8 and from 0.07 to 0.2 mmol/I respectively. The electromyography showed changes indicative of a myopathy. In the muscle biopsy there were no ragged red fibres in the trichrome staining (performed in West Germany by Prof. Schroeder in the Department of Neuropathology at the University of Aachen). However, electronmicroscopy showed an increased number of otherwise normal mitochondria in the biopsy. The polarographic studies revealed an elevated basic respiration of the isolated mitochondria with different substrates (Figure 2 and Figure 3). The increased state 4 respiration caused respiratory control indices of 1.5 to 2 but the ade-

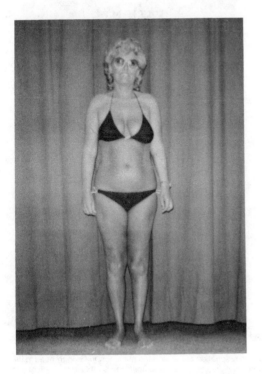
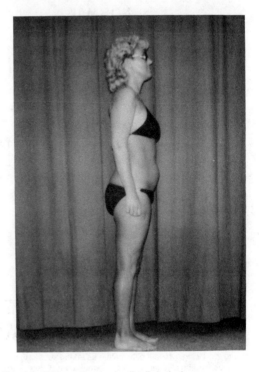

Figure 1.   The first patient at the age of 38 years. Note the slight muscle atrophy distally in the legs.

50   Mortier, Noack, and Scholte

Table 6.   Luft's syndrome

Extreme sweating
Dyspnoe at rest
Polydipsia
Increased temperature
Irritability
Tachycardia
Muscle atrophy (slight)

nosine diphosphate (ADP): 0 quotients were normal, for example: indices of 1.6 for succinate and 2.4 for glutamate were obtained. The homogenate from frozen/thawed muscle showed a lowered total carnitine level of 2.42 μmol/g wet weight, decreased activities of rotenone-sensitive NADH oxidase (to 31%), of cytochrome c oxidase (to 37%), of succinate dehydrogenase (to 42%), while the activities of the other mitochondrial enzymes were barely normal. Adenosine triphosphate (ATP) synthetase activity was measured as $Mg^{2+} - ATP$-

ase. Uncoupler stimulated the activity to 199% versus 433% in controls. The uncoupler stimulated activity was not inhibited by oligomycin, while it reduced the activity to 40% in controls (Table 7). The final data for the mitochondrial calcium metabolism as well as the P^{31} MRI-spectra under and after ischemia and exercise are not yet available, but the spectra at rest looked normal.

The life threatening episodes were treated first with chloramphenicol; transient improvement was seen in the patient published by Haydar et al. in 1971. Our patient, however, became subjectively worse and was treated subsequently with a combination of menadione (10 mg/day), ascorbate (1 g/day), and coenzyme Q_{10} (120 mg/day). She has not experienced a crisis for 6 months, up to the present time.

In summary, the patient suffered for almost 20 years from a mitochondrial dysfunction,

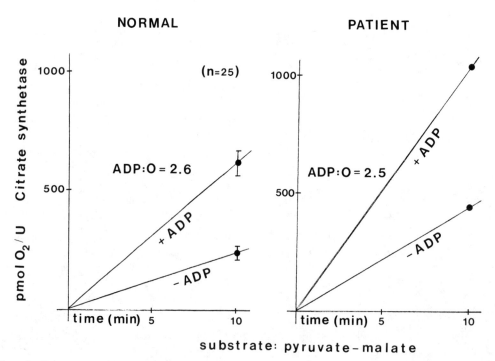

Figure 2.   Using pyruvate plus malate as added substrates, the basic respiration of the isolated mitochondria is increased in the first patient (right) compared to the "normal" control (left). The phosphorylative efficiency is almost comparable in the patient and in the control.

RESPIRATION

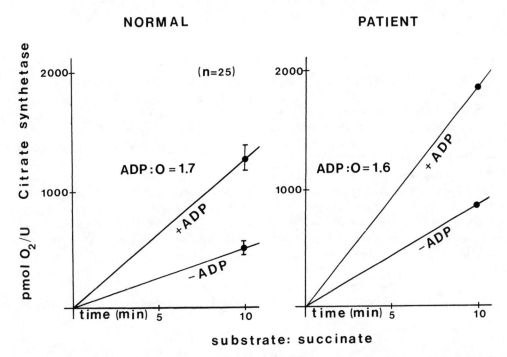

substrate: succinate

Figure 3. Using succinate as added substrate. As with other substrates, the basic respiration of the isolated mitochondria is increased in the first patient (right), while the phosphorylative efficiency is normal.

Table 7. Muscle homogenate assays in the patient with Luft's syndrome[a,b]

	Patient	Controls	(*n*)
Protein (mg)	164	174	(53)
Total carnitine (μmol)	2.42	3.96	(59)
Rotenone-insensitive NADH oxidase (U)	1.00	3.19	(10)
Succinate dehydrogenase (mU)	305	723	(58)
Antimycin-sensitive succinate-cytochrome *c* reductase (U)	2.00	3.99	(21)
Cytochrome oxidase (min^{-1})	33	90	(16)
Carnitine palmitoyltransferase I (mU)	68	77	(55)
Carnitine palmitoyltransferase II (mU)	51	96	(57)
Mg^{2+}-ATPase without additions (mU)	13	7	(5)
,, plus uncoupler (mU)	25	28	(5)
,, plus oligomycin (mU)	10	6	(5)
,, plus uncoupler and oligomycin (mU)	25	11	(5)

[a]Barth, Scholte, Berden, van der Klei-van Moorsel, Luyt Houwen, van't Veer Korthof, van der Harten, & Sobotka-Plojhar (1983); Scholte, Busch, Luyt-Houwen, Vaandrager-Verduin, Przyrembel, and Arts (in press).

[b]Activities and amounts per gram wet tissue weight.

Luft's syndrome. Possible benefit from a rational preventive therapeutic regimen has resulted.

The Second Patient

The patient is a 14-year-old girl with small stature and slight kyphoscoliosis (Figure 4). The patient had normal development, but at the age of 10 years she complained about headache, nausea, and vomiting from which she recovered. Within 3 years she suffered increasingly from alternating stroke-like episodes, hemianopsia on the right side, focal and generalized seizures, bilateral sensorineural impairment, and rapid intellectual deterioration, with alexia and agraphia (Table 8). In addition, a non-obstructive hypertrophic cardiomyopathy was diagnosed by echocardiogram and heart catheterization. Since the patient was found to have normal protein content in the cere-

brospinal fluid, and since negative viral titers for measles and rubella ruled out the possibility of a brain tumor, the girl was referred to our hospital for further evaluation. From the patient's history and data in hand, we suspected a distinct syndrome of a mitochondrial myopathy in combination with encephalomyopathy, lactate acidosis, and stroke-like episodes, specifically: MELAS-syndrome (Pavlakis, Phillips, Di Mauro, De Vivo, & Rowland, 1984). Our hypothesis was supported by the following results: lactate and pyruvate levels were increased in the blood (3.5 and 0.1 mmol/l) and in the cerebrospinal fluid (4.0 and 0.2 mmol/l), with elevated ratios of 34 and 18 respectively, indicating the dysfunction of the respiratory chain and involvement of the brain. After fasting for 24 hours, the ratio of β-hydroxybutyrate to acetoacetate rose to 6. The muscle biopsy revealed only a few ragged red fibers (Figure 5); electronmicroscopy revealed an increased

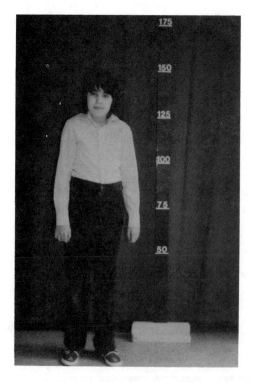 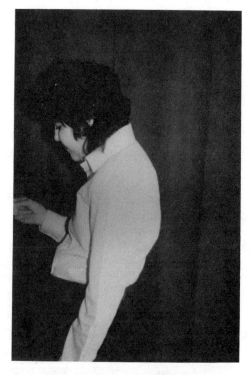

Figure 4.   The second patient at the age of 14 years. Note the small stature and the kyphoscoliosis.

Table 8. MELAS-syndrome; patient

1971	Birth of Sandra Pf.
1981	Headache, vomiting, CT scan: Atrophy of cerebellum Neurosurgeons suspect a brain tumor.
1984	Hemiparesis left side, ataxia CT scan = Focal defect right temporal-parietal, disappearing within days (CT scan control) Angiogram = normal. A brain tumor is still suspected.
1985	(January) Headache, drowsiness, ataxia NMR: Pathol. right temporal-parietal A brain tumor is unlikely.
1985	(February) Hemiparesis right side, ataxia CT scan = hypodensity left hemisphere Myoclonic jerks right leg, dementia Alexia, agraphia
1985	(April) Diagnosis of the MELAS-syndrome

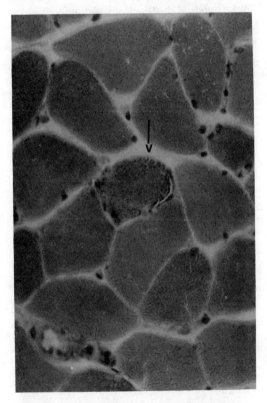

Figure 5.   In the second patient with the MELAS-syndrome, the muscle biopsy showed clearly, but only a few ragged red fibers were visible (arrow). Trichrome stain, original magnification × 40.

number of very elongated mitochondria. Oxydative phosphorylation studies showed a decreased basic respiration and lowered respiratory control indices as well as ADP:0 ratios, with glutamate and pyruvate plus malate. The indices for succinate and palmitoyl-carnitine looked normal (Table 9). The biochemical analysis in this patient has not yet been finished, but a pyruvate- or α-ketoglutarate dehydrogenase is possible. A therapeutic trial with carnitine, medium chain triglycerides, and glutamate had an impressive positive effect but lasted for only 4 weeks; this therapy was discontinued. A therapeutic trial with steroids (2mg/kg/day) over a period of 3 months was ineffective; the patient worsened progressively and finally died. In summary, the patient's tests were extensive; they included five computerized tomography scans, one magnetic resonance imaging test, an angiogram of the brain, and several cerebrospinal taps. The patient was found to have one of the most distinctive syndromes of the encephalomyopathies (Di Mauro et al., 1985). The chances for recovery are doubtful in such a case, but a specific diagnosis may be important for future genetic counseling.

Table 9. Oxidative phosphorylation in skeletal muscle of a patient with MELAS

	Succinate	Glutamate	Pyruvate + malate	Palmitoyl-carnitine
Resp. 4[a]	38.2 (52.2)	12.6 (21.0)	14.2 (24.4)	80.3 (6.8)
Resp. 3[a]	110.9 (129.1)	18.4 (52.3)	25.9 (4.8)	160.9 (90.8)
RCI	2.8 (2.3)	1.7 (2.1)	1.6 (2.3)	1.8 (4.1)
ADP : O	1.4 (1.7)	1.9 (2.6)	2.0 (2.6)	———
O : Pc[b]	———	———	———	20.8 (14.4)

[a]Values expressed as pmol O_2/min/U citrate synthetase.
[b]Palmitoyl-carnitine.

Findings In Other Diseases

Our systematic study revealed other results: in three patients with a Kearns-Sayre syndrome, no defect could be detected in the polarographic studies (Table 9) but we are aware of the reported positive therapeutic effect with coenzyme Q_{10} by Ogasahara et al. (1986).

While the majority of patients with myogenic or neurogenic changes, and those with a disposition toward malignant hyperthermia, had normal function of the oxidative phosphorylation, six boys with the Duchenne type of muscular dystrophy showed loose coupling or a decrease of the respiratory control indices (Table 10). This is consistent with earlier findings in Duchenne patients by Scholte et al. (1980). These results probably indicate secondary changes in the mitochondria due to the basic dystrophic process; they should not be confused with the loose coupling observed in Luft's disease combined with hypermetabolism.

COMMENTS AND SUMMARY

The results shown above indicate that many patients with neuromuscular diseases have no detectable mitochondrial dysfunctions. However, an increasing number of patients from neonatal stages to adulthood are manifesting mitochondrial dysfunctions and defects which have the following consequences. First, the clinician has to be aware of the possibility that mitochondrial disease may be present, especially in patients with multiple or ill-defined diagnoses, as with our patient with Luft's syndrome, and in those patients with the unexplained symptoms mentioned above (Table 1). Second, the diagnosis should be substantiated for a possible therapeutic trial, for genetic counseling, and for the purpose of avoiding unnecessary diagnostic procedures, as in the case of the girl with the MELAS-syndrome mentioned above.

Table 10. Oxidative phosphorylation in skeletal muscle (glutamate)

		Oxygen uptake rates				
		Resp. 4[a]	Resp. 3[a]	RCI	ADP : O	Citrate synthetase (U/mg protein)
Controls	(n[b]= 25)	21.0	52.3	2.1	2.6	296.8
Duchenne muscular atrophy	(n = 6)	15.9	34.9	1.6	2.2	149.2
Spinal muscular atrophy (Kugelberg-Welander)	(n = 3)	18.5	31.3	1.4	3.7	230.6
Myositis	(n = 3)	25.5	45.0	1.9	3.3	241.4
Malignant hyperthermia (at risk)	(n = 18)	21.3	51.4	2.4	2.2	228.9
Kearns-Sayre syndrome	(n = 3)	18.5	36.8	2.3	2.5	318.2

[a]Oxygen uptake rates were expressed as pmol O_2/min/U Citrate synthetase.
[b]n = sample size.

Certainly all the patients have to be carefully selected before starting detailed enzymatic determinations or other highly specialized diagnostic techniques.

REFERENCES

Barth, P.G., Scholte, H.R., Berden, J.A., van der Klei-van Moorsel, J.M., Luyt Houwen, I.E.M., van't Veer-Korthof, E.Th., van der Harten, J.J., & Sobotka-Plojhar, M.A. (1983). An X-linked mitochondrial disease affecting cardiac muscle, skeletal muscle and neutrophil leucocytes. *Journal of the Neurological Sciences, 62,* 327–355.

Di Mauro, S., Bonilla, E., Zeviani, M., Nakagawa, M., & De Vivo, D.C. (1985). Mitochondrial myopathies. *Annals of Neurology, 17,* 521–538.

Haydar, N.A., Conn, H.L., Afifi, A., Wakid, N., Ballas, S., & Fawaz, K. (1971). Severe hypermetabolism with primary abnormality of skeletal muscle mitochondria. *Annals of Internal Medicine, 74,* 548–558.

Luft, R., Ikkos, D., Palmieri, G., Ernster, L., & Afzelius, B. (1962). A case of severe hypermetabolism of nonthyroid origin with a defect in the maintenance of mitochondrial respiratory control. A correlated clinical, biochemical and morphological study. *Journal of Clinical Investigation, 41,* 1776–1804.

McKay, N., Petrova-Benedict, R., Thoene, J., Bergen, B., Wilson, W., & Robinson, B. (1986). Lacticacidaemia due to pyruvate dehydrogenase deficiency, with evidence of protein polymorphism in the a-subunit of the enzyme. *European Journal of Pediatrics, 144,* 445–450.

Mortier, W. (1981). Congenitale myopathien und muskelhypotoni (Congenital myopathies and muscle hypotonia). In H.Ch. Hopf, K. Poeck, & H. Schliak (Eds.), *Neurologie in Praxis und Klinik* (Vol. II) (1.3–1.33). New York: Thieme Stuttgart.

Noack, E., & Mortier, E. (1984). Mitochondrienfunktionsstörungen bei myopathien. (Mitochondrial dysfunction in myopathies). In W. Mortier (Ed.), *Moderne diagnostik und therapie bei kindern* (pp. 203–216). Berlin: Grosse.

Ogasahara, S., Nishikawa, Y., Yorifuji, S., Soga, F., Nakamura, Y., Takahashi, M., Hashimoto, S., Kono, N., & Tarui, S. (1986). Treatment of Kearns-Sayre syndrome with coenzyme Q_{10}. *Neurology, 36,* 45–53.

Pavlakis, St.G., Phillips, R.C., Di Mauro, S., De Vivo, D.C., & Rowland, L.P. (1984). Mitochondrial myopathy, encephalopathy, lactic acidosis, and strokelike episodes: A distinctive clinical syndrome. *Annals of Neurology, 16,* 481–488.

Scholte, H.R., Busch, H.F.M., Luyt-Houwen, I.E.M., Stinis, J.T., Jennekens, F.G.J., & Mortier, W. (1980). Muscle carnitine in Duchenne muscular dystrophy. In C. Angelini, G.A. Danieli, & D. Fontanari (Eds.), *Muscular dystrophy research advances and new trends* (pp. 303–304). Amsterdam: Excerpta Medica.

Scholte, H.R., Busch, H.F.M., Luyt-Houwen, I.E.M., Vaandrager-Verduin, M.H.M., Przyrembel, H., & Arts, W.F.M. (in press). Defects in oxidative phosphorylation. Biochemical investigations in skeletal muscle and expression of the lesion in other cells. *Journal of Inherited Metabolic Diseases.*

Chapter 7

Application of Ultrastructural Studies of Muscle in Diagnosis

Victor Dubowitz and Caroline A. Sewry

ELECTRON MICROSCOPY HAS A LIMITED BUT important role in the diagnosis of neuromuscular disorders. This procedure should never be undertaken in isolation but should always be seen as an extension of a full clinical assessment of the patient. This should be followed by screening investigations such as serum creatine kinase, electromyography, ultrasonography, and full light microscopy assessment of muscle biopsy with histology and enzyme histochemistry. As sample preparation for observation by electron microscopy is time-consuming, it is also impractical to undertake as a routine procedure in every biopsy. It has been the authors' policy to always fix and embed part of our needle muscle biopsy samples for electron microscopy, but to prepare sections for further analysis only in selected cases after assessment of the light microscopy.

ELECTRON MICROSCOPY AS A DIAGNOSTIC TOOL

Electron microscopy has no place in the routine diagnosis of dystrophies or spinal atrophies, but it is an especially important imaging technique for the diagnosis of certain neuromuscular disorders.

Congenital and Metabolic Myopathies

Electron microscopy is useful in those instances where specific pathology is suspected after examination by light microscopy and where pathology can be confirmed by ultra-

structural examination. This applies particularly to the congenital myopathies with structural abnormalities, such as nemaline myopathy, central core disease, minicore disease, tubular aggregates, and cytoplasmic bodies. It also embraces the metabolic myopathies where an excess of glycogen or lipid storage may be suspected upon examination by light microscopy. It also includes situations where abnormality of mitochondria may be suspected by the presence of ragged red fibers on trichrome stain or fibers with excess oxidative activity on the oxidative enzyme reactions (Dubowitz, 1985; Sewry, 1985).

The following cases were included to illustrate these disorders:

Case Number 1 The first case involved a 1-year-old floppy infant who manifested delay in motor activity, and whose muscle biopsy showed the presence of rods after trichrome staining. Electron microscopy confirmed the presence of electron-dense rod structures connected to the Z-lines of the myofibrils.

Case Number 2 The second case involved a 6-year-old floppy infant who had hypotonia from birth and who also had associated cardiomegaly and hepatic enlargement. It was also suspected that the infant had type II glycogenosis (Pompe's disease); the infant's muscle biopsy showed a very marked vacuolar myopathy on routine staining and revealed excess glycogen with the PAS stain. Electron microscopy confirmed there was marked loss of muscle structure and replacement by glycogen,

some of which was membrane-bound (lysosomal in location). The diagnosis was further
confirmed biochemically by the demonstration
of a complete absence of acid maltase in the
biopsy.

Case Number 3   The third case involved an
example of the classic Kearns-Sayre syndrome
in an adolescent boy who manifested mild limb
weakness and fatigability, but who also presented marked ptosis, external ophthalmople-
gia, and associated cardiomyopathy. A muscle
biopsy showed abnormal fibers with a more
granular appearance on routine staining, and
excess oxidative activity. There was an increased number of mitochondria, and ultrastructurally, many of them were abnormal.

Case Number 4   The fourth case provided
an additional example of mitochondrial abnormality in a floppy infant whose biopsy showed
a vacuolar myopathy with associated marked
destruction of muscle fibers. The biopsy also
revealed an excess of glycogen, lipid, and oxidative activity upon examination by light microscopy; the presence of excessive mitochondria, as well as glycogen and lipids were
revealed upon examination by electron microscopy. This is a case of the so-called mitochondria–lipid–glycogen storage myopathy, which
may in some instances be associated with a
Fanconi syndrome of renal involvement and a
poor prognosis. Some cases have been shown
to have an associated cytochrome oxidase deficiency. It should be noted that the structural
changes of the mitochondria upon viewing by
electron microscopy are nonspecific and are
similar in different metabolic and clinical disorders affecting the mitochondria.

ELECTRON MICROSCOPY IN MINIMAL CHANGE AND VACUOLAR MYOPATHIES

In some biopsies, the light microscopy picture
is not entirely normal, but the abnormality is
not specific. Electron microscopy may be helpful in trying to establish a more definitive diagnosis. In cases of "minimal change myopathy" wherein the main change is variation in

fiber size or in the presence of internal nuclei or
other such nonspecific changes, electron microscopy may show evidence of some dysfunction of fibers, or the presence of some specific
subcellular abnormality of organelles. In other
instances, light microscopy may show the presence of vacuoles, which can be further examined by electron microscopy. Vacuolar myopathy is particularly associated with periodic
paralysis; the changes observed with electron
microscopy may be fairly specific, and may
include a high incidence of tubular aggregates
as a fairly consistent feature, together with
structural abnormalities related to the vacuolation. So-called rimmed vacuoles with a
basophilic staining around the vacuoles on
light microscopy are found in oculopharyngeal
myopathy; upon examination by electron microscopy, characteristic inclusions in a small
proportion of the nuclei are revealed. These
inclusions are thought to be of viral origin, but
their exact nature has not been determined.
Similar rimmed vacuoles, together with
cytoplasmic and nuclear inclusions, are also
found in inclusion body myositis, where the
intranuclear inclusions are slightly larger and
are thought to be different from those of
oculopharyngeal myopathy. The clinical presentation is also different, usually with limb
weakness presenting as a limb girdle type of
syndrome.

As an example of vacuolar myopathy, a case
was described of a 7-year-old boy, referred as a
possible limb girdle dystrophy, with a 1-year
history of mild limb weakness and a positive
Gower sign on getting up from the floor. His
creatine kinase (CK) was moderately elevated
(247 iu/l). Upon examination by light microscopy, a degenerative myopathy with necrosis
and phagocytosis of fibers was observed; in
addition, rimmed vacuoles were present in
many of the fibers. Electron microscopy revealed the presence of myelin bodies in relation
to the vacuoles and the intranuclear inclusions
characteristic of inclusion body myositis. A recent report (Chou, 1986) has suggested inclusion body myositis may be caused by a mumps
virus.

ELECTRON MICROSCOPY AND ABNORMALITIES IN SUBCELLULAR ORGANELLES

Some patients with overt neuromuscular clinical problems do not have pronounced pathological changes under light microscopy, but under electron microscopy, specific structures are revealed. These structures include zebra-body myopathy, fingerprint body myopathy, and sarcoplasmic body myopathy. Whereas some of these ultrastructural abnormalities may occur as an incidental feature in other myopathies, they appear to be the only feature and may be of some significance in these cases.

TOMORROW'S MYOPATHIES

Finally, as an illustration of the value of electron microscopy, we would like to discuss a few cases which one may look upon as "tomorrow's myopathies." These are myopathies about which clinical diagnoses have not yet been established but which may, in the future, prove to signal specific disorders and new syndromes.

A Case Involving a New X-linked Autophagic Vacuolar Myopathy

The case involved a 2½-year-old boy who presented with a 2-month history of difficulty with running and climbing stairs; he also manifested gait abnormality. Clinical assessment showed he had a mild weakness of the limbs with a waddling gait, had difficulty going up steps, and manifested a Gower sign when getting up from the floor. He was unable to jump. There was no associated facial weakness. His CK was moderately elevated at 615 iu/l (N < 170), and his electromyography (EMG) results were equivocal, with some focal polyphasic potentials suggestive of myopathic abnormality; the ultrasound scan of quadriceps showed a mild increase in echo that suggested abnormality.

The boy's mother had an unusual history of attacks of weakness during each of her three pregnancies; these attacks became more marked during her latest pregnancy with this child. During these attacks, which mainly occurred at night, she found herself to be completely paralyzed and unable to move. The attacks subsequently settled down spontaneously after about an hour. They were somewhat suggestive of a periodic paralysis. Clinically, she showed no evidence of any weakness, but her CK was mildly elevated at 290 iu/l. Her EMG and ultrasound were normal.

Needle biopsy of the child showed a vacuolar myopathy, with small vacuoles present in many of the fibers, whereas the mother showed a similar but less striking change with the presence of very small vacuoles, or "cracks," in many fibers (Figure 1 and Figure 2).

Electron microscopy showed a similar picture in both the child and the mother, with the presence of autophagic vacuoles and unusual dense bodies within the vacuoles (Figure 3). These were different from those in any other previously described disorder, and did not resemble those seen in periodic paralysis. There were none of the tubular aggregates present that are common in periodic paralysis.

The changes were identical to those described in abstract in a family with an X-linked pattern of inheritance by Kalimo, Paljarvin, Savontaus, Sonnigen, & Lang (1984). We have compared our biopsy material with those of Kalimo and we and they agree that the materials appear to be identical. We could thus presume that the inheritance in our cases may also be X-linked, with the mother being a manifesting carrier of the X-linked gene. It would be interesting to locate the gene on the X chromosome (which should be possible in Kalimo's extensive family) in order to establish whether it is near to the loci of Duchenne and Becker dystrophy genes (Xp21), or possibly that of Emery-Dreifuss dystrophy genes near the long arm of the X chromosome.

A Case Involving a Neuromuscular Disorder Affecting Muscle Fibers

The case involved a 2-week-old infant who was extremely floppy from birth and who had difficulty swallowing in addition to marked muscle

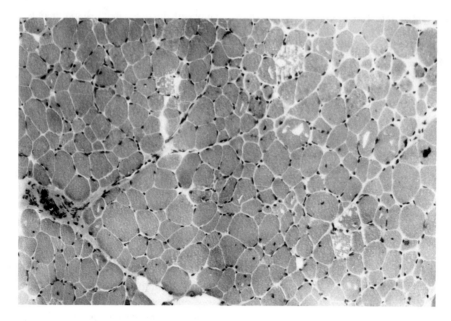

Figure 1.   Needle biopsy from the quadriceps of a 2-year-old boy with mild weakness showing variation in fiber size, internal nuclei, and several vacuolated fibers. (Haematoxylin and Eosin [H & E] × 156).

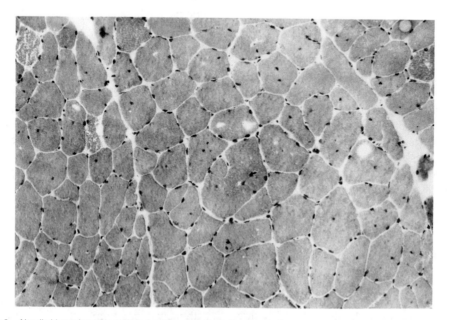

Figure 2.   Needle biopsy from the mother showing a pathological picture similar to her son (Figure 1) with variation in fiber size, internal nuclei, split fibers, and vacuolation. (H & E × 156).

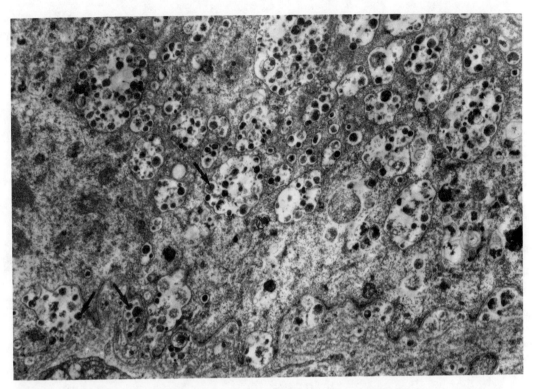

Figure 3.   Electron micrograph of a vacuolated fiber in the son's biopsy. Note the membrane-bound vacuoles containing dense bodies, and the encapsulation of dense bodies in the basement membrane (arrows). (× 98,600).

weakness. Clinically, the infant was thought to possibly have some degree of central nervous system abnormality; normal responsiveness characteristic of a full-term newborn infant was absent.

Needle biopsy of the quadriceps showed a rather unusual picture, with isolated fibers showing complete loss of structure and a hyalinised, somewhat amorphous appearance on all the routine stains. These fibers were negative for the various enzyme histochemical reactions (Figure 4). The remaining fibers seemed to show a normal histological and histochemical pattern.

Upon examination by electron microscopy, a striking degeneration of many fibers was revealed, with complete loss of structure, and an abundance of filamentous material (Figure 5 and Figure 6). These filaments were difficult to identify with certainty, but they appeared to resemble actin. Immunocytochemical studies showed that they were not desmin. Other fibers still had a structural pattern or were in the process of losing their structure.

The child continued to deteriorate, and an additional needle biopsy 2 weeks later showed an essentially similar change. The infant subsequently died within a few weeks; autopsy permission was refused.

This child appeared to have had an unusual destructive type of neuromuscular disorder that affected all components of the muscle fibers and was associated with residual filamentous material. There is some possibility the disorder had a developmental basis and could therefore be genetically determined.

Three Cases Involving Minimal Change Myopathy

Two cases were two Arab siblings, a boy of 9 years and a girl of 4 years. The two siblings presented a somewhat similar clinical picture

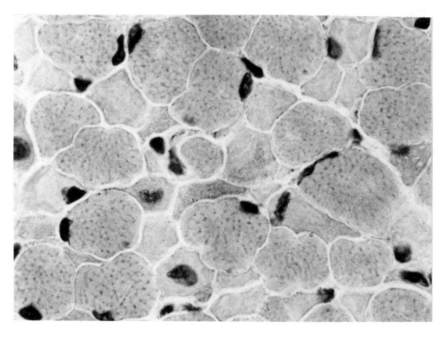

Figure 4.   Needle biopsy of the quadriceps from a 2-week-old hypotonic boy showing variation in fiber size, disruption of fibers, and several pale-staining hyaline fibers. (H & E × 1000).

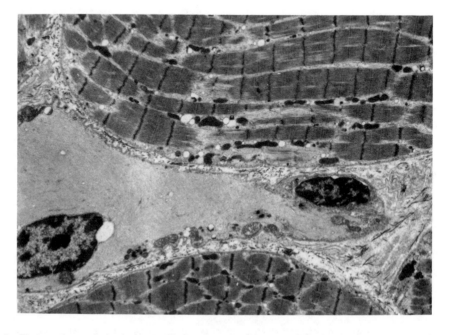

Figure 5.   Electron micrograph showing an atrophic fiber that has completely lost its striation pattern and is filled with filaments. (× 5,000).

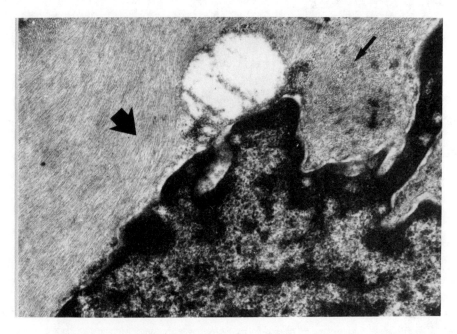

Figure 6. High power electron micrograph showing the filaments that fill some of the fibers in longitudinal (large arrow) and transverse section (small arrow). (Dense structure lower right is a nucleus.) (× 34,000).

characterized by a delay in intellectual and motor milestones, associated hypotonia, and the presence of congenital cataracts. This suggests a Marinesco-Sjögren's syndrome. Needle biopsy showed a somewhat nonspecific mild abnormality, with some variability in fiber size and occasional degenerate-looking fibers representing a "minimal change myopathy" (Figure 7). Upon examination by electron microscopy, vacuoles were found to be present, together with myelin bodies that were relatively nonspecific. In addition, there was a distinctive change in both children which we have not seen before in any other biopsy material. This was the presence of an unusual membrane in relation to some of the sarcolemmal nuclei (Figure 8). The membrane was dense and may have been a tubular structure.

We have recently investigated a 3-year-old boy with a similar clinical and pathological picture. Electron microscopy again showed the unusual membrane round nuclei and the presence of myelin whorls.

The clinical manifestations in all three cases resembled Marinesco-Sjögren's syndrome,

and we believe the dense membranous structure may be specific.

ELECTRON MICROSCOPY AND MUSCLE DISORDER RESEARCH

Apart from their potential diagnostic value, ultrastructural studies have also made significant contributions to the research investigating the pathogenesis of some of these muscle disorders, particularly the muscular dystrophies. One of the theories currently in vogue is that a primary abnormality in the muscle membrane may be responsible for the pathology of the muscle (for review see Rowland, 1980); this theory has been supported by the recognition of breaks in the muscle membrane at electron microscope level, the so-called delta lesions. The question arises as to whether these lesions are in fact primary or possibly secondary to the destructive process. The same question applies to abnormalities found in the inner or outer aspects of the plasma membrane on electron microscopic freeze fracture studies. In these

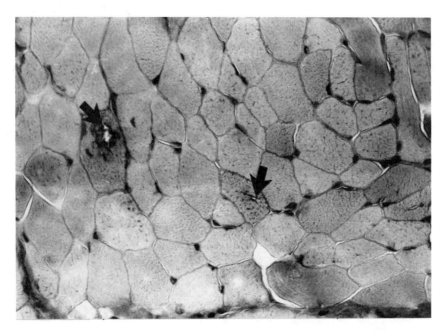

Figure 7.   Needle biopsy from one of two siblings presenting with hypotonia and congenital cataracts, showing minimal patholog-ical changes except for occasional fibers with rimmed vacuoles (arrows). (Verhoeff-VanGieson [VVG] × 430).

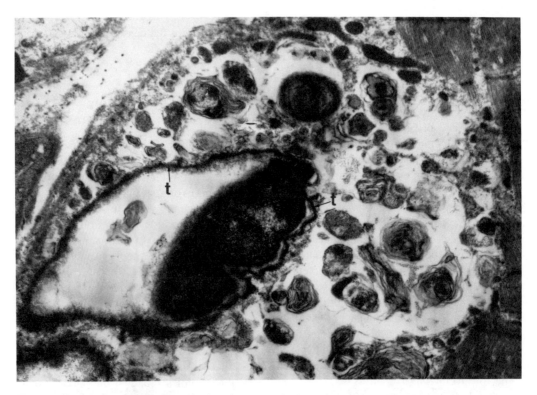

Figure 8.   Electron micrograph showing a pyknotic nucleus surrounded by an unusual dense tubule-like structure (t) and adjacent membranous whorls. (× 22,950).

studies, abnormalities were detected in the number of intramembranous particles, in the orthagonal array density, and in the caveolar density (Bonilla, Schotland, & Wakayama, 1982).

Immunocytochemical studies at electron microscope level have also helped to identify specific proteins in muscle disorders, such as alpha-actinin in the rods of nemaline myopathy, desmin, or intermediate filaments in relation to some myopathies. The further use of monoclonal antibodies will undoubtedly help to identify more of these specific abnormalities. Recent studies in our laboratory with the use of various lectins in relation to the muscle membrane have shown an absence of the lectin *Ricinus communis* agglutinin-I (RCA-I) in Duchenne and other X-linked muscular dystrophies, whereas it is usually present in normal muscle as well as in other neuromuscular disorders (Capaldi, Dunn, Sewry, & Dubowitz, 1983).

REFERENCES

Bonilla, E., Schotland, D.L., & Wakayama, Y. (1982). Freeze-fracture studies in human muscular dystrophies. In D. L. Schotland (Ed.), *Disorders of the motor unit* (pp. 475–487). New York: John Wiley & Sons.

Capaldi, M.J., Dunn, M.J., Sewry, C.A., & Dubowitz, V. (1983). Altered binding of Ricinus communis I lectin by muscle membranes in Duchenne muscular dystrophy. *Journal of the Neurological Sciences, 63,* 129–142.

Chou, S.M. (1986). Inclusion body myositis: A chronic persistent mumps myositis? *Human Pathology, 17,* 765–777.

Dubowitz, V. (1985). *Muscle biopsy: A practical approach* (2nd ed.). Philadelphia: Bailliere Tindall.

Kalimo, H., Paljarvin, L., Savontaus, M.-L., Sonnigen, V., & Lang, H. (1984). Hereditary myopathy with enhanced autophages. *Acta Neurologica Scandinavica* (Suppl.), *98,* 180–181.

Rowland, L.P. (1980). Biochemistry of muscle membranes in Duchenne muscular dystrophy. *Muscle & Nerve, 3,* 3–20.

Sewry, C.A. (1985). Ultrastructural changes in diseased muscle. In V. Dubowitz, *Muscle biopsy: A practical approach* (2nd ed., pp. 129–183). London: Bailliere Tindall.

Chapter 8

The Spectrum of Peroxisomal Disorders

*Peter G. Barth, Ruud B.H. Schutgens, Ronald J. Wanders,
and Hugo S.A. Heymans*

SINCE THE OBSERVATION THAT RECOGNIZable peroxisomes are lacking in Zellweger syndrome (Goldfischer et al., 1973), a new class of genetic disorders related to peroxisomes has been established. Most of these involve the nervous system and are therefore of significance to pediatric neurologists. On the basis of present knowledge, three groups of inherited peroxisomal disorders can be distinguished. *Group I* includes those disorders that are due to a deficiency of peroxisomes and hence to a loss of multiple peroxisomal functions. In *Group II*, only rhizomelic chondrodysplasia calcificans punctata is represented. It is characterized by involvement of a limited number of peroxisomal pathways. *Group III* is represented by disorders in which only one peroxisomal metabolic pathway is affected.

An overview of established peroxisomal disorders is given in Table 1. This review concerns the peroxisomal disorders that are presently known. We will restrict our descriptions to those that affect the nervous system.

PEROXISOMES AND PEROXISOMAL FUNCTIONS

Peroxisomes were discovered by Rhodin (1954) and later defined by De Duve and Baudhuin (1966) as membrane-bound organelles containing at least one oxidase to form hydrogen peroxide and catalase to decompose it (De Duve & Baudhuin, 1966). The name peroxisome refers to peroxide metabolism and not to peroxidases, since not all peroxidases are peroxisomal.

Table 1. Inherited peroxisomal disorders

Group I

Deficiency of peroxisomes and multiple peroxisomal dysfunction

1. Cerebrohepatorenal (Zellweger) syndrome
2. Infantile Refsum disease
3. Neonatal adrenoleukodystrophy

Group II

Impairment of a limited number of peroxisomal functions

  Rhizomelic chondrodysplasia calcificans punctata

Group III

Disorders arising from a single peroxisomal enzyme deficiency

IIIA. Disorders affecting the catabolism of very long chain fatty acid (VLCFA)

1. X-linked adrenoleukodystrophy/ adrenomyeloneuropathy complex
2. Peroxisomal acyl-CoA oxidase deficiency (pseudo-NALD)
3. Peroxisomal 3-oxoacyl-CoA thiolase deficiency (pseudo-ZS)

IIIB. Other disorders affecting a single peroxisomal enzyme

1. Phytanic acid oxidase deficiency (Refsum disease)
2. Alanine:glyoxylate aminotransferase deficiency (Hyperoxaluria type I)
3. Acatalasemia

Presumptive peroxisomal disorders

1. Cerebrotendinous xanthomatosis
2. Joubert syndrome

The morphological appearance of peroxisomes varies considerably. They are bounded by a single membrane, appear spherical, and range in diameter from 0.1 μm to 0.5 μm. Their matrix has a homogenous appearance, at least in man. The large variety is found in hepatocytes and tubular epithelial cells of the kidney. Their identification may be aided by the application of histochemical staining for catalase (Roels & Goldfischer, 1979). The small variety, also called microperoxisomes, has been identified in rat brain, with a preponderance in oligoglial cells, ependymal cells, and neuroblasts (Arnold & Holtzman, 1978; Holtzman, 1982). Microperoxisomes have been identified in cultured human skin fibroblasts (Santos, Ojeda, Garrido, & Leighton, 1985). Catalase positive particles have also been identified biochemically in cultured human muscle (Wanders, Barth, et al., 1987).

The biogenesis of peroxisomes is partly known. Peroxisomes appear to arise by budding from preexisting ones, rather than from endoplasmic reticulum, as previously thought (Lazarow & Fujiki, 1985). Peroxisomes—unlike mitochondria—contain no DNA. Peroxisomal enzyme proteins are synthesized on free ribosomes. The translation products are transported through the cytosol and are taken up by peroxisomes. Posttranslational processing of a number of enzyme proteins, their cytosolic transport, their targeting mechanisms, and their uptake by peroxisomes are under study. These processes will not be discussed in this review.

The following metabolic pathways have been assigned to peroxisomes:

1. Catabolism of very long chain fatty acids (VLCFA). Chain shortening of fatty acids with more than 22 carbon atoms takes place in peroxisomes prior to further catabolism in the mitochondria. The process takes place through peroxisomal β-oxidation. This involves the following 5 steps: 1) activation by acyl-CoA synthetase, 2) oxidation by acyl-CoA oxidase, 3) and 4) hydration and dehydrogenation by so-called bifunctional enzyme, and 5) thio-

lytic cleavage by 3-oxoacyl-CoA thiolase. Fatty acids of intermediate chain length are preferentially oxidized in mitochondria. Short chain fatty acids of C8 and less cannot be oxidized further in peroxisomes, and are oxidized only in mitochondria.

Peroxisomal β-oxidation is not linked to the respiratory chain as in mitochondria. Therefore, hydrogen peroxide molecules generated in the oxidase step are dissipated by the catalase reaction that involves the formation of peroxide. Individual β-oxidation enzymes have been isolated from rat liver. Antibodies have been raised against peroxisomal acyl-CoA oxidase, bifunctional enzyme, and thiolase. These enzymes are immunologically different from their mitochondrial counterparts (Hashimoto, 1982).

2. Breakdown of dicarboxylic acids (Mortensen, Gregersen, & Rasmussen, 1983; Vamecq & Van Hoof, 1984) generated by ω-oxidation

3. Bile acid synthesis via the conversion of the normal intermediates trihydroxycoprostanoic acid (THCA) and dihydroxycoprostanoic acid (DHCA) into cholic acid and chenodeoxycholic acid, respectively (Hagey & Krisans, 1982; Kase, Björkhem, & Pedersen, 1983)

4. Biosynthesis of ether-phospholipids (plasmalogens, alkyl-glycerophospholipids) (Hajra & Bishop, 1982)

5. Peroxisomal glyoxylate metabolism via alanine: glyoxylate aminotransferase (Takada & Noguchi, 1982)

6. Oxidation of polyamines (spermidine and spermine) (Hoeltta, 1977)

7. Catabolism of pipecolic acid

8. Catabolism of phytanic acid

In the case of pipecolic acid and phytanic acid, the evidence for peroxisomal involvement in the catabolism of these metabolites is still incomplete and derives mainly from their accumulation in peroxisomal disorders of group I.

GROUP I: INHERITED PEROXISOMAL DISORDERS

Deficiency of Peroxisomes and Multiple Peroxisomal Dysfunction

The three syndromes that will be discussed are: 1) Cerebrohepatorenal (Zellweger) syndrome (ZS), 2) Infantile Refsum disease (IRD), and 3) Neonatal adrenoleukodystrophy (NALD).

Cerebrohepatorenal (Zellweger) Syndrome (ZS)

Zellweger syndrome is a multi-system disorder resulting from at least one autosomal recessive gene defect, and involving both embryofetopathy and regressive changes that continue into postnatal life. It was first described in 1964 (Bowen, Lee, Zellweger, & Lindenberg, 1964).

Clinical and Pathological Features Early death of the affected patients is usual. Eighty-three percent of the patients described in the literature die during the first 6 months of life (Heymans, 1984). Facial dysmorphia is both striking and characteristic. From an analysis of over 100 published cases (Heymans, 1984) it was concluded that high forehead, large anterior fontanel, hypoplastic supraorbital ridges, epicanthal folds, and deformed ear lobes are present in over 90% of the cases. Impaired hearing (Govaerts, Colon, Rotteveel, & Monnens, 1985) and retinopathy (Garner, Fielder, Primavesi, & Stevens, 1982) are regular features. Cataracts are often found. Liver disease resulting from fibrosis or cirrhosis, calcific stippling of the epiphyses, and small renal cysts are reported in the large majority. Brain abnormalities (De Leon et al., 1977; Evrard, Caviness, Pratts-Vinas, & Lyon, 1978; Gilchrist et al., 1976; Mei Liu, Bangaru, Kidd, & Boggs, 1976; Opitz et al., 1969; Volpe & Adams, 1972) in ZS uniquely combine malformations such as gyral abnormalities, neuronal heterotopia, pachymicrogyria, and regressive changes such as neutral fat storage in astrocytes, granulomas, and germinolytic cysts. Hypomyelination is seen rather than demyelination.

Gross delay in the attainment of milestones is found in each case of ZS. Blindness and hearing deficit may contribute to the gross development delay. Muscular hypotonia and weakness are striking in ZS. Myopathy with abnormal mitochondria has been reported (Mueller-Hoecker, Walther, Bise, Pongratz, & Huebner, 1984; Sarnat, Machin, Darwish, & Rubin, 1983) indicating a true neuromuscular involvement. Ultrastructural studies in ZS liver have revealed the absence of recognizable peroxisomes (Brun, Gilboa, Meeuwisse, & Nordgren, 1978; Goldfischer et al., 1973; Mooi et al., 1983; Pfeifer & Sandhage, 1979). Moreover, abnormal mitochondria were found in hepatocytes (Goldfischer et al., 1973; Mooi et al., 1983; Pfeifer & Sandhage, 1979) and in cortical astrocytes (Goldfischer et al., 1973). Angulate lysosomes with fine double lamellae (Mooi et al., 1983) as storage material are found mainly in macrophages, and are similar to those found in macrophages in adrenoleukodystrophy (*vide infra*). Diminished adrenocortical reserve has been described in ZS (Govaerts, Monnens, Melis, & Trijbels, 1984). Striated adrenocortical cells similar to the findings in adrenoleukodystrophy have also been found in ZS (Goldfischer et al., 1983).

Biochemical Features The recorded absence of peroxisomes in ZS (Goldfischer et al., 1973) (Figure 1) has its biochemical counterpart in multiple peroxisomal dysfunction.

1. Abnormal pipecolic acid catabolism (Danks, Tippett, Adams, & Campbell, 1975; Trijbels, Monnens, Bakkeren, van Raay-Selten, & Corstiaensen, 1979) results in increased levels of pipecolic acid in blood, urine, and cerebrospinal fluid (CSF) (Govaerts, Monnens, Tegelaers, Trijbels, & van Raay-Selten, 1982).

2. Impaired catabolism of very long chain fatty acids (VLCFA) results in increase of $C24:0$, $C26:0$, and $C26:1$ esters of fatty acids in tissues, plasma, and cultured skin fibroblasts. The elevated ratio $C26:0/C22:0$ is a useful expression for impaired peroxisomal β-oxidation (Moser, Singh, et al., 1984). The peroxisomal β-oxida-

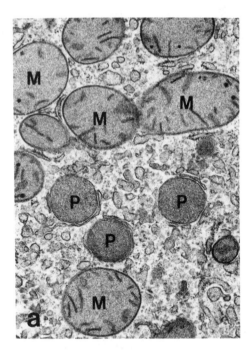 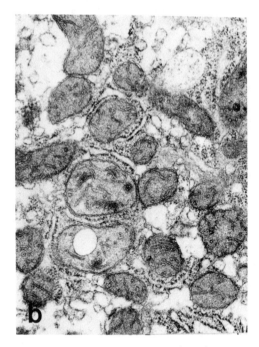

Figure 1. a) Electronmicroscopy of normal hepatocyte showing normal sized and normal structured mitochondria (M) and peroxisomes (P) (× 32.040). b) Similar preparation from Zellweger patient shows abnormal mitochondria and absence of detectable peroxisomes (× 32.040). (Courtesy Dr. K. P. Dingemans, Dept. of Pathology, University Hospital Amsterdam, with permission.)

tion enzyme proteins acyl-CoA oxidase, bifunctional protein and 3-oxoacyl-thiolase were found to be absent in liver, kidney, and cultured fibroblasts by immunoblot analysis (Suzuki, Orii, Mori, Tatibana, & Hashimoto, 1986; Tager et al., 1985) and peroxisomal β-oxidation was found to be impaired (Suzuki et al., 1986; Wanders, van Roermund, et al., 1986).

3. Impaired biosynthesis of plasmalogens (glycerophospholipids with an ether linkage instead of an ester linkage at carbon 1 of glycerol) results in decreased levels of plasmalogens in various tissues including erythrocytes (Heymans, Schutgens, Tan, van den Bosch, & Borst, 1983; Heymans et al., 1984). Impaired *de novo* biosynthesis of plasmalogens was found in cultured skin fibroblasts (Schrakamp et al., 1985). Moreover, a deficient activity of two of the enzymes involved in the biosynthesis of plasmalogens: acylCoA:-dihydroxyacetone phosphate acyltransferase

(DHAPAT) (Datta, Wilson, & Hajra, 1984; Schutgens et al., 1984) and alkyl dihydroxyacetone phosphate synthase (alkyl DHAP synthase) (Schrakamp et al., 1985) was found in liver and in cultured skin fibroblasts. It has been found that levels of plasmalogen in erythrocytes in ZS patients are age related (Wanders, Purvis, et al., 1986), which makes this test less reliable in ZS patients over 20 weeks of age.

4. Impaired biosynthesis of bile acids results in increased levels of trihydroxycoprostanoic acid (THCA) and dihydroxycoprostanoic acid (DHCA) in urine, serum/plasma, and duodenal fluid (Clayton et al., 1987; Hanson, Szczepanik-van Leeuwen, Williams, Grabowski, & Sharp, 1979; Monnens et al., 1980) which is probably due to impaired cholesterol side chain cleavage activity (Wanders, Schutgens, & Heymans, 1987).

5. Medium and long chain dicarboxylic acid-

uria can be found in ZS patients (Rocchic-cioli, Aubourg, & Bougneres, 1986).

6. Catalase latency. Catalase is a peroxisomal enzyme. In ZS patients, the percentage of particle (e.g., peroxisome) bound catalase activity in cultured fibroblasts is less than 5%, whereas it is over 65% in control fibroblasts (Wanders et al., 1984). Catalase normally is a soluble matrix enzyme of peroxisomes like L-α-hydroxyacid oxidase and D-amino acid oxidase. These activities are not deficient in ZS liver either (Wanders et al., 1984). However, the enzyme activities of DHAPAT and the peroxisomal β-oxidation enzymes are deficient in ZS (Datta et al., 1984; Schutgens et al., 1984; Suzuki et al., 1986).

7. Phytanic acid oxidase activity has been found deficient in ZS (Poulos, Sharp, & Whiting, 1984). Phytanic acid accumulates in patients with ZS, but an abnormal phytanic acid concentration in blood is a less reliable indicator in very young patients with ZS (Wanders, Smith, et al., 1987), since the accumulation is age-dependent.

Prenatal Diagnosis The various distinct biochemical abnormalities described above afford a wide range of possibilities for prenatal diagnosis on cultured amniocytes or on chorion villus biopsies. Successful approaches have been made through determination of VLCFA (Moser et al., 1984), *de novo* biosynthesis of plasmalogen (Schutgens, Heymans, Wanders, van den Bosch, & Schrakamp, 1985; Schutgens, Schrakamp, et al., 1985), the catalase latency test (Wanders, Schrakamp, van den Bosch, Tager, & Schutgens, 1986), and peroxisomal β-oxidation (Wanders, van Wijland, et al., 1987).

Infantile Refsum Disease (IRD)

Infantile Refsum disease was first described as a phytanic acid storage disease (Scotto et al., 1982) before multiple peroxisomal dysfunction became apparent.

Clinical and Pathological Features The first cases described showed hepatomegaly, mental retardation, facial dysmorphia, reti-nopathy, neurosensory deafness, osteopenia, growth retardation, hypocholesterolemia, and ultrastructural abnormalities in the liver that consisted of lamellar lipid profiles. Furthermore, levels of vitamins A and E were noticeably low, as were alpha-lipoprotein levels. High levels of serum phytanic acid were found in each case. Further cases (Boltshauser et al., 1982; Budden, Kennaway, Buist, Poulos, & Weleber, 1986; Roels et al., 1986) confirmed the characteristic clinical profile. Intracranial hemorrhage due to vitamin K deficiency was found in two cases (Budden et al., 1986). Punctate chondrodysplasia was not seen in IRD.

Biochemical Features Further studies revealed the absence of hepatic peroxisomes in three out of four cases in the study by Roels et al. (1986). The remaining case had abnormal catalase containing particles, and was subsequently reclassified as pseudo-NALD (*vide infra*). Multiple peroxisomal dysfunction was discovered (Poll-Thé, Ogier, et al., 1986; Poll-Thé, Saudubray, et al., 1986; Poulos & Sharp, 1984; Poulos, Sharp, & Whiting, 1984; Wanders, Schutgens, Schrakamp, van den Bosch, et al., 1986): impairment of the catabolism of VLCFA, absence of peroxisomal β-oxidation enzymes, impairment of *de novo* biosynthesis of plasmalogens, deficiency of peroxisomal enzymes catalyzing plasmalogen biosynthesis, deficiency of phytanic acid oxidase, increased blood levels of pipecolic acid, and of abnormal bile acids, and absence of catalase containing particles in fibroblasts. This is comparable to findings in ZS.

Neonatal Adrenoleukodystrophy (NALD)

NALD was documented for the first time in 1978 (Ulrich, Herschkowitz, Heitz, Sigrist, & Baerlocher, 1978).

Clinical and Pathological Features At least 18 autopsy proven cases are reported in the literature (Aubourg, Scotto, Rocchiccioli, Feldmann-Pautrat, & Robain, 1986; Benke, Reyes, & Parker, 1981; Haas, Stidworthy, & Farrell, 1982; Jaffe, Crumrine, Hashida, & Moser, 1982; Kelley et al., 1986; Manz, Schuelein, McCullough, Kishimoto, & Eiben,

1980; Mobley et al., 1982; Ulrich et al., 1978). Family data are consistent with autosomal recessive inheritance. Clinical expression is characteristic. Truncal hypotonia, gross motor delay, seizures (starting in the neonatal period in roughly half of the cases), and clinical regression after delayed attainment of some developmental milestones represent the main neurological features. Poor vision is related to retinopathy and, in some cases, to cataracts. Facial dysmorphia is noted quite often, though no consistent picture emerges from the descriptions and photographs presented. Adrenal insufficiency is present in a latent form, but is rarely symptomatic. The liver may be enlarged and fibrotic or cirrhotic. Severe growth failure has been noted in some cases. Half of the cases die before 3 years, while survival beyond 10 years is rare. Peripheral neuropathy is exceptional. Abnormal mitochondria have been been found in muscle in a case exhibiting severe weakness and hypotonia (Wolff et al., 1986). Contrast enhancement around demyelinated areas may be revealed by CT scanning, just as in X-linked adrenoleukodystrophy. The main neuropathological finding in deceased patients is demyelination of the cerebral hemispheres, cerebellum, and brain stem. Demyelinated areas may cavitate in some instances. Storage takes the form of neutral fat containing PAS-positive macrophages surrounding blood vessels. Perivascular lymphocytic infiltrates may be present. Ultrastructurally, the stored material consists of stacks of paired lamellae. Similar storage material may be found in the liver (mainly Kupffer cells), lymph nodes, thymus, spleen, and adrenal cortex. Some cases exhibit hydrocephalus; this may be due to intracranial hemorrhage in the neonatal period (bleeding diathesis). In addition to demyelination, neocortical microgyria is regularly found, suggesting prenatal onset of the pathological process. Embryofetopathy is not found in other tissues; for example, cortical renal cysts are not seen in NALD. Punctate chondrodysplasia, often seen in ZS, is not a feature of NALD.

Biochemical Features The absence of recognizable peroxisomes in the liver of two siblings with NALD was recorded in 1983

(Partin & McAdams, 1983). Multiple peroxisomal dysfunction similar to previous findings in ZS and IRD was found subsequently (Aubourg et al., 1986; Goldfischer et al., 1985; Kelley et al., 1986; Kelley & Moser, 1984; Vamecq et al., 1986; Wanders, Schutgens, Schrakamp, Tager, et al., 1987). This includes hyperpipecolic acidemia, abnormal bile acids, deficient biosynthesis of plasmalogens, impaired catabolism of VLCFA, increased phytanic acid in serum, and absence of catalase-containing particles in fibroblasts.

Hyperpipecolic Acidemia Hyperpipecolic acidemia was described for the first time by Gatfield et al. (1968); other studies were subsequently conducted (Burton, Reed, & Remy, 1981; Challa, Geisinger, & Burton, 1983; Thomas et al., 1975). This condition exhibits the features of retinopathy, liver disease, mental retardation, and progressive brain disease, as well as mild dysmorphia, and increased serum levels of pipecolic acid. Neuropathological findings in two cases differed: disseminated demyelination of cerebral white matter was found in the first case described by Gatfield et al. (1968), and PAS-positive storage in astrocytes and macrophages were found in the other case (Challa et al., 1983). Peroxisomes were reported in the liver in the last case. A later study of fibroblasts in the case of Thomas et al. (1975) revealed absence of catalase-containing particles, decreased activity of DHAPAT, and decreased peroxisomal β-oxidation (Wanders, van Roermund, van Wijland, Schutgens, Tager, et al., in press). The different findings in the few cases described makes one hesitant to devise a separate category. The clinical features of liver disease, retinopathy, and brain disease with predominant white matter affection also make it probable that this disorder belongs to the multiple peroxisomal deficit disorders.

The Genetic Relationship of Zellweger Syndrome, Infantile Refsum Disease, and Neonatal Adrenoleukodystrophy

Are Zellweger syndrome, infantile Refsum disease, and neonatal adrenoleukodystrophy genetically separate disorders? The extraordinary tetrad of retinopathy, brain disease, liver disease with fibrosis/cirrhosis, and sensorineural deafness is part of each of the three entities. Moreover, recognizable peroxisomes are severely deficient in each of them. In one study by Goldfischer et al. (1985), a few very small peroxisomes could be detected in the liver of a NALD patient. The same investigators had previously failed to detect any peroxisomes in the livers of ZS patients tested by the same method (Goldfischer et al., 1973).

Pathological differentiation between ZS and NALD is stressed by emphasis on the progressive demyelination, systemic infiltration by lipid laden macrophages and adrenal atrophy in NALD, and chondrodysplasia, dysmyelination (rather than demyelination), and renal cysts in ZS (Kelley et al., 1986). The last authors emphasized high levels of monounsaturated VLCFA, C26:1, in plasma and fibroblasts of ZS patients, whereas only minor elevation of C26:1 was found in NALD. Values found in fibroblasts of confirmed NALD were 0.38 ± 0.14 vs. 1.33 ± 0.14 in ZS, 0.15 ± 0.03 in X-linked ALD and 0.07 ± 0.02 in controls (values as mean $\pm$ SD in $\mu g/mg$ protein). In another study (Wanders, Schutgens, Schrakamp, Tager, et al., 1987), the catabolism of VLCFA in fibroblasts from ZS and from NALD patients was studied by its turnover. No difference was found.

We studied two siblings with a mild variant of ZS who were very similar in appearance and follow-up to the patients previously described under the heading of IRD (Figure 2), and found values of C26:1 in fibroblasts in the range of classical ZS (Barth et al., 1987). The outward appearance of patients with NALD and IRD is mostly described as mild dysmorphia, but this dysmorphia is rarely compared in detail to classical ZS. In five cases of multiple peroxisomal dysfunction that fulfilled the criteria of IRD, we found the high forehead, wide open fontanel with delayed closure, and posterior rotation of the earlobes with absent lobules to be very similar to the dysmorphic profiles of ZS patients. The series includes three published cases (Barth et al., 1983; Barth et al., 1987). The final answer to the genetic relationship

of ZS, NALD, and IRD must come from complementation analysis, now in progress. Preliminary data (Tager et al., 1987) on somatic cell fusion experiments on ZS, IRD, and NALD fibroblast lines indicate that ZS and IRD belong to one complementation group, but NALD belongs to another group. More data will be needed for a final answer.

GROUP II: IMPAIRMENT OF A LIMITED NUMBER OF PEROXISOMAL FUNCTIONS

Rhizomelic Chondrodysplasia Calcificans Punctata (RCDP)

RCDP is the only representative of this group so far. This autosomal recessive disorder is characterized by severe dysplastic skeletal disease resulting in shortening of long bones, vertebral anomalies, and periarticular calcification. The affected patients are grossly retarded and spastic. Their neurological and neuropathological abnormalities have thus far scarcely been studied. Cataracts are common. The resemblance of the periarticular calcification in this disease to the periarticular calcification that is often seen in ZS prompted a study for peroxisomal dysfunction. Peroxisomes were present in a liver biopsy but appeared to be misshapen (Heymans et al., 1986). The biosynthesis of plasmalogens was severely abnormal in all patients studied thus far, resulting in strongly deficient plasmalogen levels in erythrocytes from the patients. Subsequent studies revealed deficiency of both DHAPAT and alkyl DHAP synthase (Heymans, Oorthuys, Nelck, Wanders, & Schutgens, 1985). Additionally, patients were found to have increased levels of phytanic acid. Other parameters studied, especially the catalase latency test in fibroblasts (Heymans et al., 1986) and the β-oxidation of VLCFA were shown to be normal. The presence of catalase-containing particles (peroxisomes) in fibroblasts combined with the limited number of peroxisomal metabolic pathways affected, places this disorder in a separate group of inherited peroxisomal diseases. Complementation analysis with cell lines from patients with ZS, IRD, and NALD places this

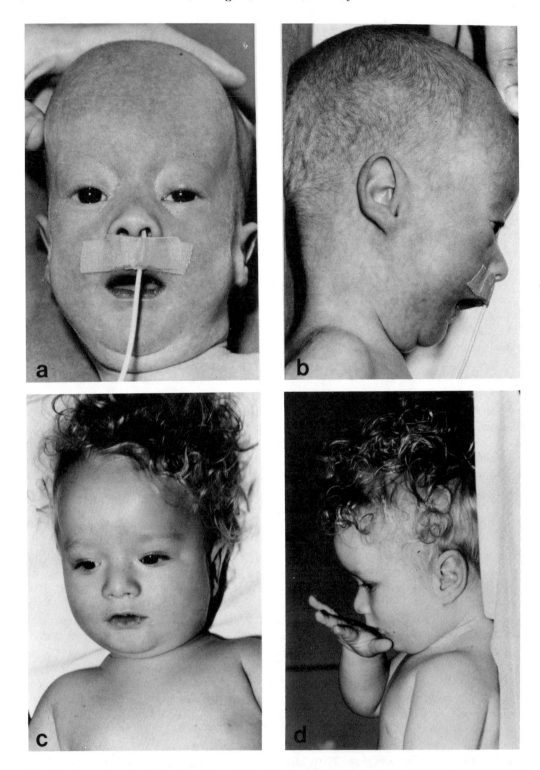

Figure 2. **a)** Frontal, and **b)** lateral views of a patient with "classical" Zellweger syndrome (copyright CIBA-GEIGY B. V. Arnhem, Netherlands, with permission). Frontal **(c)** and lateral **(d)** views of a patient with mild Zellweger syndrome or infantile Refsum disease. Notice that both patients characteristically exhibit a high forehead and posterior angulated earlobes with absent lobules. (Printed with permission, MTP Press and the Society for the Study of Inborn Errors of Metabolism.)

disorder in a separate complementation group (Tager et al., 1986). The enzyme deficiencies in RCDP present various possibilities for prenatal diagnosis.

GROUP III: DISORDERS ARISING FROM A SINGLE PEROXISOMAL ENZYME DEFICIENCY

Disorders affecting the catabolism of very long chain fatty acids (VLCFA) include: 1) X-linked adrenoleukodystrophy/adrenomyeloneuropathy complex, 2) Peroxisomal acyl-CoA oxidase deficiency (pseudo-NALD), and 3) Peroxisomal thiolase deficiency (pseudo-ZS).

Other disorders affecting a single peroxisomal enzyme include: 1) Phytanic acid oxidase deficiency (Refsum disease), 2) Hyperoxaluria type I, and 3) Acatalasemia.

X-linked Adrenoleukodystrophy/ Adrenomyeloneuropathy Complex (X-ALD/AMN)

Clinical and Pathological Features   The disorder represents an X-linked gene defect with variable expression. There is a major division between X-ALD, which presents between 4 and 8 years with disseminated demyelinated lesions in the brain, and usually ends fatally within 3 years after clinical onset, and X-AMN. An adult disorder, X-AMN involves progressive myelopathy and polyneuropathy without cerebral complications. In X-ALD, the light microscopic lesion is characterized by severe cerebral demyelination and by perivascular accumulations of lipid laden macrophages, with granular (sudanophilic) or striated appearance. Perivascular lymphocytic infiltrates arise as an immunological reaction to the lytic process. Ultrastructural findings consist of lamellar inclusions in the cytoplasm of cerebral macrophages, adrenocortical cells, Leydig cells, and Schwann cells, consisting of bileaflets with an intralamellar space, often surrounded by a membrane that is probably lysosomal (Powers, 1985). They are probably related to similar inclusions seen in lysosomes within macrophages of the liver in ZS (Mooi et

al., 1983), in IRD (Roels et al., 1986), and in systemic and CNS macrophages in NALD (Ulrich et al., 1978).

Pathological findings in X-AMN are mostly restricted to the spinal cord, with affection of the long ascending and descending tracts. Involvement of the peripheral nerves is usually mild. The initial symptoms in X-ALD are varied (Aubourg, Chaussain, Dulac, & Arthuis, 1982). Cerebral CT scan and MRI (Huckman, Wong, Sullivan, Zeller, & Geremia, 1986; Lane, Carroll, & Pedley, 1978) have proved to be useful additional diagnostic tools in X-ALD. CT scans revealed characteristic enhancement surrounding demyelinated lesions indicating blood-brain barrier destruction.

Adult males with X-AMN have signs of myelopathy with polyneuropathy, and bladder dysfunction. Addisons's disease may precede, coincide with, or follow the onset of neurological symptoms (Libber, Migeon, Brown, & Moser, 1986). Patients with X-AMN and X-ALD may belong to the same pedigree (Davis, Orth, Nicholson, Kornfeld, & Seelinger, 1979). Variants of the adult type mimicking spinocerebellar degeneration (Marsden, Obeso, & Lang, 1982), olivopontocerebellar atrophy (Kuroda, Hirano, & Yuasa, 1983), or familial spastic paraparesis (O'Neill, Swanson, Brown, Griffin, & Moser, 1985) have been reported. Female heterozygotes may clinically express the gene defect in a way that is reminiscent of AMN.

Biochemical Features   Two classic studies preceded the identification of the biochemical defect in X-ALD. One study described the clinical and pathological findings in the brain, spinal cord, adrenal glands, and testicular tissue of 17 cases (Schaumburg, Powers, Raine, Suzuki, Richardson, 1975); the second study gave an account of its histochemistry (Johnson, Schaumburg, & Powers, 1976), in this way establishing its character as a storage disease. The accumulation of VLCFA esters in the brains of X-ALD patients was established by isolation of the stored material (Igarashi et al., 1976; Menkes & Corbo, 1977). The accumulation of VLCFA in fibroblasts and in plasma of patients and most of the obligate heterozygotes was confirmed in further studies

(Moser et al., 1980; Moser et al., 1981). Furthermore, impairment of the oxidation of C26 : 0 and C24 : 0 was found in fibroblasts, while the peroxisomal oxidation of C16 : 0 and C18 : 0 was normal (Singh, Moser, Moser, & Kishimoto, 1981; Singh, Moser, Moser, & Kishimoto, 1984). An impairment of peroxisomal β-oxidation of VLCFA is now regarded as the basic abnormality in this disorder. No other peroxisomal biochemical defects have been found in X-ALD/AMN and normal peroxisomes have been identified in the liver of a patient (Goldfischer et al., 1985). Recent evidence localizes the biochemical lesion of X-ALD at the level of the activation of VLCFA, by peroxisomal VLCFA Acyl-CoA synthetase (Hashmi, Stanley, & Singh, 1986; Wanders, van Roermund, van Wijland, Nijenhuis, et al., 1987; Wanders, van Roermund, van Wijland, Schutgens, et al., 1987).

Postnatal and Prenatal Diagnosis A survey describing the experience of a single referral center for biochemical ALD diagnosis in 303 cases has provided reference data for X-ALD, X-ALD heterozygotes, NALD, and prenatal diagnosis (Moser, Moser, Singh, & O'Neill, 1984). The C26 : 0/C22 : 0 fatty acid ratio in plasma and/or fibroblasts has provided a highly reliable test for the diagnosis of X-ALD/AMN. Its application to cultured amniocytes identifies the affected fetus. Obligate carriers are identified in 93% of the cases by VLCFA analysis. Recently, linkage of X-ALD to a polymorphic DNA probe for the region Xq27-28 has provided a supplementary test which may enhance the reliability of heterozygote detection (Aubourg, Sack, Meyers, Lease, & Moser, 1987).

Therapeutic measures: A therapeutic regime has been developed for the lowering of blood VLCFA in adrenoleukodystrophy (Moser et al., 1987; Rizzo et al., 1987). The regime is based on dietary restriction of VLCFA containing foods and inhibition of endogenous synthesis by the addition of glycerol trioleate oil. Preliminary evidence is available which suggests that this regime lowers blood VLCFA levels in patients with X-AMN. Whether any clinical improvement can be induced is not yet clear.

Peroxisomal Acyl-CoA Oxidase Deficiency (Pseudo-NALD)

A brother and sister had early onset of seizures, muscle hypotonia, progressive hearing defects, and visual failure resulting from retinopathy. They had no dysmorphic features suggesting ZS. Both had latent adrenocortical insufficiency. A CT scan of one sibling showed contrast enhanced hypodense lesions at the age of 4 years. Accumulation of VLCFA in plasma and in fibroblasts was found in both patients. Other peroxisomal parameters were normal. The liver biopsy of both patients showed enlarged abnormal peroxisomes. Peroxisomal acyl-CoA oxidase deficiency was shown by immunoblotting in the liver (Poll-Thé et al., 1988).

Peroxisomal 3-Oxoacyl-CoA Thiolase Deficiency (Pseudo-ZS)

The patient was a girl from consanguineous parents; she had symptoms suggestive of ZS without chondrodysplasia and died at 11 months. At autopsy she had renal cysts, minimal liver fibrosis, demyelination in the cerebellar white matter, hypomyelination in the cerebral white matter, and foci of neuronal heterotopia. The adrenals were atrophic with striated cells. Enlarged peroxisomes were present in a liver biopsy. Accumulation of VLCFA in serum and in fibroblasts was found along with an increase of THCA in a duodenal aspirate. Other peroxisomal parameters were normal (Goldfischer et al., 1986). Further investigation revealed impaired peroxisomal β-oxidation in the liver. Also, 3-oxoacyl-CoA thiolase deficiency was shown by immunoblotting (Schram et al., 1987).

Phytanic Acid Oxidase Deficiency (Refsum Disease)

Biochemical interest in this long known autosomal recessive disorder featuring slowly progressive polyneuropathy and retinopathy has reawakened following the finding of phytanic acid elevation in disorders caused by multiple peroxisomal dysfunction: ZS, IRD, NALD, and RCDP. The biochemical basis of this disorder has been known for a long time, and treatment (phytanic acid restricted diet) is available. (For reviews, see Refsum, 1975; Refsum, Stokke, Eldjarn, & Fardeau, 1984.) Circumstantial evidence classifies phytanic acid oxidase as a peroxisomal enzyme.

Alanine: Glyoxylate Aminotransferase Deficiency

(Hyperoxaluria type I). In this autosomal recessive disorder, the enzymatic deficiency leads to increased excretion of oxalate and glycolate (Danpure & Jennings, 1986). Two phenotypes exist: a severe lethal neonatal type and a juvenile type with nephrocalcinosis.

Acatalasemia

This deficiency is not accompanied by any illness except oral infections.

Presumptive Peroxisomal Disorders

Cerebrotendinous Xanthomatosis In this disorder of bile acid synthesis, structurally abnormal peroxisomes have been described (Goldfischer & Sobel, 1981).

Joubert Syndrome A single sibship has been reported with three affected individuals combining Joubert syndrome and elevated levels of pipecolic acid in their plasma (Poll-Thé et al., 1985).

Laboratory Procedures

Biochemical tests currently used for screening and diagnosis of peroxisomal disorders are listed in Table 2.

Table 2. Diagnostic procedures in inherited peroxisomal disorders

Plasma/serum
Cholesterol
ACTH/cortisol
Pipecolic acid
Bile acids (THCA, DHCA)
VLCFA: C26:0/C22:0 and C26:1
Phytanic acid
Urine
Pipecolic acid
Bile acids (THCA, DHCA)
Dicarboxylic acids
Fibroblasts
VLCFA: C26:0/C22:0 and C26:1
Peroxisomal β-oxidation
DHAPAT activity
de novo biosynthesis of plasmalogens
Catalase latency test
Phytanic acid oxidase activity
Liver
Ultrastructure for peroxisomes
Peroxisomal β-oxidation
DHAPAT activity
De novo biosynthesis of plasmalogens
Peroxisomal β-oxidation enzyme proteins by immunoblotting procedure

REFERENCES

Arnold, G., & Holtzman, E. (1978). Microperoxisomes in the central nervous system of the postnatal rat. *Brain Research, 155,* 1–17.
Aubourg, P., Chaussain, J.L., Dulac, O., & Arthuis, M. (1982). Adrenoleucodystrophie chez l'enfant. A propos de 20 observations. *Archives Francaises de Pediatrie, 39,* 663–669.
Aubourg, P., Sack, G.H., Meyers, D.A., Lease, J.J., & Moser, H.W. (1987). Linkage of adrenoleukodystrophy to a polymorphic DNA probe. *Annals of Neurology, 21,* 349–352.
Aubourg, P., Scotto, J., Rocchiccioli, F., Feldmann-Pautrat, D., & Robain, O. (1986). Neonatal adrenoleukodystrophy. *Journal of Neurology, Neurosurgery, and Psychiatry, 49,* 77–86.
Barth, P.G., Schutgens, R.B.H., Bakkeren, J.A.J.M., Dingemans, K.P., Heymans, H.S.A., Douwes, A.C., & van der Klei-van Moorsel, J.M. (1983). A milder variant of Zellweger syndrome. *European Journal of Pediatrics, 144,* 338–342.

Barth, P.G., Schutgens, R.B.H., Wanders, R.J.A., Heymans, H.S.A., Moser, A.E., Moser, H.W., Bleeker-Wagemakers, E.M., Jansonius-Schultheiss, K., Derix, M., & Nelck, G.F. (1987). A sibship with a mild variant of Zellweger syndrome. *Journal of Inherited Metabolic Disease, 10,* 253–259.
Benke, P.J., Reyes, P.F., & Parker, J.C., Jr. (1981). New form of adrenoleukodystrophy. *Human Genetics, 58,* 204–208.
Boltshauser, E., Spycher, M.A., Steinmann, B., Briner, J., Isler, W., Kuster, T., Poulos, A., Pollard, A.C. (1982). Infantile phytanic acid storage disease: A variant of Refsum's disease? *European Journal of Pediatrics, 139,* 317–318.
Bowen, P., Lee, C.S.N., Zellweger, H., & Lindenberg, R. (1964). A familial syndrome of multiple congenital defects. *Bulletin of Johns Hopkins Hospital, 114,* 402–414.
Brun, A., Gilboa, M., Meeuwisse, G.W., & Nordgren, H. (1978). The Zellweger syndrome: Subcellular pa-

thology, neuropathology, and the demonstration of Pneumocystis carinii pneumonitis in two siblings. *European Journal of Pediatrics, 127*, 229–245.

Budden, S.S., Kennaway, N.G., Buist, N.R.M., Poulos, A., & Weleber, R.G. (1986). Dysmorphic syndrome with phytanic acid oxidase deficiency, abnormal very long chain fatty acids, and pipecolic acidemia: Studies in four children. *Journal of Pediatrics, 108*, 33–39.

Burton, B.K., Reed, S.P., & Remy, W.T. (1981). Hyperpipecolic acidemia: Clinical and biochemical observations in two male siblings. *Journal of Pediatrics, 99*, 729–734.

Challa, V.R., Geisinger, K.R., & Burton, B.K. (1983). Pathologic alterations in the brain and liver in hyperpipecolic acidemia. *Journal of Neuropathology and Experimental Neurology, 42*, 627–638.

Clayton, P.T., Lake, B.D., Hall, N.A., Shortland, D.B., Carruthers, R.A., & Lawson, A.M. (1987). Plasma bile acids in patients with peroxisomal dysfunction syndromes: Analysis by capillary gas chromatography mass spectrometry. *European Journal of Pediatrics, 146*, 166–173.

Danks, D.M., Tippett, P., Adams, C., & Campbell, P. (1975). Cerebro-hepato-renal syndrome of Zellweger. A report of eight cases with comments upon the incidence, the liver lesion, and a fault in pipecolic acid metabolism. *Journal of Pediatrics, 86*, 382–387.

Danpure, C.J., & Jennings, P.R. (1986). Peroxisomal alanine:glyoxylate aminotransferase deficiency in primary hyperoxaluria type I. *FEBS, 201*, 20–24.

Datta, N.S., Wilson, G.N., Hajra, A.K. (1984). Deficiency of enzymes catalyzing the biosynthesis of glycerol-ether lipids in Zellweger syndrome: A new category of metabolic disease involving the absence of peroxisomes. *New England Journal of Medicine, 311*, 1080–1083.

Davis, L.E., Orth, D.N., Nicholson, B.S., Kornfeld, M., & Seelinger, D.F. (1979). Adrenoleukodystrophy and adrenomyeloneuropathy associated with partial adrenal insufficiency in three generations of a kindred. *American Journal of Medicine, 66*, 342–347.

De Duve, C., & Baudhuin, P. (1966). Peroxisomes (microbodies and related particles). *Physiological Reviews, 46*, 332–57.

De Leon, G.A., Grover, W.D., Huff, D.S., Morinigo-Mestre, G., Punnett, H., & Kistenmacher, M.L. (1977). Globoid cells, glial nodules, and peculiar fibrillary changes in the cerebro-hepato-renal syndrome of Zellweger. *Annals of Neurology, 2*, 473–484.

Evrard, Ph., Caviness, V.S., Jr., Pratts-Vinas, J., & Lyon, G. (1978). The mechanism of arrest of neuronal migration in the Zellweger malformation: An hypothesis based upon cytoarchitectonic analysis. *Acta Neuropathologica, 41*, 109–117.

Garner, A., Fielder, A.R., Primavesi, R., & Stevens, A. (1982). Tapetoretinal degeneration in the cerebro-hepato-renal (Zellweger's) syndrome. *British Journal of Ophthalmology, 66*, 422–431.

Gatfield, P.D., Taller, E., Hinton, G.G., Wallace, A.C., Abdelnour, G.M., & Haust, M.D. (1968). Hyperpipecolatemia: A new metabolic disorder associated with neuropathy and hepatomegaly. *Canadian Medical Association Journal, 99*, 1215–1233.

Gilchrist, K.W., Gilbert, E.F., Goldfarb, S., Goll, U., Spranger, J.W., & Opitz, J.M. (1976). Studies of mal-

formation syndromes in man. XIb: The cerebro-hepato-renal syndrome of Zellweger: Comparative pathology. *European Journal of Pediatrics, 121*, 99–118.

Goldfischer, S., Collins, J., Rapin, I., Coltoff-Schiller, B., Chang, C.H., Nigro, M., Black, V.H., Javitt, N.B., Moser, H.W., & Lazarow, P.B. (1985). Peroxisomal defects in neonatal-onset and X-linked adrenoleukodystrophy. *Science, 227*, 67–70.

Goldfischer, S., Collins, J., Rapin, I., Neumann, P., Neglia, W., Spiro, A.J., Ishii, T., Roels, F., Vamecq, J., & van Hoof, F. (1986). Pseudo-Zellweger syndrome: Deficiencies in several peroxisomal oxidative activities. *Journal of Pediatrics, 108*, 25–32.

Goldfischer, F., Moore, C., Johnson, A., Spiro, A., Valsamis, M.P., Wisniewski, H., Ritch, R., Norton, W., Rapin, I., & Gartner, L. (1973). Peroxisomal and mitochondrial defects in the cerebro-hepato-renal syndrome. *Science, 182*, 62–64.

Goldfischer, S., Powers, J.M., Johnson, A.B., Axe, S., Brown, F.R., & Moser, H.W. (1983). Striated adrenocortical cells in cerebro-hepato-renal (Zellweger) syndrome. *Virchow's Archiv. A, Pathological Anatomy and Histopathology, 44*, 355–361.

Goldfischer, S., & Sobel, H.J. (1981). Peroxisomes and bile-acid synthesis. *Gastroenterology, 81*, 196–197.

Govaerts, L., Colon, E., Rotteveel, J., & Monnens, L. (1985). A neurophysiological study of children with the cerebro-hepato-renal syndrome of Zellweger. *Neuropediatrics, 16*, 185–190.

Govaerts, L., Monnens, L., Melis, T., & Trijbels, F. (1984). Disturbed adrenocortical function in cerebro-hepato-renal syndrome of Zellweger. *European Journal of Pediatrics, 143*, 10–12.

Govaerts, L., Monnens, L., Tegelaers, W., Trijbels, F., & van Raay-Selten, A. (1982). Cerebro-hepato-renal syndrome of Zellweger: Clinical symptoms and relevant laboratory findings in 16 patients. *European Journal of Pediatrics, 139*, 125–128.

Haas, J.E., Stidworthy, J., & Farrell, D.L. (1982). Neonatal-onset adrenoleukodystrophy in a girl. *Annals of Neurology, 12*, 449–457.

Hagey, L.R., & Krisans, S.K. (1982). Degradation of cholesterol to propionic acid by rat liver peroxisomes. *Biochemical and Biophysical Research Communications, 107*, 834–841.

Hajra, A.K., & Bishop, J.E. (1982). Glycerolipid biosynthesis in peroxisomes via the acyl dihydroxyacetone phosphate pathway. *Annals of the New York Academy of Sciences, 386*, 170–182.

Hanson, R.F., Szczepanik-van Leeuwen, P., Williams, G.C., Grabowski, G., & Sharp, H.L. (1979). Defects of bile acid synthesis in Zellweger's syndrome. *Science, 203*, 1107–1108.

Hashimoto, T. (1982). Individual peroxisomal β-oxidation enzymes. *Annals of the New York Academy of Sciences, 386*, 5–12.

Hashmi, M., Stanley, W., & Singh, I. (1986). Lignoceryl-CoASH ligase: Enzyme defect in fatty β-oxidation system in X-linked childhood adrenoleukodystrophy. *FEBS, 196*, 247–259.

Heymans, H.S.A. (1984). Cerebro-hepato-renal (Zellweger) syndrome. Clinical and biochemical consequences of peroxisomal dysfunction. Ph.D. thesis, University of Amsterdam.

Heymans, H.S.A., Oorthuys, J.W.E., Nelck, G., Wanders, R.J.A., Dingemans, K.P., & Schutgens, R.B.H. (1986). Peroxisomal abnormalities in rhizomelic chondrodysplasia punctata. *Journal of Inherited Metabolic Disease, 9,* 329–331.

Heymans, H.S.A., Oorthuys, J.W.E., Nelck, G., Wanders, R.J.A., & Schutgens, R.B.H. (1985). Rhizomelic chondrodysplasia punctata: Another peroxisomal disorder (letter). *New England Journal of Medicine, 313,* 187–188.

Heymans, H.S.A., Schutgens, R.B.H., Tan, R., van den Bosch, H., & Borst, P. (1983). Severe plasmalogen deficiency in tissues of infants without peroxisomes (Zellweger syndrome). *Nature, 306,* 69–70.

Heymans, H.S.A., van den Bosch, H., Schutgens, R.B.H., Tegelaers, W.H.H., Walther, J.U., Mueller-Hoecker, J., & Borst, P. (1984). Deficiency of plasmalogens in the cerebro-hepato-renal (Zellweger) syndrome. *European Journal of Pediatrics, 142,* 10–15.

Hoeltta, E. (1977). Oxidation of spermidine and spermine in rat liver purification and properties of polyamine oxidase. *Biochemistry, 16,* 91–100.

Holtzman, E. (1982). Peroxisomes in nervous tissue. *Annals of the New York Academy of Sciences, 386,* 523–525.

Huckman, M.S., Wong, P.W.K., Sullivan, Th., Zeller, P., & Geremia, G.K. (1986). Magnetic resonance imaging compared with computed tomography in adrenoleukodystrophy. *American Journal of Diseases of Children, 140,* 1001–1003.

Igarashi, M., Schaumburg, H.H., Powers, J., Kishimoto, Y., Kolodny, E., & Suzuki, K. (1976). Fatty acid abnormality in adrenoleukodystrophy. *Journal of Neurochemistry, 25,* 851–860.

Jaffe, R., Crumrine, P., Hashida, Y., & Moser, H.W. (1982). Neonatal adrenoleukodystrophy. Clinical, pathologic, and biochemical delineation of a syndrome affecting both males and females. *American Journal of Pathology, 108,* 100–111.

Johnson, A.B., Schaumburg, H.H., & Powers, J.M. (1976). Histochemical characteristics of the striated inclusions of adrenoleukodystrophy. *Journal of Histochemistry and Cytochemistry, 24,* 725–730.

Kase, F., Björkhem, I., & Pedersen, J.I. (1983). Formation of cholic acid from 3α, 7α, 12α-trihydroxy-5β-cholestanoic acid by rat liver peroxisomes. *Journal of Lipid Research, 24,* 1560–1567.

Kelley, R.I., Datta, N.S., Dobyns, W.B., Hajra, A.K., Moser, A.B., Noetzel, M.J., Zackai, E.H., & Moser, H.W. (1986). Neonatal adrenoleukodystrophy: New cases, biochemical studies, and differentiation from Zellweger and related peroxisomal polydystrophy syndromes. *American Journal of Medical Genetics, 23,* 869–901.

Kelley, R.I., & Moser, H.W. (1984). Hyperpipecolic acidemia in neonatal adrenoleukodystrophy. *American Journal of Medical Genetics, 19,* 791–795.

Kuroda, S., Hirano, A., & Yuasa, S. (1983). Adrenoleukodystrophy-cerebello-brainstem dominant case. *Acta Neuropathologica, 60,* 49–52.

Lane, B., Carroll, B.A., & Pedley, T.A. (1978). Computerized cranial tomography in cerebral diseases of white matter. *Neurology, 28,* 534–544.

Lazarow, P.B., & Fujiki, Y. (1985). Biogenesis of peroxisomes. *Annual Review of Cellular Biology, 1,* 489–530.

Libber, S.M., Migeon, C. J., Brown, F.R., III, & Moser, H.W. (1986). Adrenal and testicular function in 14 patients with adrenoleukodystrophy or adrenomyeloneuropathy. *Hormone Research, 24,* 1–8.

Manz, H.J., Schuelein, M., McCullough, D.C., Kishimoto, Y., & Eiben, R.M. (1980). New phenotypic variant of adrenoleukodystrophy. Pathologic ultrastructural and biochemical study in two brothers. *Journal of the Neurological Sciences, 45,* 245–260.

Marsden, C.D., Obeso, J.A., & Lang, A.E. (1982). Adrenoleukomyeloneuropathy presenting as spinocerebellar degeneration. *Neurology, 32,* 1031–1032.

Mei Liu, H., Bangaru, B.S., Kidd, J., & Boggs, J. (1976). Neuropathological considerations in cerebro-hepato-renal syndrome (Zellweger's syndrome). *Acta Neuropathologica, 34,* 115–123.

Menkes, J.H., & Corbo, L.M. (1977). Adrenoleukodystrophy. Accumulation of cholesterol esters with very long chain fatty acids. *Neurology, 27,* 928–932.

Mobley, W.C., White, C.L., Tennekoon, G., Clark, A.W., Cohen, S.R., Green, W.R., & Moser, H.W. (1982). Neonatal adrenoleukodystrophy. *Annals of Neurology, 12,* 204–205.

Monnens, L., Bakkeren, J., Parmentier, G., Janssen, G., van Haelst, U., Trijbels, F., & Eyssen, H. (1980). Disturbances in bile acid metabolism of infants with Zellweger (cerebro-hepato-renal) syndrome. *European Journal of Pediatrics, 133,* 31–35.

Mooi, W.J., Dingemans, K.P., van den Bergh Weerman, M., Joebsis, A.C., Heymans, H.S.A., & Barth, P.G. (1983). Ultrastructure of the liver in the cerebrohepatorenal syndrome of Zellweger. *Ultrastructural Pathology, 5,* 135–144.

Mortensen, P.B., Gregersen, N., Rasmussen, K. (1983). The β-oxidation of dicarboxylic acids in isolated mitochondria and peroxisomes. *Journal of Inherited Metabolic Disease,* [suppl 2] *6,* 123–124.

Moser, A.E., Borel, J., Odone, A., Naidu, S., Cornblath, D., Sanders, D.B., & Moser, H.W. (1987). A new dietary therapy for adrenoleukodystrophy: Biochemical and preliminary clinical results in 36 patients. *Annals of Neurology, 21,* 240–249.

Moser, H.W., Moser, A.B., Frayer, K.K., Chen, W., Schulman, J.D., O'Neill, B.P., & Kishimoto, Y. (1981). Adrenoleukodystrophy: Increased plasma content of saturated very long chain fatty acids. *Neurology, 31,* 1241–1291.

Moser, H.W., Moser, A.B., Kawamura, N., Murphy, J., Suzuki, K., Schaumburg, H., & Kishimoto, Y. (1980). Adrenoleukodystrophy: Elevated C 26 fatty acid in cultured skin fibroblasts. *Annals of Neurology, 7,* 542–549.

Moser, H.W., Moser, A.E., Singh, I., & O'Neill, B. P. (1984). Adrenoleukodystrophy. Survey of 303 cases: Biochemistry, diagnosis and therapy. *Annals of Neurology, 16,* 628–641.

Moser, A.E., Singh, I., Brown, F.R., Solish, G.I., Kelley, R.I., Benke, P.J., & Moser, H.W. (1984). The cerebrohepatorenal (Zellweger) syndrome. Increased levels and impaired degradation of very-long-chain fatty acids and their use in prenatal diagnosis. *New England Journal of Medicine, 310,* 1141–1146.

Mueller-Hoecker, J., Walther, J.U., Bise, K., Pongratz, D., & Huebner, G. (1984). Mitochondrial myopathy with loosely coupled oxidative phosphorylation in a case of Zellweger syndrome. *Virchows Archiv. B, Cell Pathology, 45,* 125–138.

O'Neill, B.P., Swanson, J.W., Brown, F.R., III, Griffin, J.W., & Moser, H.W. (1985). Familial spastic paraparesis: An adrenoleukodystrophy phenotype? *Neurology, 35,* 1233–1235.

Opitz, J.M., ZuRhein, G.M., Vitale, L., Shahidi, N.T., Howe, J.J., Chou, S.M., Shanklin, D.R., Sybers, H.D., Dood, A.R., & Gerritsen, Th. (1969). The Zellweger syndrome (cerebro- hepato- r enal s yndrome). *Birth Defects, 5*(2), 144–158.

Partin, J.S., & McAdams, J. (1983). Absence of hepatic peroxisomes in neonatal onset adrenoleukodystrophy. *Pediatric Research, 17,* 294.

Pfeifer, U., & Sandhage, K. (1979). Licht - und elektronenmikroskopische Leberbefunde beim Cerebrohepato-renalen Syndrom nach Zellweger (Peroxisomen-Defizienz). (Light- and electronmicroscopic findings in the liver in the cerebro-hepato-renal syndrome of Zellweger [deficiency of peroxisomes]). *Virchows Archiv. A, Pathology, Anatomy, and Histopathology, 384,* 269–284.

Poll-Thé, B.T., Ogier, H., Saudubray, J.M., Schutgens, R.B.H., Wanders, R.J.A., van den Bosch, H., & Schrakamp, G. (1986). Impaired plasmalogen metabolism in i nfantile Refsum's disease. *European Journal of Pediatrics, 144,* 513–514.

Poll-Thé, B.T., Perignon, J.L., Parvy, P., Lombes, A., Trijbels, J., Schutgens, R.B.H., Wanders, R.J.A., & Saudubray, J.M. (1985). Joubert's syndrome associated with hyperpipecolic acidemia. Three siblings. In K.W.A. Wirtz & J.M. Tager (Eds.), *Peroxisomes and their metabolites in cellular functions.* UNESCO-TUB Workshop, Zeist, The Netherlands.

Poll-Thé, B.T., Roels, F., Ogier, H., Scotto, J., Vamecq, J., Schutgens, R.B.H., Wanders, R.J.A., van Roermund, C.W.T., van Wijland, M.J.A., Schram, A.W., Tager, J.M., & Saudubray, J.-M. (1988). A new peroxisomal disorder with enlarged peroxisomes and a specific deficiency of acyl-CoA oxidase (pseudo neonatal adrenoleukodystrophy). *American Journal of Human Genetics, 42,* 422–434.

Poll-Thé, B.T., Saudubray, J.M., Ogier. H., Schutgens, R.B.H., Wanders, R.J.A., Schrakamp, G., van den Bosch, H., Trijbels, F., Poulos, A., Moser, H.W., van Eldere, J., & Eyssen, H. (1986). Infantile Refsum's disease: Biochemical findings suggesting multiple peroxisomal dysfunction. *Journal of Inherited Metabolic Disease, 9,* 169–174.

Poulos, A., & Sharp, P. (1984). Plasma and skin fibroblast C26 fatty acids in infantile Refsum's disease. *Neurology, 34,* 1606–1608.

Poulos, A., Sharp, P., & Whiting, M. (1984). Infantile Refsum's disease (phytanic acid storage disease): A variant of Zellweger's syndrome? *Clinical Genetics, 25,* 579–586.

Powers, J.M. (1985). Adreno-leukodystrophy (Adreno-testiculo-leuko-myelo-neuropathic complex). Review article. *Clinical Neuropathology, 4,* 181–199.

Refsum, S. (1975). Heredopathia atactica polyneuritiformis (Refsum disease). In P.J. Vinken & G.W. Bruyn (Eds.), *Handbook of Clinical Neurology* (Vol. 21). Amsterdam: North-Holland.

Refsum, S., Stokke, O., Eldjarn, L., & Fardeau, M. (1984). Heredopathia atactica polyneuritiformis (Refsum disease). In P.J. Dyck, P.K. Thomas, E.H. Lambert, & R. Bunge (Eds.), *Peripheral neuropathy* (Vol. II, pp. 1680–1703). Philadelphia: W.B. Saunders.

Rhodin, A.G. (1954). Doctoral Thesis, Karolinska Institute Stockholm.

Rizzo, W.B., Phillips, M.W., Dammann, A.L., Leshner, R.T., Jennings, S.S., Avigan, J., & Proud, V.K. (1987). Adrenoleukodystrophy: Dietary oleic acid lowers hexacosanoate levels. *Annals of Neurology, 21,* 232–239.

Rocchiccioli, F., Aubourg, P., & Bougneres, P.F. (1986). Medium and long chain dicarboxylic aciduria in patients with Zellweger syndrome and neonatal adrenoleukodystrophy. *Pediatric Research, 20,* 62–66.

Roels, F., Cornelis, A., Poll-Thé, B.T., Aubourg, P., Ogier, H., Scotto, J., & Saudubray, J.M. (1986). Hepatic peroxisomes are deficient in infantile Refsum's disease. *American Journal of Medical Genetics, 25,* 257–271.

Roels, F., & Goldfischer, S. (1979). Cytochemistry of human catalase. The demonstration of hepatic and renal peroxisomes by a high temperature procedure. *Journal of Histochemistry and Cytochemistry, 27,* 1471.

Santos, M.J., Ojeda, J.M., Garrido, J., & Leighton, F. (1985). Peroxisomal organization in normal and cerebrohepatorenal (Zellweger) syndrome fibroblasts. *Proceedings of the National Academy of Sciences of the United States of America, 82,* 6556–6560.

Sarnat, H.B., Machin, G., Darwish, H.Z., Rubin, S.Z. (1983). Mitochondrial myopathy of cerebro-hepato-renal (Zellweger) syndrome. *Canadian Journal of Neurological Sciences, 10,* 170–177.

Schaumburg, H.H., Powers, J.M., Raine, C.S., Suzuki, K., Richardson, E.P., Jr. (1975). Adrenoleukodystrophy. A clinical and pathological study of 17 cases. *Archives of Neurology, 32,* 577–591.

Schrakamp, G., Rosenboom, C.F.P., Schutgens, R.B.H., Wanders, R.J.A., Heymans, H.S.A., Tager, J.M., & van den Bosch, H. (1984). Alkyl dihydroxyacetone phosphate synthase in human fibroblasts and its deficiency in Zellweger (cerebro-hepato-renal) syndrome. *Biochemical and Biophysical Research Communications, 120,* 179–184.

Schrakamp, G., Schutgens, R.B.H., Wanders, R.J.A., Heymans, H.S.A., Tager, J.M., & van den Bosch, H. (1985). The cerebro-hepato-renal (Zellweger) syndrome: Impaired *de novo* biosynthesis of plasmalogens in cultured skin fibroblasts. *Biochimica et Biophysica Acta, 833,* 170–174.

Schram, A.W., Goldfischer, S., van Roermund, C.W.T., Brouwer-Kelder, E.M., Collins, J., Hashimoto, T., Heymans, H.S.A., van den Bosch, H., Schutgens, R.B.H., Tager, J.M., & Wanders, R.J.A. (1987). Human peroxisomal 3-oxoacyl-coenzyme A thiolase deficiency. *Proceedings of the National Academy of Sciences of the United States of America, 84,* 2494–2496.

Schutgens, R.B.H., Heymans, H.S.A., Wanders, R.J.A., van den Bosch, H., & Schrakamp, G. (1985). Prenatal diagnosis of the cerebro-hepato-renal (Zellweger) syndrome by detection of an impaired plasmalogen biosynthesis. *Journal of Inherited Metabolic Disease, 8,* 153–154.

Schutgens, R.B.H., Romeyn, G.J., Wanders, R.J.A., van den Bosch, H., Schrakamp, G., & Heymans, H.S.A. (1984). Deficiency of acyl-CoA: Dihydroxyacetone phosphate acyltransferase in patients with Zellweger (cerebro-hepato-renal) syndrome. *Biochemical and Biophysical Research Communications, 120,* 179–184.

Schutgens, R.B.H., Schrakamp, G., Wanders, R.J.A., Heymans, H.S.A., Moser, H.W., Moser, A.E., Tager, J.M., van den Bosch, H., & Aubourg, P. (1985). The cerebro-hepato-renal (Zellweger) syndrome: Prenatal diagnosis based on impaired biosynthesis of plasmalogens. *Prenatal Diagnosis, 5,* 337–344.

Scotto, J.M., Hadchouel, M., Odievre, M., Laudat, M.H., Saudubray, J.M., Dulac, O., Beucler, I., & Beaune, P. (1982). Infantile phytanic acid storage disease, a possible variant of Refsum's disease: Three cases, including ultrastructural studies of the liver. *Journal of Inherited Metabolic Disease, 5,* 83–90.

Singh, I., Moser, H.W., Moser, A.B., & Kishimoto, Y. (1981). Adrenoleukodystrophy. Impaired oxidation of long chain fatty acids in cultured skin fibroblasts and adrenal cortex. *Biochemical and Biophysical Research Communications, 102,* 1223–1229.

Singh, I., Moser, A.B., Moser, H.W., & Kishimoto, Y. (1984). Adrenoleukodystrophy: Impaired oxidation of very long chain fatty acids in white blood cells, cultured skin fibroblasts and amniocytes. *Pediatric Research, 18,* 286–289.

Suzuki, Y., Orii, T., Mori, M., Tatibana, M., & Hashimoto, T. (1986). Deficient activities and proteins of peroxisomal β-oxidation enzymes in infants with Zellweger syndrome. *Clinica Chimica Acta, 156,* 191–196.

Tager, J.M., Ten Harmsen van der Beek, W., Wanders, R.J.A., Hashimoto, T., Heymans, H.S.A., van den Bosch, H., Schutgens, R.B.H., & Schram, A.W. (1985). Peroxisomal β-oxidation enzyme proteins in the Zellweger syndrome. *Biochemical and Biophysical Research Communications, 126,* 1269–1275.

Tager, J.M., Westerveld, A., Strijland, A., Schram, A., Schutgens, R.B.H., van den Bosch, H., & Wanders, R.J.A. (1987). Complementation analysis of peroxisomal diseases by somatic cell fusion. In H. Fahimi & H. Sies (Eds.), *Peroxisomes in biology and medicine* (pp. 353–357). New York: Springer Verlag.

Takada, Y., & Noguchi, T. (1982). The evolution of peroxisomal and mitochondrial alanine:glyoxylate aminotransferase I in mammalian liver. *Biochemical and Biophysical Research Communications, 108,* 153–157.

Thomas, G.H., Haslam, R.H.A., Batshaw, M.L., Capute, A.J., Neidengard, L., & Ransom, J.L. (1975). Hyperpipecolic acidemia associated with hepatomegaly, mental retardation, optic nerve dysplasia and progressive neurological disease. *Clinical Genetics, 8,* 376–382.

Trijbels, J.M.F., Monnens, L.A.H., Bakkeren, J.A.J.M., van Raay-Selten, A.H.J., & Corstiaensen, J.M.B. (1979). Biochemical studies in the cerebro-hepato-renal syndrome of Zellweger: A disturbance in the metabolism of pipecolic acid. *Journal of Inherited Metabolic Disease, 2,* 39–42.

Ulrich, J., Herschkowitz, N., Heitz, Ph., Sigrist, Th., & Baerlocher, P. (1978). Adrenoleukodystrophy. Preliminary report of a connatal case. Light- and electron micro-scopical, immunohistochemical and biochemical findings. *Acta Neuropathologica, 43,* 77–83.

Vamecq, J., Draye, J.P., van Hoof, F., Misson, J.P., Evrard, Ph., Verellen, G., Eyssen, H.J., van Eldere, J., Schutgens, R.B.H., Wanders, R.J.A., Roels, F., & Goldfischer, S.L. (1986). Multiple peroxisomal enzymatic deficiency disorders: A comparative biochemical and morphologic study of Zellweger cerebrohepatorenal syndrome and neonatal adrenoleukodystrophy. *American Journal of Pathology, 125,* 524–535.

Vamecq, J., & van Hoof, F. (1984). Implication of a peroxisomal enzyme in the catabolism of glutaryl-CoA. *Biochemical Journal, 221,* 203–211.

Volpe, J.J., & Adams, R.D. (1972). Cerebro hepato-renal syndrome of Zellweger: An inherited disorder of neuronal migration. *Acta Neuropathologica, 20,* 175–198.

Wanders, R.J.A., Barth, P.G., van Roermund, C.W.T., Ofman, R., Wolterman, R., Schutgens, R.B.H., Tager, J.M., van den Bosch, H., & Bolhuis, P. (1987). Peroxisomes and peroxisomal functions in muscle. Studies with muscle cells from controls and a patient with the cerebro-hepato-renal (Zellweger) syndrome. *Experimental Cell Research, 170,* 147–152.

Wanders, R.J.A., Kos, M., Roest, B., Meijer, A.J., Schrakamp, G., Heymans, H.S.A., Tegelaers, W.H.H., van den Bosch, H., Schutgens, R.B.H., & Tager, J.M. (1984). Activity of peroxisomal enzymes and intracellular distribution of catalase in Zellweger syndrome. *Biochemical and Biophysical Research Communications, 123,* 1054–1061.

Wanders, R.J.A., Purvis, Y.R., Heymans, H.S.A., Bakkeren, J.A.J.M., Parmentier, G.G., van Eldere, J., Eyssen, H., van den Bosch, H., Tager, J.M., & Schutgens, R.B.H. (1986). Age related differences in plasmalogen content of erythrocytes from patients with the cerebro-hepato-renal (Zellweger) syndrome: Implications for postnatal detection of the disease. *Journal of Inherited Metabolic Disease, 9,* 335–342.

Wanders, R.J.A., Schrakamp, G., van den Bosch, H., Tager, J.M., & Schutgens, R.B.H. (1986). A prenatal test for the cerebro-hepato-renal (Zellweger) syndrome by demonstration of the absence of catalase-containing particles (peroxisomes) in amniotic fluid cells. *European Journal of Pediatrics, 145,* 136–138.

Wanders, R.J.A., Schutgens, R.B.H., & Heymans, H.S.A. (1987). Deficient cholesterol side chain oxidation in patients without peroxisomes (Zellweger syndrome): Evidence for the involvement of peroxisomes in bile acid synthesis in man. *Clinica Chimica Acta, 162,* 295–301.

Wanders, R.J.A., Schutgens, R.B.H., Schrakamp, G., Tager, J.M., van den Bosch, H., Moser, A.B., & Moser, H.W. (1987). Neonatal adrenoleukodystrophy. Impaired plasmalogen biosynthesis and peroxisomal β-oxidation due to a deficiency of catalase-containing particles (peroxisomes) in cultured skin fibroblasts. *Journal of the Neurological Sciences, 77,* 331–340.

Wanders, R.J.A., Schutgens, R.B.H., Schrakamp, G., van den Bosch, H., Tager, J.M., Schram, A.W., Hashimoto, T., Poll-Thé, B.T., & Saudubray, J.M. (1986). Infantile Refsum disease: Deficiency of catalase containing particles (peroxisomes), alkyldihydroxyacetone phosphate synthase and peroxisomal β-oxidation enzyme proteins. *European Journal of Pediatrics, 145,* 172–175.

Wanders, R.J.A., Smit, W., Heymans, H.S.A., Schutgens, R.B.H., Barth, P.G., Schierbeek, H., Smit, G.P.A., Berger, R., Przyrembel, H., Eggelte, T.A., Tager, J.M., Maaswinkel-Mooy, P.D., Peters, A.C.B., Monnens, L.A.H., Bakkeren, J.A.J.M., Trijbels, J.M.F., Lommen, E.J.P., & Beganovic, N. (1987). Age-related accumulation of phytanic acid in plasma from patients with the cerebro-hepato-renal (Zellweger) syndrome. *Clinica Chimica Acta, 166,* 45–56.

Wanders, R.J.A., van Roermund, C.M.T., de Vries, C.T., van den Bosch, H., Schrakamp, G., Tager, J.M., Schram, A.W., & Schutgens, R.B.H. (1986). Peroxisomal β-oxidation of palmitoyl-CoA in human liver homogenates and its deficiency in the cerebro-hepato-renal (Zellweger) syndrome. *Clinica Chimica Acta, 159,* 1–10.

Wanders, R.J.A., van Roermund, C.W.T., van Wijland, M.J.A., Nijenhuis, A.A., Tromp, A., Schutgens, R.B.H., Brouwer-Kelder, E.M., Schram, A.W., Tager, J.M., van den Bosch, H., & Schalkwijk, C. (1987). X-linked adrenoleukodystrophy: Defective peroxisomal oxidation of very long chain fatty acids but not of very long chain fatty acyl-CoA esters. *Clinica Chimica Acta, 165,* 321–329.

Wanders, R.J.A., van Roermund, C.W.T., van Wijland, M.J.A., Schutgens, R.B.H., Heikoop, J., van den Bosch, H., Schram, A.W., & Tager, J.M. (1987). Peroxisomal fatty acid β-oxidation in relation to the accumulation of very long chain fatty acids in cultured skin fibroblasts from patients with Zellweger syndrome and other peroxisomal disorders. *Journal of Clinical Investigation, 80,* 1778–1783.

Wanders, R.J.A., van Roermund, C.W.T., van Wijland, M.J.A., Schutgens, R.B.H., Tager, J.M., van den Bosch, H., Thomas, G.H. (in press). Peroxisomes and peroxisomal functions in hyperpipecolic acidaemia. *Journal of Inherited Metabolic Disease, 11* (Suppl. 2).

Wanders, R.J.A., van Wijland, M.J.A., van Roermund, C., Schutgens, R.B.H., van den Bosch, H., Tager, J.M., Nijenhuis, A., & Tromp, A. (1987). Prenatal diagnosis of Zellweger syndrome by measurement of very long chain fatty acid (C26:0) β-oxidation in cultured chorionic villous fibroblasts: Implications for early diagnosis of other peroxisomal disorders. *Clinica Chimica Acta, 165,* 303–310.

Wolff, J., Nyhan, W.L., Powell, H., Takahashi, D., Hutzler, J., Hajra, A.K., Datta, N.S., Singh, I., & Moser, H.W. (1986). Myopathy in an infant with a fatal peroxisomal disorder. *Pediatric Neurology, 2,* 141–146.

Chapter 9

Motor Phenomena during Sleep
Its Significance in Basal Ganglia Disorders of Childhood
Natan Gadoth, Hanan Costeff, Shaul Harel, and Perez Lavie

THE USE OF RESTRICTION FRAGMENT length polymorphisms (RLFPs) to identify genetic markers of inherited neurological diseases requires identification of large affected families. Many dominantly inherited neural diseases are associated with variations in severity, and *forme fruste* patients in the same family may be missed on clinical examination. Thus, finding a genetic marker that is objective and establishing its presence in phenotypically healthy family members may assist in delineating appropriate lineages for molecular genetic study. We have used this approach in the study of families afflicted with L-dopa responsive juvenile dystonia and have established the presence of a specific motor disorder during sleep in a significant number of "healthy" family members of our patients.

BODY MOVEMENTS AND PERIODIC LEG MOVEMENTS DURING SLEEP

Body Movements during Sleep (BMS)

Body movements during sleep (BMS) are a stable and predictable phenomenon that are independent of environmental precipitants. Their number and distribution within the various sleep stages are fairly constant and independent of the methods of estimation (Fukumoto, Mochizuki, Takeishi, Nomura, & Segawa, 1981). The number of movements has been shown to decrease with age during normal development. This decrease is significant from birth to 12 months of age and subsequently plateaus. Body movements during sleep are most frequent in sleep stage 1 (S1). The frequency gradually decreases during REM, S2, S3, and S4, in the stated order (Hashimoto, Hiura, Suzue, Kobayashi, Kawano, Fukuda, Endo, Kokawa, & Miyao, 1979).

We have scored the number of BMS for each REM period in 10 adults. They were studied in our laboratory for various sleep disorders. Four of the adults suffered from chronic insomnia, two had excessive daytime sleep, and two had periodic leg movements during sleep (PMS); two had no sleep abnormality. A mean of 3.8 gross movements were present for each REM period (Table 1).

Abnormal BMS patterns (e.g., increased BMS) occur in a number of neurological disorders. An increase in BMS is seen, for example, in Gilles de la Tourette syndrome (GTS), Huntington's chorea, and L-dopa treated Parkinson's disease. Additionally, a decrease in BMS has been reported in untreated Parkinson's disease, in GTS treated with haloperidol, in a small number of patients with the hereditary dystonia of Segawa (HPD-ST), in primary and acquired forms of torsion dystonia, and in athetosis (Endo et al., 1981; Hashimoto et al., 1981). Also, BMS measurements have been suggested as predictors of the prognosis of childhood epilepsy (Iwakawa et al., 1986).

It was suggested that the study of BMS is useful when evaluating the pathophysiology of basal ganglia disease (Segawa et al., 1985).

Table 1. Motor phenomena during sleep in three patients and their 11 otherwise healthy siblings

	Patients			Fathers			Mothers			Siblings				
	16y	19y	10y	40y	47y	46y	39y	41y	41y	67y[a]	14y	6y	5y	4y
Grade of increased BMS[b] in REM sleep	+++	++	++	−	+	−	−	+	−	−	−	−	−	−
PMS							c						c	
No. per night	−	−	−	115	114	127	50	193	72	333	−	120	51	72

[a]Parental grandfather.
[b]BMS = Body movements during sleep.
[c]Borderline PMS (periodic leg movements during sleep).

As the central catecholaminergic system may be analyzed by scoring BMS (Iwakawa et al., 1986), it is of great importance to note that some researchers have not been paying special attention to body movements, and seem to miss them in their observations. In a study of sleep in 14 patients with GTS, special attention was paid to the recording of tics, while body movements "were recorded by technicians' observations via closed-circuit TV and by video tape monitoring" (Glaze, Frost, & Jankovic, 1983). Observations conducted in this manner could easily miss a variety of movements.

Periodic Leg Movements during Sleep (PMS)

Periodic leg movements during sleep (PMS) are stereotyped, repetitive movements of the lower extremities that are triggered by sleep. They last from 2–15 seconds and occur with remarkable periodicity (Coleman, Pollack, & Weitzman, 1980). More than 40 PMS per night are considered abnormal. Coleman et al. (1983) have shown that in a population of 409 patients with various sleep-wake disorders, PMS was found in 13% of the cases. In another study of 708 patients suffering from disordered sleep, it was found that the prevalence of PMS increases steadily with age. Thus, in patients over 65 years of age, 18% had PMS (Coleman, Miles, Guilleminault, Zarcone, Van der Hoed, & Dement, 1981). It is not surprising that we could not find data on the prevalence of PMS in children, as in our own experience, we have not seen children with this disorder. Familial cases of "primary PMS" have not been re-

ported. However, the association of PMS with the restless leg syndrome has been found in members of two unrelated families (Boghen & Peyronnard, 1976; Montplaisir et al., 1985). In the family described by Montplaisir et al. (1985), one member (the propositus) had high concentrations of free norepinephrine and dopamine and their main metabolites, MHPG and HVA, in the cerebrospinal fluid (CSF). Recently, a family with PMS and nocturnal cramping was reported (Jacobsen, Rosenberg, Huttenlocher, & Spire, 1986). Based on electrophysiological studies, it was suggested that PMS may be caused by increased segmental excitability at spinal levels (Wechsler, Stakes, Shahani, & Busis, 1986). It is generally agreed that the etiology of PMS is yet unknown, although a variety of hypotheses exist. Theories of cause range from epilepsy to the suggestion that a central nervous system "pacemaker" may be responsible for the remarkable periodicity of PMS similar to that of periodic sleep apnea, periodic breathing caused by acute brain trauma, heart rate, spinal fluid pressure, or arterial blood pressure (Coleman, 1982).

BODY MOVEMENTS DURING SLEEP IN HEREDITARY DYSTONIA WITH MARKED DIURNAL FLUCTUATIONS (HPD-ST)

Hereditary dystonia with marked diurnal fluctuation, Segawa type (HPD-ST) was described by Segawa as a familial disorder in 1971 (Segawa, Ohmi, Itoh, Aoyama, & Hayakawa, 1971). This functional disorder of basal ganglia was examined in repeated studies by Segawa on a few of his patients; the studies have shown a decrease in the number of BMS. Segawa distinguished between twitch movements (phasic movements shorter than 0.5 seconds) and gross movements; the main finding in his studies is a decrease of twitch movements during REM sleep, with a gradual increase in twitch movements toward REM stages in later sleep cycles. After L-dopa treatment, the dystonia dramatically dissolved, and the number of twitch movements returned to normal (Segawa, Nomura, Shinomiya, Hosaka, & Suzuki, 1981; Suzuki et al., 1980). Thus, further evidence was obtained relating body movements during sleep with central dopaminergic pathways. Furthermore, low CSF dopamine and HVA levels were also found in his patients prior to L-dopa treatment (Segawa, Hosaka, Miyagawa, Nomura, & Imai, 1976). Although familial cases have been reported in HPD-ST, only 10 out of 27 reported patients showed definite autosomal dominant inheritance (Costeff, Gadoth, Mendelson, Harel, & Lavie, 1987). However, no attempt was made to study unaffected family members in order to detect abnormal motor phenomena during sleep.

For the last 7 years, the authors have closely followed one girl with classical features of HPD-ST; in addition, we have diagnosed two additional unrelated female patients. In all three patients, gross body movements were increased during each REM period. In control patients who suffered from various forms of sleep disorders, we recorded a mean of 3.4 movements per REM period; in one of the patients, there were 58 movements per REM period, and in another patient there were 14 movements. Other than those movements, sleep structures were normal. Repeated studies of patients who were receiving L-dopa and who were in complete clinical remission showed that there was no significant change in the severity or distribution of the abnormal body motility.

Eleven healthy close relatives of the patients, consisting of three pairs of parents, four young siblings, and one elderly paternal grandfather, had repeated polysomnograms with special emphasis on body motility. In one pair of parents, increased body movements during REM sleep were present. In all three fathers, in two mothers, in the grandfather, and in two female siblings, an abnormal number of PMS were recorded. The third mother and one sibling were considered borderline cases of PMS because they had 50 PMS per night. Thus, 10 out of the 11 healthy close relatives of the patients had PMS, while two of the relatives had BMS.

The data on motor phenomena during sleep in the examined patients are shown in Table 1, while the family tree is given in Figure 1. As the grandfather suffered from insomnia, with sleep efficiency of 63 percent, treatment with clonazepam 1 mg at bedtime was given. This

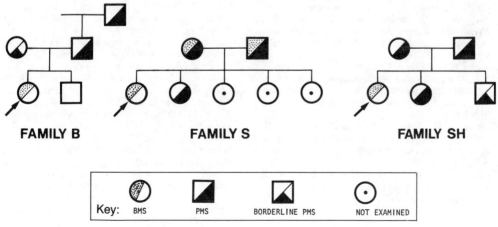

FAMILY B   FAMILY S   FAMILY SH

Key: BMS   PMS   BORDERLINE PMS   NOT EXAMINED

Figure 1.   Family trees of the three families.

resulted in dramatic clinical and laboratory improvements in the patient.

COMMENT

The data presented are unique for several reasons. It was shown on repeated polysomnograms that for all three patients, the number of gross body movements was increased during REM sleep; these numbers were not reduced by the administration of L-dopa. We are unable to explain the difference between our observations and those made by Segawa and colleagues. However, the disturbed sleep cycle that was manifested by patients as an unresistable need to fall asleep at early afternoon only to get up at early dawn (4 a.m.) responded dramatically to treatment with L-dopa (Gadoth, Bechar, & Lavie, 1981). BMS were also found in one pair of parents who were otherwise entirely healthy.

The most striking finding was the presence of PMS in 8 out of 11 healthy close relatives;

borderline PMS was found in two of the relatives. The presence of PMS in two consecutive generations in all families involving both sexes suggests autosomal dominant inheritance. As no families with "pure" PMS are known, our data indicate that PMS, BMS, and HPD-ST may be related. The presence of both movement disorders in an L-dopa responsive functional disorder of basal ganglia may indicate a common dopaminergic mechanism for both forms of movements. However, their presence in healthy members of these families might serve as a marker for *forme fruste* cases. This will support the early suggestion made by Segawa et al. (1976) that this type of dystonia is inherited in an autosomal dominant fashion. The authors suggest that all families affected with HPD-ST should be studied in a similar way in order to permit clarification of the mode of inheritance. Similarly, studies for GTS are justified in which high familial incidence, wide variability in severity, and a history of sleep disturbance in about 20 percent of patients is present.

REFERENCES

Boghen, D., Peyronnard, J.M. (1976). Myoclonus in familial restless legs syndrome. *Archives of Neurology,33,* 368–370.

Coleman, R.M. (1982). Periodic movements in sleep (nocturnal myoclonus) and restless legs syndrome. In C. Guilleminault (Ed.), *Sleeping and waking disorders: Indications and techniques* (pp. 265–295). Menlo Park, CA: Addison-Wesley.

Coleman, R.M., Bliwise, D.L., Sajben, N., de Bruyn, L., Boomkamp, A., Menn, M.E., & Dement, W.C. (1983). Epidemiology of periodic movements during sleep. In C. Guilleminault & E. Lugaresi (Eds.), *Sleep/Wake disorders: Natural history, epidemiology, and long-term evolution* (pp. 217–229). New York: Raven Press.

Coleman, R.M., Miles, L.E., Guilleminault, C., Zarcone, V.P., Van Der Hoed, J., & Dement, W. (1981). Sleep-wake disorders in the elderly: A polysomnographic analysis. *Journal of the American Geriatric Society, 29,* 289–296.

Coleman, R.M., Pollack, C.P., & Weitzman, E.D. (1980). Periodic movements in sleep (nocturnal myoclonus): Relation to sleep disorders. *Annals of Neurology, 8,* 416–421.

Costeff, H., Gadoth, N., Mendelson, L., Harel, S., & Lavie, P. (1987). Fluctuating dystonia responsive to Levodopa. *Archives of Disease in Childhood, 62,* 801–804.

Endo, S., Hashimoto, T., Kawano, N., Hiura, K., Suzue,

J., Kokawa, T., Fukuda, K., & Miyao, M. (1981). Sleep polygraphic studies in patients with involuntary movements. *Brain & Development, 3,* 24.

Fukumoto, M., Mochizuki, N., Takeishi, M., Nomura, Y., & Segawa, M. (1981). Studies of body movements during night sleep in infancy. *Brain & Development, 3,* 37–43.

Gadoth, N., Bechar, M., & Lavie, P. (1981). Juvenile dystonia with marked diurnal variation and distortion of normal sleep cycle. *Excerpta Medica, 584,* 39.

Glaze, D.G., Frost, J.D., & Jankovic, J. (1983). Sleep in Gilles de la Tourette syndrome: Disorder of arousal. *Neurology, 33,* 586–592.

Hashimoto, T., Endo, S., Fukuda, K., Hiura, K., Kawano, N., Suzue, J., Kokawa, T., & Miyao, M. (1981). Increased body movements during sleep in Gilles de la Tourette syndrome. *Brain & Development, 3,* 31–35.

Hashimoto, T., Hiura, K., Suzue, J., Kobayashi, Y., Kawano, N., Fukuda, K., Endo, S., Kokawa, T., & Miyao, M. (1979). Studies on body movements during sleep. *Brain & Development, 1,* 209.

Iwakawa, Y., Ogiso, M., Suzuki, H., Kawano, Y., Koyama, J., & Shimohira, M. (1986). Polygraphic study on age dependent epileptic encephalopathy—relationship between body movements during sleep and prognosis. *Brain & Development, 8,* 433–442.

Jacobsen, J.H., Rosenberg, R.S., Huttenlocher, P.R., & Spire, J.P. (1986). Familial nocturnal cramping. *Sleep, 9,* 54–60.

Montplaisir, J., Godbout, R., Boghen, D., De Champlain, J., Young, S.N., & Lapierre, G. (1985). Familial restless legs with periodic movements in sleep: Electrophysiologic, biochemical and pharmacologic study. *Neurology, 35,* 130–134.

Segawa, M., Hosaka, A., Miyagawa, F., Nomura, Y., & Imai, H. (1976). Hereditary progressive dystonia with marked diurnal fluctuation. *Advances in Neurology, 14,* 215–233.

Segawa, M., Nomura, Y., Hakamada, S., Nagata, E., Okamura, Y., Yamashita, K., & Tanaka, S. (1985). Body movements during sleep—importance of their analysis for neurological examination. *Brain & Development, 7,* 143.

Segawa, M., Nomura, Y., Shinomiya, N., Hosaka, S., & Suzuki, Y. (1981). Hereditary progressive dystonia (HPD) with marked diurnal fluctuation. *Brain & Development, 3,* 223.

Segewa, M., Ohmi, K., Itoh, S., Aoyama, M., & Hayakawa, H. (1971). Childhood basal ganglia disease with remarkable response to L-dopa: Hereditary basal ganglia disease with marked diurnal fluctuation. *Shinryo, 24,* 667–672.

Suzuki, Y., Hosaka, S., Shinomiya, N., Muraki, N., Nomura, Y., Hachimori, K., Iwakawa, Y., Niwa, T., & Segawa, M. (1980). Body movements during sleep: The significance of childhood dystonia. *Brain & Development, 2,* 287.

Wechsler, L.R., Stakes, J.W., Shahani, B.T., & Busis, N.A. (1986). Periodic leg movements of sleep (nocturnal myoclonus): An electrophysiological study. *Annals of Neurology, 19,* 168–173.

Chapter 10

Pathogenesis of Virus-Induced and Autoimmune Nervous System Injuries

Richard J. Kascsak and Henryk M. Wisniewski

ACUTE VIRAL INFECTIONS HAVE LONG been a major cause of human disease resulting in sequela and death. The classical description of these viral infections involves agent replication at the site of entry and subsequent spread to secondary sites of replication. Destruction of cells at these primary and secondary sites leads to disease and a host response designed to limit infection. The response limits infection nonspecifically by phagocytosis and interferon induction and specifically by humoral and cellular immune responses. In patients who survive this acute infectious process, the infectious agent is cleared from the host and the host is protected from subsequent infections by immune surveillance. An understanding of mechanisms of virus spread and transmission, and of effective patient care and treatment combined with the implementation of vaccination programs, have helped to control or eliminate many of these infections. Viruses have, however, evolved a variety of strategies that have permitted them to alter the above scenario and to establish chronic, latent, or persistent infections. These strategies involve various interactions between host, virus, and immune system (Table 1) that allow the virus to remain within the host for extended periods of time.

VIRAL PERSISTENCE

Viral genetic information can remain within the host in an integrated or episomal form. Retroviruses (e.g., HIV-I) use reverse transcriptase to insert their DNA proviral form into the host cell DNA; this integration step is a prerequisite for replication of these RNA viruses (Mahry, 1985). Herpes simplex virus, which resides in sensory ganglion cells, integrates its viral DNA directly into host nuclear DNA (Johnson, 1982). The DNA of other DNA viruses, such as Epstein-Barr virus, or JC agent, a polyoma virus responsible for progressive multifocal leukoencephalopathy, remain latent in a nonintegrated episomal form (Johnson, 1980). Viruses may also use a combination of integration, antigenic variation, and replication in cells of the immune system to establish persistence. Retroviruses such as visna (Narayan, Griffin, & Silverstein, 1977) and equine infectious anemia virus can persist in the presence of neutralizing antibody and can

We thank Drs. R.I. Carp and J. French and also Mrs. H. Brown for their assistance and comments in preparation of this manuscript. We also thank Lucille Olsen for typing the manuscript and Richard Weed and Anne Erickson for preparation of the figures and illustrations.

Table 1. Organism's response to infection

1. The infectious agent is destroyed by the host immune response.
   a. Recovery takes place.
   b. Host is protected from subsequent infection.

2. Agent is not destroyed but remains in a latent or persistent form.
   a. Viral genetic information remains within the host in an integrated or episomal form.
   b. Viral genetic expression is reduced or altered.
   c. Immune surveillance is avoided.

change their antigenic properties (see later discussion).

Persistence may also occur without integration, provided that there is an alteration in normal viral gene expression (Table 1). Mutation (Holland, 1984) and generation of defective interfering particles (Welsh, Lampert, & Oldstone, 1977) have been implicated in such infections. Subacute sclerosing panencephalitis (SSPE) is a chronic degenerative CNS disease resulting from a persistent measles virus (MV) infection of brain cells. Persistence involves the inability to generate complete virions due to a defect in the expression of an MV gene product, the matrix protein (Sheppard, Raine, Bornstein, & Udam, 1985). This protein is thought to mediate the organization of viral structural components at the host plasma membrane, resulting in virion formation. Mutation in the matrix protein gene has led to an unstable product that undergoes rapid posttransitional degradation and renders the virus unable to generate a complete infectious virus. Cells persistently infected with Sendai virus, another paramyxovirus, appear to demonstrate a similar mechanism (Roux & Waldvogel, 1982). Production of infectious virus can also be inhibited by the generation of defective interfering particles (DIPS) (Welsh et al., 1977). These noninfectious particles compete with infectious virus both at extracellular and intracellular levels. The infectious process is slowed and altered, affecting host response to, and interaction with, the virus. Replicating RNA viruses frequently mutate their genomic RNA; these mutant genomes increase the capacity of these agents to survive during persistent infection. Genomic heterogeneity has been established as a characteristic of persistent infection with HIV-I (Hahn et al., 1986). Repeated isolation of virus cells from individual AIDS patients has confirmed the rapid rate of genetic change for these viruses and the parallel evolution of viral variants within each patient. The extreme heterogeneous nature of this virus population has important implications in the design of immune and non-immune defenses against these agents.

VIRUSES AND THE CNS

The site of these latent or persistent infections is often the central nervous system (CNS). Viruses may enter the CNS by a variety of mechanisms (Figure 1). Agents present in the bloodstream can enter by replication in the endothelial cells which line the vessels or may be carried in within lymphocytes and macrophages. They can then infect peripheral neurons at such sites as the neuromuscular junction and can be axonally transported toward the CNS (see Figure 1). Once within the CNS, viruses encounter a differentiated cell population with complex, functionally integrated cell-to-cell interactions. The highly specialized cytoplasmic membranes of the diversified cell population within the CNS allow for great variation in viral receptor sites and in the abilities of cells to support virus replication. Viral tropism to cells within the CNS involves both cell and viral receptor proteins (Figure 2 and Figure 3). Surface receptors on susceptible cells that attach to viruses are considered to be the determinants of both species and cellular virus specificity. Receptors for poliovirus are known to confer susceptibility upon human and some primate cells, while cells from other species lack these receptors and are resistant to infection (Johnson, 1982). The resistance of certain strains of mice to mouse hepatitis virus is a classic example of the importance of the host genotype in determining susceptibility to viral infection (Boyle, Weismuller, & Holmes, 1987). Resistant animals lack a specific virus

VIRAL ENTRY INTO CNS

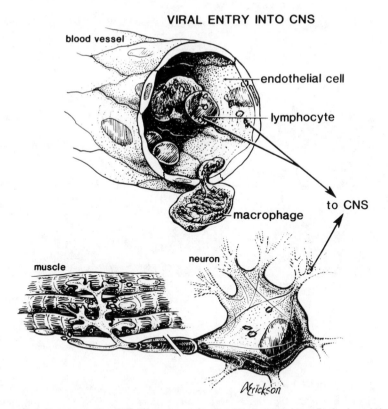

Figure 1.   Mechanism of viral entry into CNS. Viruses may enter from blood vessels by replication in endothelial cells and by being transported within macrophages or lymphocytes. Viruses may also enter at the neuromuscular junction and be axonally transported.

Interaction between Virus and Host

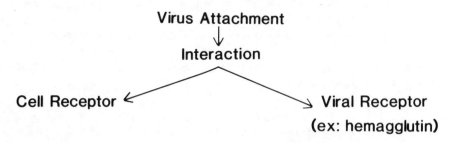

Figure 2.   Interaction between virus and host. Virus attachment is the end result of the interaction of the receptors present on the virus and of the receptors present on the surface of host cells.

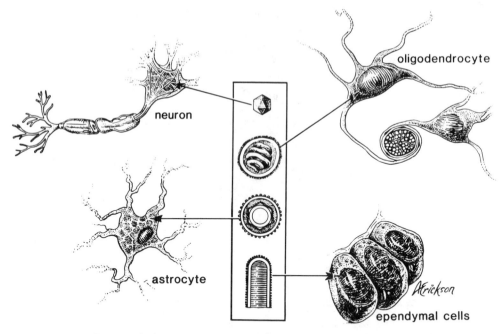

Figure 3. Cell types within the CNS that can be specifically infected by viruses.

receptor which is present on the plasma membrane of target cells from genetically susceptible animals.

Viruses may show a specificity for certain cell types within the CNS (Figure 3). While viruses may replicate in several cell types—either peripherally or within the CNS—their lytic or disruptive effect (i.e., neuropathic effect) can be directed toward one cell type. Polioviruses display a particular affinity for anterior horn motor neurons, while rabies virus normally prefers neurons of the limbic system (Johnson, 1982). Experimental infections with orthomyxo- or paramyxovirus usually involve the selective infection of ependymal cells (Johnson, 1980). The JC virus, the causative agent of progressive multifocal leukoencephalopathy, produces a lytic infection of oligodendrocytes and a nonpermissive infection of astrocytes, while neurons are not susceptible to infection (Johnson, 1982). The Ia antigen receptors, present on a variety of cells within the CNS, have also been implicated as viral receptors. Lactic dehydrogenase-elevating virus appears to have a selective affinity of Ia receptors (Inada & Mims, 1985). Cells undergoing dif-

ferentiation may alter their expression of viral receptors thereby modulating their ability to be infected. The specific affinity of rabies virus to acetylcholine receptors serves to facilitate uptake and transfer of the virus to the CNS, and also to determine neuronal specificity (Lentz & Burrage, 1982). Normally, the CNS is a sheltered environment providing limited access for viruses. However, the peripheral nervous system is exposed to the microenvironment at the neuromuscular junction. Viruses such as rabies can use their affinity for specific neuronal receptors (e.g., neurotransmitter receptors) to circumvent these normal host barriers and gain access to the CNS.

Specific viral proteins have also been implicated in cell and tissue tropism and in altering virulence (Figure 2 and Figure 3). Studies of the neurovirulence and neurotropism of reoviruses indicate that the major surface glycoprotein of the virus, the hemagglutinin, confers this specificity (Fields & Greene, 1982). Intracerebral inoculation of newborn mice with type 3 reovirus leads to the development of an acute encephalitis that is uniformly fatal and is associated with specific viral replication in neurons but not in ependymal cells. In contrast, inoculation of type 1 reovirus causes a nonfatal acute ependymitis without involvement of neurons. Localization in both cases is determined by the hemagglutinin protein encoded by the S1 gene. Substitution of the type 3 S1 gene by the alternative allelic form of type 1 S1 gene attenuates the virus by channeling the virus to less lethal sites. This attenuation also involves an alteration in the host immune response to this protein. The hemagglutinin epitope recognized by neurons also appears to be important both in neutralization of the virus and in the cytotoxic T cell response (Rubin, Werner, Fields, & Greene, 1981). The presence of viral coded hemagglutinin proteins on the surface of a wide spectrum of RNA viruses suggests that this or similar proteins may play a major role in the neurotropism of these viruses.

As discussed earlier, the classic result of CNS virus infection is cell destruction represented by necrosis and inflammatory reaction (Table 2). Persistent or latent infections often do not yield these familiar footprints, and in many instances fail to demonstrate the presence of morphologically identifiable viruses, or even the expression of viral gene products. In these noncytopathic viral infections, infectious agents may alter specific cell functions with no obvious effect on the morphologic integrity of the cell. These alterations can lead to loss of specialized functions, inhibition of mitotic activity, or even premature senescence.

Persistent infection of neuroblastoma cells with lymphocytic choriomeningitis virus

(LCMV) can result in a lower production of choline acetyl transferase and acetylcholine esterase (Oldstone, Holmstoen, & Welsh, 1977). These cellular "luxury" functions may be turned off without observable alteration in vital functions such as growth or synthesis of nucleic acid and protein in these cells. Similar phenomena have been observed in lymphocytes infected with cytomegalovirus or measles virus in which infection aborted specialized functions of IgG production or diminished the ability of these cells to act as cytotoxic effectors (Mahry, 1985). Infection with HIV-I affects the cloning efficiency of persistently infected T cells. *In vivo* studies have confirmed these observations. Persistent infection of the anterior lobe of the pituitary gland with LCMV results in diminished production of growth hormone (Oldstone & Sinha, 1982). Animals display retarded growth and hypoglycemia with no morphologic evidence of cell necrosis or inflammation. These studies suggest that persistent or latent infection can impair differentiated or specialized cell functions, and can thus disrupt homeostasis and interaction of entire cell groups, such as the nervous, immune, and endocrine cell systems.

ANTIBODY MEDIATED ANTIGENIC MODULATION

The immune system is one of the human body's primary defenses against viral infection; its primary function is the removal of these foreign antigens from the host (Table 3). However, many viruses are able to persist in spite of an active immune response directed against them. One mechanism by which this may occur has

Table 2. Consequences of virus replication on brain cells

1. Cytopathic effects
   a. lysis
   b. cell fusion (syncytia formation)
   c. viral inclusions
   d. immune mediated cell destruction
2. Noncytopathic effects
   a. transformation
   b. cellular dysfunction, loss of "luxury functions"
   c. disruption of cell interactions and system to system interactions

Table 3. Immune mediated consequences of virus infection

1. Antibody and cell mediated inflammation and cell lysis
2. Immune-complex formation
3. Antibody induced antigenic modulation
4. Autoimmune responses
   a. molecular mimicry
   b. polyclonal lymphocyte activation
   c. autosensitization

been termed *antibody mediated antigenic modulation*. In one test, the incubation of measles virus-infected cells with specific antibody caused the removal or stripping of measles virus antigens expressed on the surface of these cells (Fujinami & Oldstone, 1984). These infected cells were then protected from immune lysis mediated either through antibody or immune lymphocytes. Removal of the antibody allowed the re-expression of these viral antigens and a renewed susceptibility to immune mediated lysis. It has also been shown that the presence of an antibody can alter the expression of some intracellular viral polypeptides (Fujinami & Oldstone, 1980). Anti-measles virus antibody-induced modulation caused changes in the synthesis and phosphorylation of viral P and M proteins. Antibody-induced modulation has been suggested to play a role in persistent infections of herpes simplex virus and certain retroviruses (Oldstone, Fujinami, & Lampert, 1980). Evidence suggests that this mechanism is also operational *in vivo*. Persistent measles infections of hamsters and monkeys are fostered in the presence of anti-measles antibody (Albrecht, Burnstein, Klutch, Hicks, & Ennis, 1977). Persistent measles infection of mice was established employing a monoclonal antibody to measles hemagglutination (Rammohan, McFarland, & McFarlin, 1982).

The immune system, in addition to aiding the establishment of persistence (as described earlier) can also lead to immune-mediated cell injury and disease (Sissons & Borysiewicz, 1985). Many viruses can establish noncytolytic infections that lead to neither cell damage nor dysfunction. The immune system, in an attempt to clear away these nonpathological agents, generates a virus specific immune response. Components of the immune system act either against viral antigens or against neoantigens expressed on the surface of cells, eventually destroying those cells. Virus-antibody immune complexes can become trapped in certain tissues, notably: brain (choroid plexus), kidney (glomeruli), spleen, lymph nodes, and the circulatory system. This normal process, when pushed to excess due to the continu-

ous expression of virus antigen, leads to dysfunction and disease at these sites. Persistent infection with LCMV or hepatitis B viruses results in immune-complex formation. During persistent infection of mice with lactic dehydrogenase elevating virus, not only are immune complexes formed in the mice, but these complexes remain infectious, thus facilitating virus spread and replication (Notkins, Mahar, Scheele, & Goffman, 1966).

The host immune response to virus infection may also lead to virus-induced autoimmunity. Disease may result from a mechanism known as molecular mimicry (Jahnke, Fisher, & Alvord, 1985). Viral antigens may share amino acid sequences in common with host antigens so that antiviral antibodies may bind to self antigens as well as to those of the virus. The 140 residue polypeptide encoded by one of the early genes of vaccinia virus is related closely to epidermal growth factor and transforming growth factor (Brown, Twardzik, Marquardt, & Todaro, 1985). Computer searches have revealed homologues with decapeptides in two human myelin proteins and a variety of viruses known to infect humans (Jahnke et al., 1985). These viruses include measles, adeno, influenza A, and Epstein-Barr. Postinfectious or postvaccinal demyelinating encephalomyelitis and neuritis may be due to cross reactions evoked by viral epitopes homologous to regions in the target tissue.

VIRUSES AND AUTOIMMUNE RESPONSE

Numerous reports have indicated that certain viruses are capable of inducing polyclonal lymphocyte activation (Wisniewski, Schuller-Levis, Mehta, Madrid, & Lassmann, 1983). The consequence of infection can be the activation of forbidden clones of autoimmune cells. There are a large number of human diseases of undetermined etiology that possess autoimmune components. Diseases such as systemic lupus erythrematosus, insulin dependent diabetes, myasthenia gravis, or multiple sclerosis (Wisniewski et al., 1983) involve autoantibodies directed against various host antigens.

SJL/J mice infected with type 1 reovirus develop an autoimmune polyendocrine disease characterized by mild diabetes and retarded growth (Ondera et al., 1981). Spleen cells from these mice were fused with myeloma cells, and the resulting hybridomas were screened for autoantibodies reactive with normal tissue (Haspel et al., 1983). These autoantibodies were directed against the islets of Langerhans, the anterior pituitary, the gastric mucosa, and several hormones, including growth hormone and insulin. Neonatal infection with murine leukemia virus can lead to the expression of autoreactive T cells (Proffitt, Kozak, dela Motte, & Caulfield, 1985). These studies suggest that viral infection is one of the mechanisms that triggers autoimmune response in a number of diseases.

NEW TECHNOLOGIES FOR DIAGNOSIS: MONOCLONAL ANTIBODIES

A diversity of new technologies is being developed to assist in diagnosing, combating, and treating viral infections (see Table 4 and Table 5). For example, the sensitivity and specificity of monoclonal antibodies and molecular probes are ideally suited for diagnosis of viral infections. Monoclonal antibodies can be designed to react with specific epitopes determined by conformation or primary amino acid sequence. These reagents can be used in conjunction with highly sensitive immunological assays such as RIA, ELISA, or Western Blot. Blood screening is already commonplace for HIV-I, hepatitis, and CMV. As researchers learn more about other infectious conditions such as those caused by unconventional agents,

Table 4. New technologies for prevention and treatment of viral infections

1. Recombinant DNA technology
   a. Sub-unit vaccines (synthetic, expression vector)
   b. Multiple vaccine carrier (ex: vaccinia)
2. Hybridoma technology
   a. Monoclonal antibodies for immune therapy
   b. Anti-idiotypes as surrogate antigens

Table 5. New technologies for diagnosis

1. Antigen screening
   Use of specific polyclonal and monoclonal antibodies (ex: AIDS, unconventional slow virus diseases)
2. *In Situ* hybridization
   Use of nucleic acid probes to identify and locate viral genetic information.

analogous tests may be introduced. *In situ* hybridization technology now possesses the sensitivity to detect in the range of a single copy of even small viral genomes (Haase, 1986). Due to the limited or intermittent expression of viral antigens, this may be, in many instances, the only means of detecting viruses. *In situ* hybridization can define sites of viral persistence or latency and can thereby suggest modes to combat or eliminate the virus.

Monoclonal antibody technology has generated two new strategies to combat infection (Table 4). The first is the production of human hybridomas. Human hybridomas producing antibodies to measles virus have been generated using peripheral lymphocytes from a patient with SSPE (Croce, Linnenback, Hall, Steplewski, & Koprowski, 1980). Potential antibodies can be generated to epitopes associated with any known virus. *In vitro* fusion procedures now allow the human lymphocytes to be sensitized *in vitro* to the viral epitope of choice. These human hybridomas offer an unlimited supply of specific anti-viral reagents that can be given by passive immunization when necessary. The second new strategy has been the use of monoclonal antibodies to generate anti-idiotype molecules that can serve as viral vaccines (Kennedy & Dreesman, 1985). An idiotypic determinant defines the variable (V) region of the antibody molecule directed against a viral determinant. The anti-Id is the internal or mirror image of the Id, thus serving to mimic the viral antigen. The generation of idiotypic antibodies of predefined antigen specificity by immunization with anti-idiotype antibodies has been reported for a number of experimental systems. Neutralizing antibody response in mice against poliovirus type II has been produced using monoclonal anti-idiotypic antibodies (Uytdehagg & Osterhaus, 1985). Monoclonal anti-idiotypic antibodies can mimic the antigenic structure of rabies virus glycoprotein, and can induce antibodies that are capable of neutralizing viral infectivity in tissue culture (Reagen, Wunner, Wiktor, & Koprowski, 1983). As technology advances, human-hybridoma anti-idiotypic antibodies could serve as cost-effective, safe, and highly potent vaccines.

The age of molecular biology has led to the production of genetically engineered vaccines. The most important aspect of this technology is its ability to produce viral antigens without infectious virus or to manufacture the complete complement of viral genetic information. Problems encountered with attenuation, inactivation, or presence of potential oncogenic material are eliminated. The desired fragment of viral genetic information is cloned and inserted into an expression vector system. Antigen is purified from this system and used as immunogen to protect against viral infection. A vaccine produced in this manner to Cro-gD protein of HSV was able to induce antibodies that neutralized the infectivity of both HSV-1 and HSV-2 and to immunoprecipitate viral surface glycoproteins (Watson & Enquist, 1985). The development of vaccinia virus as a eukaryotic cloning vector has fostered an additional alternative to conventional vaccines (Paoletti, Lipinskas, Samsonoff, Mercer, & Panicali, 1984). The large size of the genome of vaccinia virus allows the insertion of cloned fragments of other viruses, thus creating a recombinant vaccinia vaccine. Insertions have been made of DNA fragments that encode for proteins of hepatitis B, herpes simplex, influenza, and vesicular stomatitis virus. Recombinant vaccinia vaccine has yielded neutralizing antibodies and protection from lethal infection. The large capacity of vaccinia virus for foreign DNA raises the possibility of multivalent vaccines containing cloned fragments of many different infectious agents. An individual could be vaccinated against many diverse agents at one time.

CONCLUSION

Despite many advances in the field of neurovirology, virus infections of the CNS continue to be of major concern, especially to researchers in the areas of mental retardation and developmental disabilities. New concepts of persistent, latent, or unconventional infections by a wide range of viruses have placed increased emphasis on virus mediated metabolic and molecular changes within the CNS, and on their roles in neuronal disorganization and dysfunction. Viruses such as cytomegalovirus continue to be the leading cause of damage to the CNS in the fetus and young infant. It has now become apparent that the retrovirus of acquired immunodeficiency syndrome is able to produce neurological dysfunction and developmental delay in young children. The long-term effects of the latent and carrier states of these and other viruses, especially in children, are unknown. In order to understand conditions that lead to viral mediated neurological disease, it is important to gain an understanding of virus-host interactions within the CNS. Susceptibility to and the consequences of virus infection, as discussed earlier, are the end result of many contributing factors. Parameters such as age, genetic background, and immune status of the host, as well as class, genotype, and cell specificity of the infecting virus play important roles in the outcome of infection. Knowledge of the mechanisms of pathogenesis, involving complex interactions among many cell systems and viruses, is necessary to formulate an effective means of treatment and prevention.

Current trends in neurovirology emphasize the use of molecular probes and molecularly engineered reagents for the study, diagnosis, and control of viral infection. Cloned segments of viral genomic information can be used to probe for virus in the absence of replication or expression. Hybridoma technology, examining both the B and the T cell responses to viral infection, has afforded new insights into the involvement of specific virus epitopes in disease, in immune mediated pathogenesis, in the cloning of specific virus genes, and in the sensitive and rapid diagnosis of infection using monoclonal antibodies.

The convergence of recent advances in molecular biology, immunology, and animal virology and pathogenesis marks a new era in understanding the role of virus infection in autoimmune and chronic degenerative neurological diseases. This convergence holds promise for the future control and prevention of these diseases.

REFERENCES

Albrecht, P., Burnstein, T., Klutch, M.J., Hicks, J.T., & Ennis, F.A. (1977). Subacute sclerosing panencephalitis after passive immunization and natural measles infection. *Neurology, 32,* 390–394.

Boyle, J.F., Weismuller, D.G., & Holmes, K.V. (1987). Genetic resistance to mouse hepatitis virus correlates with absence of virus binding activity on target tissues. *Journal of Virology, 61,* 185–189.

Brown, J.P., Twardzik, D.R., Marquardt, H., & Todaro, G.T. (1985). Vaccinia virus encodes a polypeptide homologous to epidermal growth factor and transforming growth factor. *Nature, 313,* 491–492.

Croce, C.M., Linnenback, A., Hall, W., Steplewski, Z., & Koprowski, H. (1980). Production of human hybridomas secreting antibodies to measles virus. *Nature, 288,* 448–491.

Fields, B.N., & Greene, M.I. (1982). Genetic and molecular mechanisms of viral pathogenesis: Implications for prevention and treatment. *Nature, 300,* 19–23.

Fujinami, R.S., & Oldstone, M.B.A. (1980). Alterations in expression of measles virus polypeptide by antibody: Molecular events in antibody induced antigenic modulation. *Journal of Immunology, 125,* 78–85.

Fujinami, R.S., & Oldstone, M.B.A. (1984). Antibody initiates virus persistence: Immune modulation and measles virus infection. In A.L. Notkins & M.B.A. Oldstone (Eds.), *Concepts in viral pathogenesis* (pp. 187–193). New York: Springer-Verlag.

Haase, A.T. (1986). The pathogenesis of slow virus infections: Molecular analyses. *Journal of Infectious Disease, 153,* 441–447.

Hahn, B.H., Shaw, G.M., Taylor, M.E., Redfield, R.R., Markham, P.D., Salahuddin, S.Z., Wong-Staal, F., Gallo, R.G., Parks, E.S., & Parks, W.P. (1986). Genetic variation in HTLV III/LAV over time in patients with AIDS or at risk for AIDS. *Science, 232,* 1548–1553.

Haspel, M.V., Onodera, T., Prabhakar, B.S., Horita, M., Suzuki, H., & Notkius, A.L. (1983). Virus induced autoimmunity: Monoclonal antibodies that react within endocrine tissues. *Science, 218,* 304–306.

Holland, J.J. (1984). Continuum of change in RNA viruses genomes. In A.L. Notkins & M.B.A. Oldstone (Eds.), *Concepts of Viral Pathogenesis* (pp. 137–143). New York: Springer-Verlag.

Inada, T., & Mims, C.A. (1985). Ia antigen and Fc receptors of mouse peritoneal macrophages as determinants of susceptibility to lactic dehydrogenase virus. *Journal of General Virology, 66,* 1469–1477.

Jahnke, U., Fisher, E.H., & Alvord, E.C., Jr. (1985). Sequence homology between certain viral proteins and proteins related to encephalomyelitis and neuritis. *Science, 229,* 282–284.

Johnson, R.T. (1980). Selective vulnerability of neural cells to viral infections. *Brain, 103,* 447–472.

Johnson, R.T. (1982). Selective vulnerability of neural cells to viral infections. In L.P. Roland (Ed.), *Human motor neuron diseases* (pp. 331–335). New York: Raven Press.

Kennedy, R.C., & Dreesman, G.R. (1985). Immunoglobulin idiotypes: Analysis of viral antigen-antibody systems. *Progress in Medical Virology, 31,* 168–182.

Lentz, T.L., & Burrage, T.G. (1982). Is the acetycholine receptor a rabies virus receptor? *Science, 215,* 182–185.

Mahry, B.W.J. (1985). Strategies of virus persistence. *British Medical Bulletin, 41,* 50–56.

Narayan, O., Griffin, D.E., & Silverstein, A.M. (1977). Slow virus infection: Replication and mechanisms of persistence of visna virus in sheep. *Journal of Infectious Disease, 135,* 800–806.

Notkins, A.L., Mahar, S., Scheele, C., & Goffman, J. (1966). Infectious virus antibody complex in blood of chronically infected mice. *Journal of Experimental Medicine, 24,* 81–97.

Oldstone, M.B.A., Fujinami, R.S.F., & Lampert, P.W. (1980). Membrane and cytoplasmic changes in virus infected cells induced by interactions of antiviral antibody with surface viral antigen. *Progress in Medical Virology, 26,* 45–93.

Oldstone, M.B.A., Holmstoen, J., & Welsh R.M., Jr., (1977). Alterations of acetylcholine enzymes in neuroblastoma cells persistently infected with LCMV. *Journal of Cellular Physiology, 91,* 459–472.

Oldstone, M.B.A., & Sinha, Y.N. (1982). Virus induced alterations in homeostasis: Alterations in differentiated functions of infected cells *in vivo. Science, 218,* 1125–1127.

Ondera, T., Toniolo, A., Ray, U.R., Jenson, A.B., Knazel, R.A., & Notkins, A.L. (1981). Virus-induced diabetes mellitus XX. Polyendocrinopathy and autoimmunity. *Journal of Experimental Medicine, 153,* 1457–1473.

Paoletti, E., Lipinskas, B.L., Samsonoff, C., Mercer, S., & Panicali, D. (1984). Construction of live vaccines using genetically engineered poxviruses. *Proceedings of the National Academy of Sciences, 81,* 193–197.

Proffitt, M.R., Kozak, C., dela Motte, C., & Caulfield, M.J. (1985). Immunologic mechanisms in the pathogenesis of virus induced leukemia. *Journal of Immunology, 134,* 4244–4249.

Rammohan, K.W., McFarland, H.F., & McFarlin, D.E. (1982). Subacute sclerosing panencephalitis after passive immunization and maternal measles infection. *Neurology, 32,* 390–394.

Reagen, K.J., Wunner, W.H., Wiktor, T.J., &

Koprowski, H. (1983). Anti-idiotypic antibodies induce neutralizing antibodies to rabies virus glycoprotein. *Journal of Virology, 48,* 660–666.

Roux, L., & Waldvogel, F.A. (1982). Instability of viral M protein in BHK-21 cells persistently infected with Sendai virus. *Cell, 28,* 293–297.

Rubin, D., Werner, H.L., Fields, B.N., & Greene, M.I. (1981). Immunologic tolerance after oral administration of reovirus: Requirement for two gene products for tolerance induction. *Journal of Immunology, 127,* 1697–1701.

Sheppard, R.D., Raine, C.S., Bornstein, M.B., & Udem, S.A. (1985). Measles virus matrix protein synthesized in a subacute sclerosing panencephalitis cell line. *Science, 228,* 1219–1221.

Sissons, J.G.P., & Borysiewicz, L.K. (1985). Viral immunopathology. *British Medical Bulletin, 41,* 34–40.

Uytdehagg, F.G., & Osterhaus, A.D. (1985). Induction of neutralizing antibody in mice against poliovirus type 11 with monoclonal anti-idiotypic antibody. *Journal of Immunology, 134,* 1225–1229.

Watson, R.J., & Enquist, L.W. (1985). Genetically engineered herpes simplex virus vaccines. *Progress in Medical Virology, 31,* 84–108.

Welsh, R.M., Lampert, P.W., & Oldstone, M.B.A. (1977). Prevention of virus induced cerebellar disease by defective interfering LCMV. *Journal of Infectious Disease, 136,* 391–398.

Wisniewski, H.M., Schuller-Levis, G.B., Mehta, P.D., Madrid, R.E., & Lassmann, H. (1983). Pathogenetic aspects of multiple sclerosis and experimental models of inflammatory demyelination. *Concepts in Immunopathology, 2,* 128–150.

Chapter 11

Immune Determinants
of Myelinopathies

Oded Abramsky and Israel Steiner

DESTRUCTION OF MYELIN CONSTITUTES the hallmark of several acute inflammatory nervous system conditions. The clinical, histopathological, and immunological features of these demyelinating disorders suggest that an immune mediated mechanism may be responsible in part for their pathogenesis (Leibowitz & Hughes, 1983; Steiner & Abramsky, 1985; Waksman, Yonezawa, & Lassman, 1983). The central nervous system (CNS) syndromes involving myelin destruction are: acute disseminated encephalomyelitis (ADE), acute hemorrhagic leukoencephalitis (AHL), acute transverse myelitis (ATM), and optic neuritis. In the peripheral nervous system (PNS), the diseases are: Guillain-Barre syndrome (GBS, acute inflammatory demyelinating neuropathy), brachial and lumbo-sacral plexitis, and mononueritis (such as idiopathic facial paralysis, i.e., Bell's palsy). Two experimental animal models serve to investigate the autoimmune pathogenesis of the human disorders; experimental allergic encephalomyelitis (EAE) is a model for CNS demyelination, and experimental allergic neuritis (EAN) is its PNS counterpart.

EXPERIMENTAL ALLERGIC ENCEPHALOMYELITIS (EAE)

Experimental allergic encephalomyelitis is an acute demyelinating disease induced by immunizing animals with whole nervous tissue with myelin or myelin components (Paterson, 1980). In 1885, Louis Pasteur introduced the first vaccine against rabies. The vaccine was prepared from the dried and preserved brain of an infected rabbit; treatment involved repeated injections over a period of weeks and months. It soon became apparent that this was a hazardous procedure, and many of the patients were protected from rabies only to develop severe neurological disease as a result of the treatment (Arnason, 1987). Similarly, Rivers, Sprunt, and Berry (1933) showed that repeated injections of aqueous solutions of rabbit brain tissue into monkeys produced a diffuse encephalomyelitis. The introduction of complete Freund's adjuvant (CFA) greatly facilitated the study of this model. It became possible to induce EAE with regularity in a wide range of animals, and it seems that there are certain animal species and strains that are highly susceptible to disease induction, while others are resistant. Susceptibility to EAE has recently been shown to be under the control of immune response genes closely linked to the major histocompatibility locus (Hughes, 1984). Encephalitogenic factors are necessary to produce the inflammatory demyelinating lesions in EAE. Most of them are antigens that are present in the brain and spinal cord within the oligodendrocyte-myelin unit. A brief consideration of the structure and antigenic composition of CNS myelin is therefore needed (Hashim, 1980; Leibowitz & Hughes, 1983).

In the CNS, myelin is formed and maintained by oligodendrocytes. The oligodendrocytes may be regarded as extensions of myelin, a plasma membrane that expands and flattens into a broad sheet to envelop the axons in a tightly packed spiral. Like other biological membranes, myelin is composed mainly of protein and lipids. The main proteins and glycolipids of the myelin are all potentially antigenic. The main protein antigens are: proteolipid protein, myelin basic protein (MBP), the Wollfgram fraction, and myelin associated glycoprotein (MAG) (which may also be of importance in several PNS conditions). The glycolipids are incomplete antigens (haptens) which are capable of eliciting an immune response when combined with a protein carrier; they include galactocerebroside (GalC), sulphatide, and GM1 and GM4 gangliosides. When myelin is injected into experimental animals to induce EAE, antibodies are produced that are directed mainly against GalC. The antibodies are capable of causing demyelination *in vitro* if they are added to cultures of CNS or PNS tissues (Bornstein & Appel, 1961). *In vivo*, however, GalC is not encephalitogenic, but it may play a role in peripheral demyelinating disorders. The myelin component responsible for EAE induction is MBP. Its physiochemical properties have been well described, and the structure and amino acid sequence in several species have been determined (Hashim, 1980). MBP constitutes 30%–40% of myelin proteins, is made of about 170 amino acids, and has a molecular weight of 18,000. The essential determinant for EAE production on the MBP is different for each species.

Clinically and histopathologically, EAE shares several common features with ADE, AHL, and ATM. Nine to twenty days following immunization, experimental animals develop a variety of neurological signs, including weakness and paralysis of the hind limbs, incontinence, loss of righting reflexes, and torticolis (Simmons, Barnard, Kerlero de Rosbo, & Carnegie, 1984). Histologically, the lesions are confined to the CNS and consist of perivascular accumulation of mononuclear cells in the brain, spinal cord, and meninges. This is accompanied by vascular leak consisting of fibrin, C3, immunoglobulins, albumin, and other serum proteins. Demyelination, varying

in degree from minimum to extensive myelin destruction, is present. In these instances, the myelin sheath is removed and phagocytosed, and myelin debris are degraded (Alvord, 1970).

The development of EAE seems to depend largely upon T cells. It can be transferred by T lymphocytes (Paterson, 1960), but not by serum, and it can be produced in bursectomized chickens, but not in thymectomized chickens (Blaw, Cooper, & Good, 1967; Jankovic & Isvaneski, 1963). Antibodies to MBP and myelin lipids are produced; sera obtained from EAE are able to destroy myelin in tissue cultures (Jankovic & Isvaneski, 1963). The humoral arm in EAE, however, seems of lesser importance, if it is important at all, in the pathogenesis of the disease. EAE is presently considered to be a cell mediated disease.

The analogy between postvaccine and postinfectious encephalomyelitis and EAE has already been mentioned. Several studies have demonstrated cell mediated immune response to MBP in patients with ADE and ATM (Abramsky & Teitelbaum, 1977; Lisak & Zwiman, 1977). If this signifies the basic immune mechanism responsible for these conditions (in addition to the clinical and pathological similarities), then they may be the human counterpart of EAE. EAE can be treated by administering immunosuppressive agents and by employing specific measures (such as desensitization with synthetic copolimers resembling MBP). Similarly, immunosuppressive agents seem to be beneficial in limiting the spread of the inflammatory process in ADE, AHL, and ATM, in promoting clinical remission, and in reducing sequelae (Walton, 1985).

EXPERIMENTAL ALLERGIC NEURITIS (EAN)

Experimental allergic neuritis was first described in 1955 by Waksman and Adams, who produced a monophasic inflammatory disease of peripheral nerves in animals by immunizing them with peripheral nerve tissues emulsified in CFA. Clinically, EAN is an acute disease appearing 2 weeks following immunization and consisting of ataxia and ascending limb weakness. In nonfatal cases, symptomatology progression is usually arrested after a week and is followed by gradual recovery. The cerebrospinal fluid of the ill animals contains elevated protein levels and evinces little or no cellular response. This clinical picture resembles the human GBS in many respects (Arnason, 1984). Similarly, the pathologic appearance is that of lymphocytic and macrophagic inflammatory reaction with segmental demyelination; the sequence of histologic events in the peripheral nerve is identical to that of GBS (Prineas, 1981; Waksman & Adams, 1955).

The components of the peripheral nerve capable of inducing EAN were isolated, purified, and characterized. Three proteins account for approximately 70% of PNS myelin (Abramsky et al., 1975): 1) P0—of 28,000 molecular weight, is restricted to the PNS, and is immunogenic but does not have neuritogenic properties, 2) P1—(also denoted as P_2 or P_2L) (Abramsky, Teitelbaum, & Arnon, 1977) is probably identical to MBP, and 3) P2—(also P_1L or P_1) (Brostoff, Levit, & Powers, 1977), of a molecular weight of about 15,000, is a specific PNS neuritogenic protein capable of producing EAN. Adjuvants are necessary for rapid and constant production of EAN. The disease induced by injection of P2 is usually rather mild when compared to the EAN provoked by whole peripheral nerve myelin. It was speculated, therefore, that production of the allergic response may be initiated by the neuritogenic protein but requires reaction against antigenic determinants of other PNS components. Sufficient information is available to indicate that the neuritogenic determinant of P2 (like MBP and EAE) varies from one species to another. Moreover, a peptide containing amino acids 1 to 20 from the amino terminal of P2 is neuritogenic in rabbits and encephalitogenic in guinea pigs (Brostoff et al., 1977; Brostoff, Powers, & Weiss, 1980). EAN induced by bovine P2 was enhanced when combined with gangliosides from the same source, indicating that they may serve as natural adjuvants in the production of EAN (Nagai, Uchida, Takeda, & Ikuta, 1978). It is generally accepted that the most important, or perhaps the only, patho-

genetic mechanism in EAN is one of cell mediated immunity. Evidence includes *in vivo* sensitivity of peripheral blood lymphocytes to crude myelin extracts in EAN animals, destruction of myelin in tissue cultures by lymphocytes obtained from these animals, and chronology of events in the damaged nerve. In addition, it is possible to transfer EAN either by lymphocytes immunized with peripheral nerve myelin antigen or by lymphocytes taken from animals with EAN and with P2 reactive T cell lines (Abramsky & Teitelbaum, 1977; Astrom & Waksman, 1962; Rostami, Burns, Brown, et al., 1983). The neuritogenic protein P2 may also be an antigen important in GBS pathogenesis. For example, it is capable of inducing proliferation of lymphocytes obtained from peripheral blood of patients (Abramsky, Webb, Teitelbaum, & Arnon, 1975); these lymphocytes are also capable of attacking and destroying myelin *in vitro* (Arnason, 1970).

Some work on the humoral arm of the immune response in EAN and GBS has been reported. Of note is the experimental model reported by Saida and colleagues (Saida, Saida, Brown, et al., 1978; Saida, Saida, Silberberg, et al., 1978). When serum obtained from animals with peripheral nerve induced EAN was injected directly into peripheral nerves of experimental animals *in vivo*, it caused acute demyelination of the nerve. The antigen GalC may play an important role in this model. Several studies suggested that anti-GalC antibodies are responsible for the tissue damage in this model (Lisak, Saida, Kennedy, et al., 1980), but their relevance to human GBS remains an open question.

CONCLUSION

In conclusion, it appears that several acute inflammatory demyelinating disorders may have autoimmune pathogenesis. Further understanding of the relevant experimental models, as well as exploration of possible immune mechanisms acting in human disorders, may enable researchers to elucidate the autoantigen of this condition, as well as its etiology and pathogenesis.

REFERENCES

Abramsky, O., & Teitelbaum, D. (1977). The autoimmune features of acute transverse myelopathy. *Annals of Neurology, 2,* 36–40.

Abramsky, O., Teitelbaum, D. & Arnon, R. (1977). Experimental allergic neuritis induced by a basic neuritogenic protein (P_1L) of human peripheral origin. *European Neurology, 7,* 214–217.

Abramsky, O., Teitelbaum, D., Webb, C., & Arnon, R. (1975). Neuritogenic and encephalitogenic properties of the peripheral nerve basic proteins. *Journal of Neuropathology and Experimental Neurology, 34,* 36–45.

Abramsky, O., Webb, C., Teitelbaum, D., & Arnon, R. (1975). Cell mediated immunity to neural antigens in idiopathic polyneuritis and myeloradiculitis. *Neurology, 25,* 1154–1159.

Alvord, E.C. (1970). Acute disseminated encephalomyelitis and "allergic" neuroencephalopathies. In P.I. Vinken & G.W. Bruyn (Eds.), *Handbook of clinical neurology* (Vol. 9, pp. 500–571).

Arnason, B.G.W. (1970). The inflammatory lesion in idiopathic polyneuritis compared to that in experimental allergic neuritis. In Masson & Cie (Eds.), *Proceedings of the sixth international congress of neuropathologists,* Paris.

Arnason, B.G.W. (1984). Acute inflammatory demyelinating polyradiculineuropathy. In P.J. Dyck, P.K. Thomas, E.H. Lambert, & R. Bunge (Eds.), *Peripheral neuropathy* (2nd ed., pp. 2050–2100). Philadelphia: W.B. Saunders.

Arnason, B.G.W. (1987). Neuroimmunology. *New England Journal of Medicine, 316,* 406–408.

Astrom, K.E., & Waksman, B.H. (1962). The passive transfer of experimental allergic encephalomyelitis and neuritis with living lymphoid cells. *Journal of Pathology and Bacteriology, 83,* 89–106.

Blaw, M.E., Cooper, M.D., & Good, R.A. (1967). Experimental allergic encephalomyelitis in agammaglobulinic chickens. *Science, 158,* 1198–1200.

Bornstein, M.B., & Appel, S.H. (1961). The application of tissue cultures to the study of experimental allergic encephalomyelitis. One pattern of demyelination. *Journal of Neuropathology and Experimental Neurology, 20,* 141–160.

Brostoff, S.W., Levit, S., & Powers, J.M. (1977). Induction of experimental allergic neuritis with a peptide from myelin P_2 basic protein. *Nature, 268,* 752–753.

Brostoff, W.S., Powers, J.M., Weiss, M.J. (1980). Allergic encephalomyelitis induced in guinea pigs by a peptide from the NH_2-terminus of bovine P_2 protein. *Nature, 285,* 103–104.

Hashim, G.A. (Ed.). (1980). *Myelin: Chemistry and biology.* New York: Alan R. Liss.

Hughes, R.A.C. (1984). Immunological aspects of multiple sclerosis. In M.J.G. Harrison (Ed.), *Contemporary neurology* (pp. 282–292). London: Butterworth.

Jankovic, B.D.. & Isvaneski, M. (1963). Experimental allergic encephalomyelitis in thymectomized, bursectomized and normal chickens. *International Archives of Allergy and Applied Immunology, 23,* 188–206.

Leibowitz, S., & Hughes, R.A.C. (1983). *Immunology of the nervous system.* London: Edward Arnold.

Lisak, R.P., Saida, T., & Kennedy, P.G.E., et al. (1980). EAE, EAN and galactocerebroside sera bind to oligodendrocytes and Schwann cells. *Journal of the Neurological Sciences, 48,* 287–296.

Lisak, R.P., & Zwiman, B. (1977). In vitro cell-mediated immunity of cerebrospinal fluid lymphocytes to myelin basic protein in primary demyelinating diseases. *New England Journal of Medicine, 297,* 850–853.

Nagai, Y., Uchida, T., Takeda, S., & Ikuta, F. (1978). Restoration of activity for induction of experimental allergic peripheral neuritis by a combination of myelin basic protein P_2 and gangliosides from peripheral nerve. *Neuroscience Letter, 8,* 247–254.

Paterson, P.Y. (1960). Transfer of allergic encephalomyelitis in rats by means of lymph node cells. *Journal of Experimental Medicine, 11,* 119–136.

Paterson, P.Y. (1980). The immunopathology of experimental allergic encephalomyelitis. In A.H. Davison & M.L. Cuzner (Eds.), *The suppression of experimental allergic encephalomyelitis and multiple sclerosis* (pp. 11–30). London: Academic Press.

Prineas, J.W. (1981). Pathology of the Guillain-Barre syndrome. *Annals of Neurology, 9* (suppl), 6–19.

Rivers, T.M., Sprunt, D.H., & Berry, G.P. (1933). Observations on attempts to produce acute disseminated encephalomyelitis in monkeys. *Journal of Experimental Medicine, 58,* 39–54.

Rostami, A., Burns, J.B., Brown, M.J., et al. (1983). Transfer of experimental allergic neuritis with P_2 reactive T cells. *Annals of Neurology, 14,* 108.

Saida, K., Saida, T., Brown, M.J., et al. (1978). Antiserum-mediated demyelination in vivo—a sequential study using intraneural injection of experimental neuritis serum. *Laboratory Investigation, 39,* 449–462.

Saida, T., Saida, K., Silberberg, D.H., et al. (1978). Transfer of demyelination with experimental allergic neuritis serum by intraneural injection. *Nature, 272,* 639–641.

Simmons, R.D., Barnard, C.C.A., Kerlero de Rosbo, N., & Carnegie, P.R. (1984). Criteria for an adequate explanation of typical clinical signs of EAE in rodents. In E.C. Alvord, M.W. Kies, & A.J. Suckling (Eds.), *Experimental allergic encephalomyelitis. A useful model for multiple sclerosis* (pp. 23–29). New York: Alan R. Liss.

Steiner, I., & Abramsky, O. (1985). Immunology of Guillain-Barre syndrome. *Springer Seminars in Immunopathology, 8,* 165–176.

Waksman, B.H., & Adams, R.D. (1955). Allergic neuritis: Experimental disease of rabbits induced by peripheral nervous tissue and adjuvants. *Journal of Experimental Medicine, 102,* 213–235.

Waksman, B.H., Yonezawa, T., Lassmann, H. (Eds.). (1983). Inflammation and demyelination in the central nervous system. *Acta Neuropathologica* (Suppl IX), 1–91.

Walton, J. (1985). *Brain's diseases of the nervous system* (9th ed.). Oxford: Oxford University Press.

Chapter 12

Cellular Mechanisms of Bilirubin Encephalopathy in the Newborn

Leo Stern and William J. Cashore

IN DEGREE OF IMPORTANCE, THE PREVA-lence of visible jaundice in the newborn constitutes a major clinical manifestation if one considers that approximately 30% of all newborn infants will have at least the appearance of icterus. It is, however, the potential neurotoxicity of these bilirubin elevations (most particularly in the central nervous system) that highlights its presence as well as justifies the means taken to attempt to control it.

The ability of bilirubin to reach the central nervous system is conditioned by factors that relate to the binding and separation of bilirubin to albumin in the plasma, the capacity for integrity of the vascular tight endothelial junctions, and the amount and distribution of cerebral blood flow. Once transported into the CNS cell the effects of the bilirubin on the cell's metabolic activity and the "lysosomal like" capacity for removal of any sequestered amounts will determine the final nature and degree of toxicity in both full term and premature infants.

MEASUREMENT OF BILIRUBIN

In 1916, Van Den Bergh and Muller observed that serum from patients with hemolytic jaundice did not react promptly with diazotized sulfanilic acid except in the presence of alcohol, whereas serum from patients with obstructive jaundice reacted immediately in aqueous solution, thus establishing the concept of "direct" and "indirect" reacting bilirubin (Van Den

Bergh & Muller, 1916). The methods currently used to record these two fractions are basically modifications of the method employed by Malloy and Evelyn (1937), which determines "direct" and "total" bilirubin, with the subtraction product designated as the "indirect" acting fraction. The "indirect" fraction represents unconjugated bilirubin, while the "direct" acting fraction is conjugated bilirubin diglucuronide.

The differences in toxicity potential of the two fractions with respect to the brain (e.g., the production of kernicterus) have classically been considered to be a function of their different physical properties. Bilirubin itself (indirect acting, unconjugated) is insoluble in water but is relatively more soluble in a lipid medium, thereby allegedly accounting for its entry into the lipid rich central nervous system. In contrast, glucuronidated bilirubin (direct acting, conjugated) is soluble in aqueous solution and is relatively insoluble in lipids. Thus, the elevation of the indirect fraction represents a potential hazard for kernicterus while even extreme elevations of the direct acting fraction (plasma is essentially an aqueous solution) are not considered hazardous.

KERNICTERUS

The toxicity of bilirubin to the central nervous system was originally described by Schmorl in 1903. The term kernicterus is a pathologic one and refers to the finding of yellow staining of brain nuclei at autopsy. The term bilirubin encephalopathy was proposed by Zetterstrom and Ernstner in 1956 as more appropriately reflective of a gradual and progressive degree of impairment, a view that would explain the occurrence of high tone deafness in premature infants as a result of the presence of bilirubin deposition at its earliest site in the auditory nucleus of the eighth cranial nerve. They proposed that the mechanism of action was an uncoupling of oxidative phosphorylation in brain mitochondria. This suggestion was refuted a decade later (Diamond & Schmid, 1967) by the use of radioactive tracer studies.

The factors that promote the occurrence of CNS toxicity of bilirubin (notably at lower levels of bilirubin in premature infants) are clinically associated with acidosis, hypothermia, hypoxia, and hypercapnea (Stern & Doray, 1968), but the precise mechanisms by which the injury is produced are still a matter of speculation.

THE BONDING OF
BILIRUBIN TO ALBUMIN

Unconjugated bilirubin is bound to albumin in plasma. The resultant complex is nondiffusible, and the binding to albumin thus has the function both of transporting bilirubin to the liver and of preventing the egress of bilirubin from serum into tissues. The amount of "free" and "bound" bilirubin at any given time is a function of the quantitative amounts of both bilirubin and albumin in the circulation, and of the albumin's capacity to bind to the bilirubin present.

This binding process is pH dependent, and the complex tends towards dissociation with acidosis. In addition to this dissociation effect on bilirubin albumin binding (Odell, 1959), acidosis also causes an increased affinity for bilirubin by brain mitochondria (Odell, 1966). Additionally, the presence of one or more anions, which may compete with bilirubin for common binding sites on the albumin molecule, may give rise to large amounts of "free" unconjugated bilirubin, despite the presence of sufficient albumin to theoretically bind all the

bilirubin in the system. By displacing bilirubin from its binding sites, these anions will promote the development of kernicterus at relatively low levels of serum bilirubin. Since Silverman (Silverman, Anderson, Blanc, & Crozier, 1956) reported that the administration of sulfisoxazole to premature infants provoked the development of kernicterus at low levels of serum bilirubin, others have identified a number of endogenous and exogenous substances that compete with bilirubin for one or more shared or proximate albumin binding sites. Hematin present in increased amounts in hemolytic situations may explain the higher risk of kernicterus in hemolytic, as compared to nonhemolytic, hyperbilirubinemias. The nonesterified (free) fatty acids are elevated in plasma under conditions of both hypothermia and hypoglycemia. In addition to sulfisoxazole, salicylates and caffeine sodium benzoate will displace bilirubin from its albumin binding sites. Other drugs, singly or in combination, may also share this capacity (Brodersen, Friis-Hansen, & Stern, 1983; Schiff, Chan, & Stern, 1971). Not only should administration of these agents to the newborn who is jaundiced be avoided, but they should also be withheld from a nursing mother who can transmit them to the newborn in her milk.

ENTRY INTO THE
CENTRAL NERVOUS SYSTEM

Whether or not there is a blood-brain "barrier" in other than an anatomical sense governing egress from the vascular tree and entry into the CNS cell is a question about which there is ongoing debate and controversy. If molecular size is a determinant of such egress, what factors may increase or protect against its occurrence? In this regard, there is evidence that the vascular tight endothelial junctions may be opened and made more porous and permeable by hypertonicity (e.g., increase in serum osmolality [Bratlid, Cashore, & Oh, 1983; Rapoport, Fredericks, Ohno, et al., 1980]). They may also be made more permeable by hypoxia, although sufficiently severe or prolonged hypoxia would ultimately result in loss of vascular integrity and nonspecific leakage from the entire vascular tree. Although it has been argued that the vessels of the immature infant should be less resistant to such adverse stimuli, there is little objective evidence to support a maturational protective effect. Given the ability to achieve sufficient elevated unconjugated bilirubin levels, cases of proven kernicterus have been shown to occur beyond the immediate newborn period and well into early childhood and young adult life (Crigler & Najjar, 1952; Naiman & Kosoy, 1964; Wolkoff, Chowdhury, Gartner, et al., 1979). Vascular factors may in addition influence the degree and locale of distribution of bilirubin pigment. Thus, CO_2, a potent cerebral vasodilator, has been shown experimentally to influence the deposition and distribution of bilirubin in the brain (Bratlid, Cashore, & Oh, 1984; Burgess et al., 1985).

CELLULAR EFFECTS OF BILIRUBIN

Studies in our department on isolated fat cell preparations have shown that the relatively lipid soluble unconjugated bilirubin has only limited ability to influence metabolic reactions within the cell itself. Almost paradoxically, the addition of bilirubin appears to enhance the rate of glucose oxidation within the cell, an effect similar to that produced by the addition of insulin. However, incubation of lipid cell membranes with bilirubin produced a striking reduction in the content of adenylate cyclase in the membranes, presumably thereby compromising membrane integrity (Sheppard, Moreno, Cashore, & Fain, 1979). Aggregation at the cell periphery of the water insoluble bilirubin could also produce cellular asphyxia from prevention of entry and/or egress of substances in either direction (Brodersen, 1986). Other studies have demonstrated the ability of bilirubin to interfere with the incorporation of ^3_H thymidine in neural cell lines, thus suggest-

ing an interference with protein synthesis within the cell itself (Schiff, Chan, & Poznansky, 1985). This effect appears to be protected against by the addition of albumin. This suggests that albumin may, in addition to its capacity to bind the bilirubin in plasma (and thus prevent its entry into the central nervous system) exert a protective effect within the cell itself. There is also evidence to suggest that the presence or absence of potentially bioenergetic or physiochemical modifying substances (e.g., carbohydrates or glycolipids) may affect the nature and degree of bilirubin toxicity to the cell (Sugita, Takayushi, Fuse, & Nakagima, 1986).

Evidence has now been obtained for an inhibitory neurotransmitter effect of bilirubin on CNS tissue with resultant effects on synaptosomes and changes in the concentrations of neurotransmitter substances (e.g., Synapsin I and II, Hansen, Walass, Bratlid, & Greengard, 1986). This would place a functional injury focus at the integrative, static perceptual, and motor levels.

Brain and other tissues contain an enzyme system, bilirubin oxidase (Brodersen & Bartels, 1969), capable of transforming considerable amounts of bilirubin into soluble colorless and presumably non-toxic products. The enzymatic process has not been studied in detail, but it would appear to be adversely affected by changes in pH and pO_2 levels. As a "cleanup" and detoxification mechanism, it is likely that such endogenous removal of any accumulated bilirubin may play a critical role in maintaining the stability of the CNS on bilirubin exposure. Such a function would also explain the clinically valid observation that prior CNS injury secondary to asphyxia, hypoxemia, intracranial hemorrhage, and/or sepsis and meningocephalitis may increase the risk for kernicterus through destruction or inactivation of the enzymatic protective removal mechanism.

REFERENCES

Bratlid, D., Cashore, W.J., & Oh, W. (1983). Effect of serum hyperosmolality on opening of the blood-brain barrier for bilirubin in rat brain. *Pediatrics, 71,* 909–912.

Bratlid, D., Cashore, W.J., & Oh, W. (1984). Effect of acidosis on bilirubin deposition in rat brain. *Pediatrics, 73,* 431–434.

Brodersen, R. (1986). Aqueous solubility, albumin binding and tissue distribution of bilirubin. In J.E. Ostrow, (Ed.), *Bile pigments and jaundice* (pp. 157–181). New York: Marcel Dekker.

Brodersen, R., & Bartels, P. (1969). Enzymatic oxidation of bilirubin. *European Journal of Biochemistry, 10,* 468–473.

Brodersen, R., Friis-Hansen, B., & Stern, L. (1983). Drug induced displacement of bilirubin from albumin in the newborn. *Developmental Pharmacology and Theraputics, 6,* 217.

Burgess, G.H., Oh, W., Bratlid, D., Brubakk, A.M., Cashore, W.J., & Stonestreet, B.S. (1985). The effects of brain blood flow on brain bilirubin deposition in newborn piglets. *Pediatric Research, 19,* 691–696.

Crigler, J.R., Jr., & Najjar, V.A. (1952). Congenital familiar non-hemolytic jaundice with kernicterus. *Pediatrics, 10,* 169–180.

Diamond, I., & Schmid, R. (1967). Oxidative phosphorylation in experimental bilirubin encephalopathy. *Science, 155,* 1288.

Hansen, T.W.R., Walass, S.I., Bratlid, D., & Greengard, P. (1986). Effects of bilirubin on phosphorylation of Synapsin I. *Pediatric Research, 20,* 462A.

Malloy, H.T., & Evelyn, K.A. (1937). Determination of Bilirubin with the Photoelectric Colormeter. *Journal of Biological Chemistry, 119,* 481.

Naiman, J.L., & Kosoy, M.H. (1964). Red cell glucose-6-phosphate dehydrogenase deficiency, a newly recognized cause of neonatal jaundice and kernicterus in Canada. *Canadian Medical Association Journal, 91,* 1243–1249.

Odell, G.B. (1959). The dissociation of bilirubin from albumin and its clinical significance. *Journal of Pediatrics, 55,* 268.

Odell, G.B. (1966). The distribution of bilirubin between albumin and mitochondria. *Journal of Pediatrics, 68,* 164.

Rapoport, S.I., Fredericks, W.R., Ohno, K., et al. (1980). Quantitative aspects of reversible opening of the blood-brain barrier. *American Journal of Physiology, 238,* R421–431.

Schiff, D., Chan, G., & Poznansky, M.J. (1985). Bilirubin toxicity in neural cell lines N-115 and NB-10A. *Pediatric Research, 19,* 908–911.

Schiff, D., Chan, G., & Stern, L. (1971). Fixed drug combinations and the binding of bilirubin to albumin. *Pediatrics, 48,* 139.

Schmorl, G. (1903). Zur kentas des icterus neonatorum. *Verhandlungen Der Deutschen Gesellschaft Fur Pathologie, 6,* 109.

Sheppard, R.E., Moreno, F.J., Cashore, W.J. & Fain, J.N. (1979). Effects of bilirubin on fat cell metabolism and lipolysis. *American Journal of Physiology, 237,* 504–508.

Silverman, W.A., Anderson, D.H., Blanc, W.A., & Crozier, D.N., (1956). A difference in mortality rate and incidence of kernicterus in premature infants allotted to two prophylatic antibacterial regimens. *Pediatrics, 18,* 614.

Stern, L., & Doray, B. (1968). *Hypothermia, acidosis and kernicterus in small premature infants* (p. 512). Proceedings of the Twelfth International Congress of Pediatrics, Mexico.

Sugita, K., Takayushi, S., Fuse, A., & Nakagima, H. (1986). The effect of glycolipids and carbohydrates on bilirubin cylotoxicity in vitro. *Biology of the Neonate, 49,* 255–260.

Van Den Bergh, A.A.H., & Muller, P. (1916). Uber eine direkte und eine indirekte diazoreaktionen auf bilirubin. *Biochemische Zeitschrift, 77,* 90.

Wolkoff, A.W., Chowdhury, J.R., Gartner, L.M., et al. (1979). Crigler Najjar syndrome (Type I) in an adult male. *Gastroenterology, 76,* 840–848.

Zetterstrom, R., & Ernstner, L. (1956). Bilirubin, an uncoupler of oxidative phosphorylation in isolated mitochondria. *Nature, 178,* 1335.

Chapter 13

Does Vitamin D Have a Role in the Developing Brain?

Shaul Harel, Dalia Somjen, Yehoshua Earon,
Abraham Tomer, Alvin M. Kaye,
Yosef Weisman, and Itschak Binderman

VITAMIN D IS A PROHORMONE FOR THE more polar metabolites, $1\alpha,25$-dihydroxyvitamin D_3 ($1,25(OH)_2D_3$) and $24,25$-dihydroxyvitamin D_3 ($24,25(OH)_2D_3$), which are the principal mediators of the biological activities originally ascribed to the parent compound. The metabolite involved principally in calcium metabolism is $1,25(OH)_2D_3$, which acts on a range of adult organs containing specific receptors (Norman, Roth, & Orci, 1982). The more recently recognized vitamin D metabolite $24,25(OH)_2D_3$, which is not implicated in calcium transport, is involved in embryonic development of endochondral bone (Corvol, Dumontier, Garabedian, & Rapaport, 1978; Endo, Kiyoki, Kawashima, Nasuchi, & Hashimoto, 1980; Malluche et al., 1980; Ornoy, Goodwin, Wolff, & Edelstein, 1978). Recently, the authors showed that an increase in activity of the brain type isoenzyme of creatine kinase (CKBB, ATP: creatine phosphotransferase, EC 2.7.3.2.) is induced in the rat kidney by the two vitamin D metabolites. This occurs at different stages of postnatal development, correlated with changes in the concentrations of $1,25(OH)_2D_3$ receptors or $24,25(OH)_2D_3$ binding proteins (Somjen et al., 1986). Here we report a parallel effect of vitamin D metabolites on the developing rabbit brain. The cerebellum, but not the cerebrum, is sequentially responsive to the two metabolites during different times in the perinatal period, suggesting a more general role for $24,25(OH)_2D_3$ in normal brain development.

Recent investigations have shown a wide tissue distribution of $1,25(OH)_2D_3$ receptors and $1,25(OH)_2D_3$ dependent calcium binding proteins. These findings suggest a function of the sterol in nonclassical target organs in animals, such as the pancreas, parathyroid, thymus, skin, placenta, mammary tissue (Norman et al., 1982; Pike, 1985) and muscle (Boland, 1986). There is increasing evidence indicating that the brain is also a target organ for vitamin D. Reports of interactions between vitamin D metabolites and the brain have described vitamin D receptors or the presence of calcium binding proteins (CaBP). Vitamin D receptors have been found in the rat pituitary gland and cerebellum, and in specific rat brain nuclei (Norman et al., 1982; Pike, 1985; Sonnenberg, Luine, Krey, & Christakos, 1985; Stumpf, Sar, Clark, & DeLuca, 1982). Immunohistochemical studies allowed detection of an antigen cross-reacting with vitamin D dependent calcium binding protein in the brain of chicks

This research was supported in part by a grant from the Rockefeller Foundation. We thank Dr. N. Kariv at the Animal Center at Tel Aviv University for his help in the surgical procedures. A. M. Kaye is the incumbent of the Joseph Moss Professorship in Molecular Endocrinology at the Weizman Institute of Science.

(Jande, Tolnai, & Lawson, 1981; Roth, Baetens, Norman, & Garcia-Segura, 1981) rats (Baimbridge, Miller, & Parkes, 1982; Jande, Maler, & Lawson, 1981) and humans (Wasserman & Feher, 1978). Evidence for its production by the brain was derived from *in vitro* translation of mRNA (Thomasset, Desplan, & Parkes, 1983).

A recent study (Pasteels et al., 1986) reported that the brain of the rat synthesizes two proteins of distinct molecular weights (29,000 and 27,000 Da), both cross-reacting with antibodies raised against chick intestinal D-CaBP. Immunogold staining with electron microscopy allowed detection of D-CaBP in Purkinje cells and in climbing fibers of the cerebellum. The immunoreactivity was found to be present in neuronal soma, in neurites, and in postsynaptic and presynaptic terminals. An increase in immunoreactive calcium binding protein was found in chick cerebellum following chronic, but not acute, administration of vitamin D to severely vitamin D deficient chicks (Taylor, 1977). Rat brain nuclei, which contain receptors for $1,25(OH)_2D_3$ and/or calcium binding proteins, showed an increase in choline acetyl transferase activity after one week of treatment with $1,25(OH)_2D_3$ (Sonnenberg et al., 1985).

PRESENT STUDY

To the best of our knowledge, the following test is the first demonstration of an acute affect of vitamin D metabolites on the brain. Specifically, this is the first demonstration that the cerebellum responds to $1,25\ (OH)_2D_3$ and $24,25(OH)_2D_3$ by increasing creatine kinase (CK) enzyme activity. The use of stimulation of CK activity as a marker for hormone action in this case parallels its use in chick (Somjen, Kaye, & Binderman, 1984), rat (Somjen et al., 1986), and human (Somjen, Binderman, Weisman, & Kaye, 1985) systems as a marker for vitamin D metabolites, and for an extremely wide range of other steroid and peptide hormone and growth factors (Somjen et al., 1986; Somjen, Binderman, et al., 1985).

The rabbit was selected for this study since,

like the human, it is a "perinatal brain developer," with its brain growth spurt occurring from 10 days before birth to 30 days after birth (Harel, Watanabe, Linke, & Schain, 1972). New Zealand white does were raised at the Tel Aviv University Animal Colony: fetuses or newborns, from 6 days before to 15 days after birth, were treated with 3 ng/g body weight of $1,25(OH)_2D_3$, 9 ng/g body weight of $24,25(OH)_2D_3$ (Somjen et al., 1986) or with vehicle (20% ethanol in saline). These doses, based on the average fetal weight from previous experiments, were the same as those used for our previous work, which showed stimulation of CK activity by vitamin D metabolites in bones and kidneys of normal rats (Somjen, Weisman, et al., 1984; Somjen et al., 1986). In order to inject the fetuses with the metabolites, cesarean sections were performed; the uterine horns were gently lifted out, avoiding unnecessary trauma. Three groups of fetuses in each female were designated for separate intraperitoneal injection of the metabolites or the vehicle into the abdomen of each fetus. The uterus was gently returned to the abdominal cavity and both muscle and skin were closed with a single stitch. Twenty-four hours later, all fetuses were removed by cesarean section, the fetus brains were excised, and the separated cerebrum and cerebellum were stored at $-20°C$. Another group of does were allowed to delivery naturally. On designated days, the pups were injected intraperitoneally with the metabolites; 24 hours later they were sacrificed, and the pup brain tissue was removed and stored at $-20°C$ for CK analysis. Samples were homogenized (Somjen et al., 1986) using a teflon-glass homogenizer; CK activity was determined using a coupled spectrophotometric assay (Somjen, Kaye, & Binderman, 1984). One unit was defined as the activity catalyzing the formation of 1 mole of ATP per minute at $30°C$.

The basal (untreated) activity of CK shows a different developmental pattern in cerebrum and cerebellum tissue during the period studied, from 6 days before birth until 15 days postnatally (Figure 1). The basal CK activity in

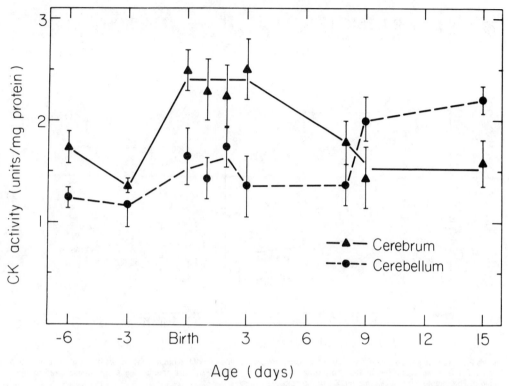

Figure 1.   Perinatal developmental changes in the specific activity of creatine kinase in brain. Portions of rabbit cerebrum and cerebellum were assayed as described previously (Somjen et al., 1984). The results are means ± SE for n = 3 –9.

embryonic cerebrum at 6 days before birth is 1.7 units/mg protein, significantly higher than the 1.2 units/mg protein in the cerebellum at this age. In both cerebrum and cerebellum tissue, CK activity rises significantly between 3 days before birth (−3d) and birth. The cerebrum maintains its high CK activity reached at birth through day 3, shows a decline by day 8, then levels off close to its activity at −3d. Cerebellar CK is also higher at birth than at −3d, declines by day 3, then shows a second rise by day 9, which is maintained to reach its highest activity at day 15, the latest day tested (Figure 1).

There is a striking difference between the cerebrum and the cerebellum in their responsiveness to $1,25(OH)_2D_3$ and $24,25(OH)_2D_3$ during the perinatal period. Neither $1,25-(OH)_2D_3$ nor $24,25(OH)_2D_3$ induces CK activity in the cerebrum (Figure 2). In the cerebellum, however, $24,25(OH)_2D_3$ significantly increases CK activity from −6d to +9d, while $1,25(OH)_2D_3$ stimulates CK activity only from +8d (Figure 2).

DISCUSSION

The intriguing regional and temporal differences in CK activity reported here may be explained by differences in the pattern of development of the cerebrum and the cerebellum during the perinatal period up to 3 weeks of age (Harel et al., 1972). At this time, the process of growth in the cerebellum is characterized predominantly by cell proliferation, while in the cerebrum increase in cell size (Harel et al., 1972) is the main characteristic.

The increase in CK activity during the stage of most rapid cell division in the cerebellum of untreated rabbits, and its stimulation by $24,25(OH)_2D_3$ to a greater extent in prenatal than in postnatal cerebellum, is reminiscent of other rat and avian systems in which CK activity parallels growth and division (Kaye et

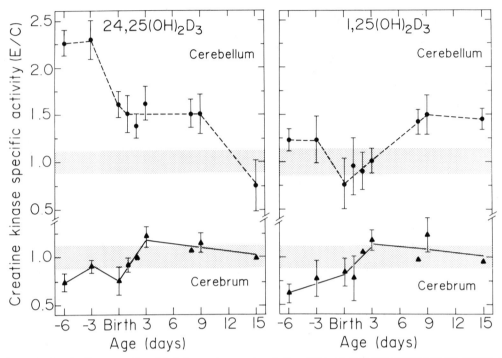

Figure 2.   Creatine kinase specific activity in the cerebrum and cerebellum of the perinatal rabbit 24 hours after i.p. injection of vitamin D metabolites. The results (E/C) are means ± SE for n = 6 −12 of experimental divided by control (vehicle injected values). The stippled bands indicate the SE of the control means.

al., 1986; Somjen, Binderman, et al., 1985). Therefore, the stimulation of CK activity, which probably accompanies, rather than causes, induction of other proteins having specific and/or controlling roles in cell division, can serve as an indicator for these more specific hormone-induced processes by helping to define the characteristic hormone responsiveness of a given tissue.

The mechanism of induction of CK in the cerebellum by vitamin D metabolites is likely to occur via transcriptional regulation, since mRNA for CK is induced by estrogen in rat uterus (Walker & Kaye, 1981), and actinomycin D prevents the stimulation of CKBB activity by parathyroid hormone in bone cells (Somjen, Kaye, et al., 1985).

The fact that these regional and temporal differences in CK basal activity and respon-siveness are correlated with differences in growth rates suggests that vitamin D metabolites may play a role in normal brain development.

CONCLUSIONS

Does vitamin D have a role in the developing brain? It is now apparent that the brain is a target for vitamin D, and that biochemical changes in the brain with distinct regional and temporal patterns can be induced by vitamin D metabolites in correlation with differences in brain growth rates. The functional correlates of these vitamin D induced biochemical responses are still unknown. Further collaboration between basic and clinical research is necessary to elucidate this issue.

REFERENCES

Baimbridge, K.G., Miller, J.J., & Parkes, C.O. (1982). Calcium binding protein distribution in the rat brain. *Brain Research, 239*, 519–525.

Boland, R. (1986). Role of vitamin D in skeletal muscle function. *Endocrine Review, 7*, 434–448.

Corvol, M.T., Dumontier, M.F., Garabedian, R., &

Rapaport, R. (1978). Vitamin D and cartilage: II. Biological activity 25-hydroxycholecalciferol and 24,25 dihydroxycholecalciferols on cultured growth plate chondrocytes. *Endocrinology, 102,* 1269–1274.

Endo, H., Kiyoki, M., Kawashima, K., Nasuchi, T., & Hashimoto, Y. (1980). Vitamin D_3 metabolites and PTH synergistically stimulate bone formation of chick embryonic femur *in vitro. Nature, 286,* 262–264.

Harel, S., Watanabe, K., Linke, I., & Schain, R.J. (1972). Growth and development of the rabbit brain. *Biology of the Neonate, 21,* 381–399.

Jande, S.S., Maler, L., & Lawson, D.E.M. (1981). Immunohistochemical mapping of vitamin D dependent calcium binding protein in brain. *Nature, 294,* 765–767.

Jande, S.S., Tolnai, S., & Lawson, D.E. (1981). Immunohistochemical localization of vitamin D dependent calcium binding proteins in duodenum, kidney, uterus and cerebellum of chickens. *Histochemistry, 71,* 99–116.

Kaye, A.M., Reiss, N.A., Weisman, Y., Binderman, I., & Somjen, D. (1986). Hormonal regulation of creatine kinase BB. In N. Brautbar (Ed.), *Myocardial and skeletal muscle bioenergetics* (pp. 83–102). New York: Plenum.

Malluche, H.H., Henry, H., Meyer-Savellek, W., Sherman, D., Massry, S.G., & Norman, A.W. (1980). Effects and interactions of 24R,25$(OH)_2D_3$ and 1,25$(OH)_2D_3$ on bone. *American Journal of Physiology, 228,* E494–E498.

Norman, A.W., Roth, J., & Orci, L. (1982). The vitamin D endocrine system: Steroid metabolism, hormone receptors and biological response. *Endocrine Reviews, 3,* 331–366.

Ornoy, A., Goodwin, D., Wolff, D., & Edelstein, S. (1978). 24,25 dihydroxy vitamin D is a metabolite of vitamin D essential for bone formation. *Nature, 276,* 517–519.

Pasteels, J.K., Pochet, R., Suradi, I., Hubeau, C., Chirnoaga, M., Parmentier, M., & Lawson, D.E.M. (1986). Ultrastructural localization of brain vitamin D-dependent calcium binding proteins. *Brain Research, 364,* 294–301.

Pike, J.W. (1985). Intracellular receptors mediate the biologic action of 1,25-dihydroxyvitamin D_3. *Nutrition Reviews, 43,* 161–168.

Roth, J., Baetens, J.D., Norman, A.W., & Garcia-Segura, L.M. (1981). Specific neurons in chick central nervous system stain with antibody against chick intestinal vitamin D dependent calcium binding protein. *Brain Research, 22,* 452–457.

Somjen, D., Binderman, I., Weisman, Y., & Kaye, A.M. (1985). Regulation of creatine kinase: A response marker for metabolites of vitamin D. In A. Ornoy, A. Harell, & J. Sela (Eds.), *Current advances in skeletogenesis,* (pp. 183–188). Amsterdam: Elsevier.

Somjen, D., Kaye, A.M. and Binderman, I. (1984). 24R,25 dihydroxy vitamin D stimulates creatine kinase BB activity in chick cartilage cells in culture. *FEBS Letters, 167,* 281–284.

Somjen, D., Kaye, A.M., & Binderman, I. (1985). Stimulation of creatine kinase BB activity by parathyroid hormone and by prostaglandin E_2 in cultured bone cells. *Biochemical Journal, 225,* 591–596.

Somjen, D., Weisman, Y., Berger, E., Earon, Y., Kaye, E., & Binderman, I. (1986). Developmental changes in the responsiveness of rat kidney to vitamin D metabolites. *Endocrinology, 118,* 354–359.

Somjen, D., Weisman, Y., Binderman, I., & Kaye, A.M. (1984). Stimulation of creatine kinase BB activity by 1,25-dihydroxycholecalciferol and 24R,25-dihydroxycholecalciferol in rat tissues. *Biochemical Journal, 219,* 1037–1041.

Sönnenberg, J., Luine, V.H., Krey, L., & Christakos, S. (1985). Administration of 1,25 dihydroxy vitam D_3 (1,25$(OH)_2D_3$) results in increased choline acetylase activity in specific brain nuclei. In A.W. Norman, K. Schaefer, H.G. Gigoleit, & D.V. Herroth (Eds.), *Vitamin D, a chemical, biochemical and clinical update* (pp. 117–118). Berlin: Walter de Gryter.

Stumpf, W.E., Sar, M., Clark, S.A., & DeLuca, H.F. (1982). Brain target sites for 1.25-dihydroxyvitamin D_3. *Science, 215,* 1403–1405.

Taylor, A.N. (1977). Chick brain calcium binding protein: response to cholecalciferol and some developmental aspects. *Journal of Nutrition, 107,* 480–487.

Thomasset, M., Desplan, C., & Parkes, O. (1983). Rat vitamin D dependent calcium binding proteins. Specificity of mRNAs coding for the 7,500 Mr protein from duodenum and the 28.000 Mr protein from kidney and cerebellum. *European Journal of Biochemistry, 129,* 519–524.

Walker, M.D., & Kaye, A.M. (1981). mRNA for the rat uterine estrogen induced protein. Translation *in vitro* and regulation by estrogen. *Journal of Biological Chemistry, 256,* 23–26.

Wasserman, R.H., & Feher, J.J. (1978). Vitamin D-dependent calcium binding proteins. In R.H. Wasserman, R.A. Corradino, E. Carafoli, R.H. Kretsinger. D.H. Mac Lennon, & F.L. Siegel (Eds.), *Calcium binding proteins and calcium functions* (pp. 233–302). New York: Elsevier/North Holland.

Chapter 14

Potential Developmental Consequences of Uncontrolled Epileptogenicity

John H. Menkes and Sophie Goldblum

FOR A LONG TIME, IT HAS BEEN THE CON-sensus among researchers that seizures during the neonatal period have grave prognostic implications for the infant's ultimate intellectual development. In part, the adverse outcome reflects the underlying neuronal abnormality that gives rise to the neonatal seizures, and in part, it reflects the deleterious effects of seizures, per se, on several structural and functional parameters of the developing brain.

Adverse effects can occur acutely or chronically. A number of chemical convulsants, notably bicuculine, pentylene tetrazol, and flurothyl, have been employed to induce prolonged seizures in neonatal animals (Wasterlain & Duffy, 1976). Such seizures are accompanied by hypoventilation and apnea, which result in hypoxemia and hypercapnia. The most significant acute affect of seizures on the brain is the marked increase in its energy requirements. There is a three- to five-fold increase in high energy phosphate utilization associated with increased glycolysis and an increase in brain lactate. Glycolysis, a relatively inefficient means of providing energy, causes a drop in brain glucose concentrations. The presence of lactate, in turn, induces vasodilation and an increased cerebral blood flow (Volpe, 1986). Impairment of vascular autoregulation, induced by a prolonged seizure, ul-timately reduces cerebral blood flow, and compromises energy delivery to the brain (Wasterlain & Graham, 1980).

Wasterlain and his co workers have shown that electroconvulsive seizures of 5 to 20 seconds duration that are repeated at 30 minute intervals have a variety of adverse effects on the brain (Dwyer & Wasterlain, 1982; Jorgensen, Dwyer, & Wasterlain, 1980; Wasterlain, 1976; Wasterlain, 1977; Wasterlain, 1978). These are summarized in Table 1. In particular, both protein and lipid levels in brain tissue were chronically reduced after animals had been subjected to brief but repetitive seizures. These changes reflect impairment in cellular prolifcration, differentiation, and myelination. Whereas the acute changes seen with seizures are undoubtedly relevant to the clinical situation, the effects of repetitive seizures on brain development of animals may not be directly applicable to the infant.

Excitatory Neurotransmitters and Cell Damage

Another route by which seizures may induce neuronal cell death involves the excitatory neurotransmitters (Rothman, 1985). Cerebral hypoxia and hypoglycemia, common accompaniments to neonatal seizures, release the excitatory neurotransmitters glutamate and N-methyl-D-aspartate (NMDA) which, in turn,

Table 1.   Effect of seizures on neonatal rat

Brain metabolism
  ATP utilization increased 3- to 5-fold (prevented
    by paralysis and cerebral oxygenation)
  Lactic acidosis resulting from increased
    glycolysis, and an elevated NADH/NAD ratio
  Fall in brain glucose
Brain structure
  Recurrent seizures:
    Retard brain growth
    Reduce brain protein synthesis
    Reduce myelin content
    Reduce synaptic protein content
    Dissociate brain polysomes

initiate a cascade of reactions culminating in injury to the neuronal cell body and its dendrites. The mechanism of this neurotoxicity is outlined in Table 2.

Glutamate is released into the perfusates in the course of seizures, and when administered either intracerebrally or systematically, both glutamate and aspartate induce seizures under experimental conditions. Conversely, valproate, a potent anticonvulsant, decreases brain aspartate concentrations (Meldrum, 1984).

In animals, the injection of such glutamate analogues as kainate, quisqualate, or quinolinate (a metabolite of tryptophan) leads to the development of sustained limbic siezures and to a pattern of brain damage that resembles the pathology of human temporal lobe epilepsy. Damage induced by glutamate or aspartate is axon-sparing. Such damage is characterized by acute swelling of dendrites and vacuolar de-

Table 2.   Neurotoxicity of excitatory amino acids

Effects of glutamate, N-methyl-D-aspartate,
quinolinic acid:

1. Cell depolarization increases intracellular
   chloride
2. Cations drawn into cell
3. Increased intracellular osmolarity
4. Water enters cell
5. Increased tension on cell membrane causes
   cell to lyse

No evidence that calcium influx is primarily
responsible for cell death.

From "The neurotoxicity of excitatory amino acids is produced by passive chloride influx" by S.M. Rothman, 1985, *Journal of Neuroscience, 5*, pp. 1483–1489. Copyright 1985 by *Journal of Neuroscience*. Reprinted by permission.

generation of neuronal soma, common features of the acute cytopathology induced by such other neurotoxic agents as kainic, ibotenic, quisqualic, or quinolinic acids (Olney, Collins, & Sloviter, 1986). The patterns of cytopathology are somewhat different for each of these. Thus, kainate induces a selective degeneration of the CA3 pyramidal hippocampal neurons, while ibotenic acid, quinolinic acid, and NMDA induce comparable lesions of both CA3 pyramidal neurons and dentate granule cells (Meldrum, 1985).

Persistent electrical stimulation of the perforant path, a major, presumably glutamatergic, excitatory input to the hippocampus, reproduces a pattern of hippocampal lesions similar to those observed in various models of induced epilepsy. In these models, brain damage occurs as a consequence of sustained seizure activity. Conversely, vulnerability to excitatory neurotransmitters is reduced by lesions of the cortico-striatal (glutamic acid) input (McGeer, McGeer, & Singh, 1978).

Amino Acid Receptor Antagonists

One hypothesis for this reduction, already proven, is that specific excitatory amino acid receptor antagonists protect against seizure-mediated brain damage. Three excitatory amino acid receptors have been demonstrated to date: NMDA, kainate, and quisqalate. Glutamic acid appears to be the agonist for the quisqualate receptors, while aspartic and quinolinic acids act preferentially at the NMDA receptors (Davies, Evans, Francis, Jones, & Watkins, 1981). Inasmuch as NMDA receptors are considered to be the most abundant in the CNS, research in the last few years has been directed toward the development of NMDA antagonists. Currently known antagonists include APV (2-amino-phosphonovalerate), AP7 (2-amino-7-phosphonoheptanoic acid), phencyclidine, and CPP (carboxypiperazine). All of these antagonists show anticonvulsant properties against audiogenic seizures (Jones, Croucher, Meldrum, & Watkins, 1984), against photosensitive seizures in the primate *papio papio*, and appear to protect against amino acid–induced brain damage (Meldrum, 1985). When administered by an intracerebral or ventricular route, they are more potent anticonvulsants than valproate and many other commonly used drugs.

The pattern of lesions resulting from cerebral ischemia or hypoglycemia, specifically, the loss of hippocampal pyramidal neurons (CA1 and CA3) can be prevented by the local or systemic injection of NMDA antagonists, provided that levels are maintained for 12 or more hours after the insult (Simon, Swan, Griffiths, & Meldrum, 1984; Wieloch, 1985). Doses required for the hypoxic and hypoglycemic sparing effects are substantially higher than seizure protective doses (Meldrum, Evans, Swan, & Simon, 1987).

It appears that even when hypoxia is prevented, the loss of high energy phosphates interferes with the re-uptake of excitatory neurotransmitters. Their continued presence induces cell death, particularly within the basal ganglia and the limbic structures of the brain. The possibility that antagonists to excitatory neurotransmitters may turn out to be useful, not only as anticonvulsants, but also as preventives for hypoxic brain damage, has only recently been explored (Foster, Gill, & Woodruff, 1987; Meldrum, 1985; Wong, Kemp, Priestley, et al., 1986).

NEONATAL SEIZURES: PROGNOSIS

The prognosis for infants with neonatal seizures has improved somewhat in terms of sur-

vival but prognosis has improved relatively little in terms of neurological sequelae (Figure 1). Clearly, the most important factor determining outcome is the underlying process responsible for the seizures (Table 3). Infants who suffer seizures as a consequence of hypoxic ischemic encephalopathy and who survive have a 50% chance of normal development. In contrast, when seizures result from an intraventricular hemorrhage, or when they are due to a developmental defect of the brain, the outlook is poor (Volpe, 1986). Although in older studies the incidence of developmental malformations responsible for neonatal seizures has been relatively infrequent, evaluations of infants with nuclear magnetic resonance scans have uncovered a significant number of otherwise unrecognized developmental malformations, notably microgyria, lissencephaly, and heterotopic gray matter.

The outlook for hypoglycemic seizures is difficult to evaluate, since in most instances, hypoglycemia renders the brain more susceptible to ischemic insults. Furthermore, factors that induce neonatal hypoglycemia are also conducive to impaired brain development. Thus, when neonatal seizures occur in small-for-gestational-age infants, the prognosis tends to be less favorable than for infants who are appropriate for gestational age (Derham, Matthews, & Clarke, 1985) (Figure 2). Less than 10% of infants who suffered seizures during the neonatal period, and whose birth weight

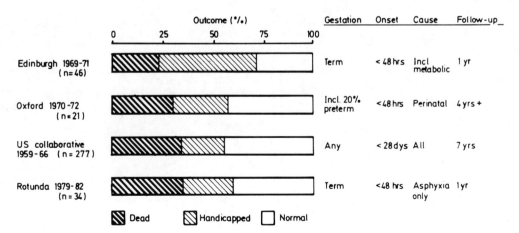

Figure 1. Outcome of neonatal seizures. (From Derham, R.J., Matthews, T.G., & Clarke, T.A. [1985]. *Archives of Disease in Childhood, 60,* 809–813).

116   Menkes and Goldblum

Table 3.   Prognosis of neonatal seizures—
Relation to neurological disease

Neurological disease[a]	Normal development
Hypoxic-ischemic encephalopathy	50%
Intraventricular hemorrhage	< 10%
Primary subarachnoid hemorrhage	90%
Hypocalcemia	
Early onset	50%
Later onset	100%
Hypoglycemia	50%
Bacterial meningitis	25–65%
Developmental defect	0

[a]Prognosis is for those cases with the stated neurological disease when seizures are a manifestation (thus, value usually will differ from overall prognosis for the disease).

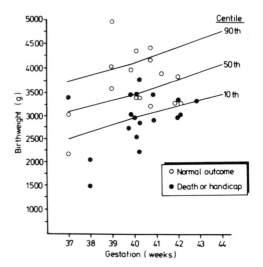

Figure 2.   Centile birth weights in relation to outcome in 34 term infants who suffered seizures in the first 48 hours of life. (From Derham, R.J., Matthews, T.G., & Clarke, T.A. [1985]. *Archives of Disease in Childhood, 60,* 809–813).

was in the 10th percentile or below, are normal when examined at 1 year of age.

In terms of immediate prognosis, the outcome tends to be more favorable if certain conditions exist: if seizures subside within 24 hours of onset, if routine feedings are tolerated by 5 days of age, and if the neurological examination is normal, specifically, abnormal eye movements are determined to be absent. The interictal EEG is also of considerable prognostic value. Low voltage burst suppression patterns or electrocerebral inactivity predict a poor outcome, as does the presence of epileptiform, multifocal discharges. The presence of

focal low frequency discharges, focal rhythmic discharges, and other electroencephalographic seizures—whether or not they are associated with clinical seizure manifestations—also predict a poor outcome (Rose & Lombroso, 1970; Rowe, Holmes, Hafford, et al., 1985).

Treatment of neonatal seizures, whether by administration of glucose, calcium, pyridoxine, or anticonvulsants, is outside the scope of this paper.

REFERENCES

Davies, J., Evans, R. H., Francis, A. A., Jones, A. W., & Watkins, J. C. (1981). Antagonism of excitatory amino acid–induced and synaptic excitation of spinal neurones by cis-2,3-peperidine dicarboxylate. *Journal of Neurochemistry, 36,* 1305–1307.

Derham, R.J., Matthews, T.G., & Clarke, T.A. (1985). Early seizures indicate quality of perinatal care. *Archives of Disease in Childhood, 60,* 809–813.

Dwyer, B.E., & Wasterlain, C.G. (1982). Electroconvulsive seizures selectively impair myelin accumulation in the immature rat. *Experimental Neurology, 78,* 616–628.

Foster, A.C., Gill, R., & Woodruff, G.N. (1987). MK-801 prevents degeneration of striatal neurones caused by intrastriatal injection of quinolinic acid. *British Journal of Pharmacology, 90,* 7P.

Jones, A. W., Croucher, M. J., Meldrum, B. S., & Watkins, J. C. (1984). Suppression of audiogenetic seizures in DBA/2 mice by two new dipeptide NMDA receptor antagonists. *Neuroscience Letters, 45,* 157–161.

Jorgensen, O.S., Dwyer, B.E., & Wasterlain, C.G. (1980). Synaptic proteins after electroconvulsive sei-

zures in immature rats. *Journal of Neurochemistry, 35,* 1235–1237.

McGeer, E.G., McGeer, P.L.. & Singh, K. (1978). Kainate-induced degeneration of neostriatal neurons: Dependency upon cortico-striatal tract. *Brain Research, 139,* 381–383.

Meldrum, B. (1984). Amino acid neurotransmitters and new approaches to anticonvulsant drug action. *Epilepsia* (Suppl.) *2,* S140–S149.

Meldrum, B. (1985). Possible therapeutic applications of antagonists of excitatory amino acid neurotransmitters. *Clinical Science, 68.* 113–122.

Meldrum, B., Evans, M. C., Swan, J. H., & Simon, R. P. (1987). Protection against hypoxic/ischaemic brain damage with excitatory amino acid antagonists. *Medical Biology, 65,* 153–157.

Olney, J.W., Collins, R.C., & Sloviter, R.S. (1986). Excitotoxic mechanisms of epileptic brain damage. In A.V. Delgado-Escueta (Ed.), *Advances in neurology* (Vol. 44, pp. 857–877). New York: Raven Press.

Rose, A.L., & Lombroso, C.T. (1970). Neonatal seizure states. A study of clinical, pathological and electroencephalographic features in 137 full-term babies with a long-term follow-up. *Pediatrics, 45,* 404–425.

Rothman, S.M. (1985). The neurotoxicity of excitatory amino acids is produced bv passive chloride influx. *Journal of Neuroscience, 5,* 1483–1489.

Rowe, J.C., Holmes, G.L., Hafford, J., et al. (1985). Prognostic value of the electroencephalogram in term and preterm infants following neonatal seizures. *Electroencephalography and Clinical Neurophysiology, 60,* 183–196.

Simon, R.P., Swan, J.H., Griffiths, T., & Meldrum, B.S. (1984). Blockade of N-methyl-D-aspartate receptors may protect against ischemic damage in the brain. *Science, 226,* 850–852.

Volpe, J.J. (1986). *Neurology of the newborn* (2nd ed). Philadelphia: W.B. Saunders.

Wasterlain, C.G. (1976). Effect of neonatal status epilepticus on rat brain development. *Neurology, 26,* 975–986.

Wasterlain, C.G. (1977). Effect of epileptic seizures on brain ribosomes: Mechanism and relationship to cerebral energy metabolism. *Journal of Neurochemistry, 29,* 707–716.

Wasterlain, C.G. (1978). Neonatal seizures and brain growth. *Neuropaediatrie, 9,* 213–228.

Wasterlain, C.G., & Duffy, T.E. (1976). Status epilepticus in immature rats. *Archives of Neurology, 33,* 821–827.

Wasterlain, C.G., & Graham, S.L. (1980). Loss of autoregulation of cerebral blood flow: An asset during single seizures, a liability during status epilepticus. *Annals of Neurology, 8,* 94.

Wieloch, T. (1985). Hypoglycemia-induced neuronal damage prevented by an N-methyl-D-aspartate antagonist. *Science, 230,* 681–683.

Wong, E.H.F., Kemp, J.A., Priestley, T., et al. (1986). The antagonist MK-801 is a potent N-methyl-D-aspartate antagonist. *Proceedings of the National Academy of Sciences of the United States of America, 83,* 7104–7108.

Chapter 15

Neuropeptides and Seizures

O. Carter Snead, III

A LARGE NUMBER OF BIOLOGICALLY AC-
tive peptides have been identified in the
central nervous system over the past ten years
(Krieger & Liotta, 1979; Krieger & Martin,
1985), and many of these compounds have
been implicated to one degree or another in
experimental epilepsy (Bajorek, Lee, & Lomax, 1984). But the most intense interest to
date concerning a role for neuropeptides in epilepsy has focused primarily on the opioid peptides. Therefore, it is this group of peptides that
will be reviewed herein.

SOURCE AND DISTRIBUTION

The intense interest in opiate peptide research
that exists today dates from 1973 with the demonstration of stereospecific opiate binding in
the CNS (Pert & Snyder, 1973). Soon after
those landmark experiments, opiate-like activity was demonstrated in brain. The pen-
tapeptides leucine- and methionine enkephalin
were isolated from brain tissue and were shown
to have an affinity for the opiate receptor. Subsequently a larger peptide, β-endorphin, was
isolated and also shown to be a potent opiate
agonist. The enkephalins and β-endorphin
have been shown to differ from one another in
terms of anatomy, biochemistry, and pharmacology (Adler, 1980; Beaumont & Hughes,
1979; Coplov & Helme, 1983; Miller, 1981;
Snyder & Innis, 1979).

Opiate peptide systems in the brain were
thought to be either enkephalinergic or en-
dorphinergic until 1979, when the isolation of
another potent opiate peptide, dynorphin, from

porcine pituitary extracts, was reported (Goldstein, Tachibana, Lowney, et al., 1979). This
compound was found to be a heptadecapeptide
{dynorphin (1-17)} (Goldstein, Fischli,
Lowney, et al., 1981) and appeared to be widely distributed in the neuronal tissue of rats. The
first five amino acids at the NH_2 terminus were
identical to leucine-enkephalin, and dynorphin
was initially postulated to be a precursor for
this compound. However, a variety of experiments utilizing recombinant DNA and immunohistochemical techniques show that these
peptides come from one of three large precursor molecules (Akil, Watson, Young, et al.,
1984). The precursor for β-endorphin/adeno-
corticotropin (ACTH) seems to be proopiomelanocortin (POMC). Although the major site of production of this peptide is the
pituitary, POMC is also found in the brain. The
main cell group containing this compound is
found in the region of the arcuate nucleus of the
basal hypothalamus. This POMC system projects throughout the limbic system and brain
stem (Abrams, Nilaver, Hoffman, et al., 1980;
Pelletier, LaClerc, Saveedra, et al., 1980;
Watson, Richard, & Barchas, 1978). Another
group of POMC-containing neurons is found in
the nucleus of the solitary tract. β-endorphin
coexists and is coreleased with ACTH at least
in the pituitary (Guillemin, Vargo, Rossier, et
al., 1977; Holtt, Przenlock, & Herz, 1978).
The only opioid peptide contained by POMC is
β-endorphin. However, the precursor for
methionine and leucine-enkephalin, proenkephalin, gave rise to seven opioid peptides. The
proenkephalin molecule is ubiquitous through-

out the brain and is also found extracerebrally in the adrenal medulla.

The precursor to dynorphin is prodynorphin or the neoendorphin/dynorphin precursor. This is found not only in the hypothalamus but also in cell groups scattered throughout the brain stem.

The processing of all these precursor molecules to their respective peptides is dependent on the genetic code for the precursor as well as on the location of the cell system in the brain or extracerebrally. It is also dependent on the biological property of a given neuron; this dictates how specific peptides are cut out of these precursors (Akil et al., 1984).

A final peptide to be considered in this discussion is corticotropin releasing factor (CRF). This is a hypothalamic releasing factor which stimulates release of both β-endorphin and ACTH. The distribution of cells containing CRF is widespread throughout the forebrain, stem, and spinal cord. CRF perikarya show a codistribution pattern with POMC fibers (Joseph, Pilcher, & Krigge, 1985).

OPIATE RECEPTORS

Much data has accumulated over the past 10 years to support the concept of multiple opiate receptors (Chang, Cooper, Hazum, et al., 1979; Chang & Cuatrecasas, 1979; Wuster, Schultz, & Herz, 1981). There are pharmacologic and biochemical data to support at least five subpopulations of opiate receptor in the brain. The μ receptor has the greatest affinity for morphine, is felt to be responsible for the analgesic properties of morphine, and is found in guinea pig ileum. The δ receptor has the highest affinity for leucine- and methionine-enkephalin, a lower affinity for naloxone than the μ receptor, and is found in mouse vas deferens (Augigier, Mazarguil, Gout, et al., 1980; Kosterlitz, Lord, Paterson, et al., 1980; Lord, Waterfield, Hughes, et al., 1977). The ε receptor is thought to be that for β-endorphin and is found in rat vas deferens (Houghton, Johnson, & Pasternak, 1984; Law, Loh, & Li, 1979; Shultz, Wuster, & Herz, 1981). The σ receptor has as its prototype agonist N-allynormetazocine (SKF 10,047). The

synthetic agonist for the κ receptor is ethylketocyclazocine (Gilbert & Martin, 1976; Harris & Sethy, 1980), but dynorphin now appears to be the naturally occurring κ agonist in brain (Brooks & Bradley, 1984; Chavkin, James, & Goldstein, 1982; Oka, Negishi, Kajiwara, et al., 1982; Quiron & Pert, 1981). Other researchers (Nishimura, Recht, & Pasternak, 1984; Pasternak, Childers, & Snyder, 1980; Pasternak, Zhany, & Tecott, 1980) have postulated that opiate receptors can be classified as high affinity sites responsible for opiate analgesia and low affinity sites responsible for respiratory depression. Another hypothesis put forth to explain opiate receptor heterogeneity is that μ and δ sites are coupled allostearically in a single receptor complex (Rothman & Westfall, 1981; Rothman & Westfall, 1982; Rothman & Westfall, 1983).

OPIATE PEPTIDES AND SEIZURES

The initial research surrounding these opiate peptides concerned their ability to produce analgesia, dependence, tolerance, and withdrawal; however, the observation was made in 1977 that both morphine and methionine-enkephalin could produce epileptiform activity when given intracerebroventricularly (ICV) to rats (Urca, Frenk, Liebeskind, et al., 1977). Similarly, it was demonstrated that this property was also found in leucine-enkephalin (Frenk, Urca, & Liebeskind, 1978), and was anatomically distinct from the analgesia produced by these substances (Frenk, McCarty, & Liebeskind, 1978). Furthermore, it has been shown that the seizures induced by leucine-enkephalin were selectively overcome by antipetit mal anticonvulsants (Snead & Bearden, 1980a). Soon after the epileptogenic properties of morphine and enkephalin were reported, Henriksen et al. observed that ICV β-endorphin in small doses also resulted in "limbic seizures," that is, subcortical hippocampal spikes associated with behavioral abnormalities but without convulsions (Henriksen, Bloom, McCoy, et al., 1978).

The observation that anti-petit mal anticonvulsants specifically aborted leucine-enkephalin-induced coupled with the fact that naloxone appeared to be effective against an animal model of generalized absence seizures (Snead & Bearden, 1980b) led to a series of experiments in which the EEG response to a number of opiate agonists was examined in rats. When given intracerebroventricularly, each type of opiate receptor agonist produced a different seizure pattern with a different naloxone dose response curve and anticonvulsant profile (Snead & Bearden, 1982). The order of convulsive potency appeared to be $\epsilon > \delta > \mu > \sigma >> \kappa$. Intracerebral administration of morphine, enkephalins, and endorphin also produces seizure activity (Cain & Corcoran, 1984; Cain & Corcoran, 1985). The κ agonist dynorphin produces grooming, barrel rolling, and catatonia when given ICV (Herman & Goldstein, 1981; Katz, 1980; Zwiers, Alogo, & Gispen, 1981) but showed little analgesia (Tulunay, Jen, Cheng, et al., 1981) and no electrographic seizure (Ehlers, 1984). The μ agonist morphine is the only opiate agonist to produce generalized convulsive seizures (Snead & Bearden, 1982; Turski, Czuczuar, Kleinrok, et al., 1983), but there is some question as to whether this is an opiate effect (Frenk, Watkins, Miller, et al., 1984). This drug is also proconvulsant against seizures induced by γ-aminobutyric acid (GABA) antagonists (Foote & Gale, 1983) and pentylenetetrazole (Foote & Gale, 1984; Mannino & Wolf, 1975). When given systemically, morphine appears to be anticonvulsant against seizures produced by ICV morphine (Urca & Frenk, 1982; Urca & Frenk, 1983).

Additional evidence of receptor-specific seizure induced by these peptides is found in experiments showing that morphine and another μ agonist, morphiceptin (Haffmans & Dzoljic, 1983) have an identical ontogeny in terms of when seizures appear, how they progress, their morphology, and reversibility by naloxone. However, enkephalin seizures differ from those produced by the specific δ agonist Tyr-D-Ser-Gly-Phe-Thr (DSLET) in terms of ontogeny, morphology, and response to the specific δ antagonist ICI 154,129 (Snead, 1985). This suggests that the enkephalin seizure is not a pure δ-mediated event (Frenk, 1983) but may require both μ and δ receptor activity.

All of the above data were derived from rodent experiments. There is little data concerning the effect of these opiate peptides in other species. Meldrum, Menini, Stutzman, and colleagues (1979) have given leucine-enkephalin, β-endorphin, and morphine in varying doses into the ventricles of the baboon (Papio Papio) and were unable to demonstrate any electrical effect. However, Shippenberg and Altshuller (1982) have reported spikes and seizures in primates receiving these neuropeptides.

In contradistinction to the work cited above, there is another body of literature concerning the anticonvulsant effect of opiate peptides and opiate agonists (Berman & Adler, 1984; Cowan, Geller, & Adler, 1979; Lewis, Caldicott-Hazard, Cannon, et al., 1981; Przewlocka, Stala, Lasou, et al., 1983; Tortella, Cowan, & Adler, 1981; Tortella, Robles, & Holaday, 1985a; Tortella, Robles, Holaday, et al., 1983). This literature deals with complex, sometimes conflicting data regarding the effect of opiate agonists and/or antagonists in various models of generalized convulsive seizures and kindling. Endogenous opiates seem to mediate the postictal depression that follows kindled seizures in some fashion (Caldecott-Hazard, Yamagata, Hedlond, et al., 1983; Frenk, Engel, Ackerman, et al., 1979; Yitzhaky, Frenk, & Urca, 1982). There are several lines of evidence to support this. Daily amygdaloid stimulation produces an elevation of pain threshold 24 hours poststimulation. This phenomenon is blocked by naloxone (Abbott & Melzack, 1978; Le Gal La Salle, Calvino, & Ben-Ari, 1977; Nabeshima, Matsuno, & Kameyama, 1985). Naloxone also diminishes the postictal depression seen after a stage five kindled seizure (Frenk, Engel, Ackerman, et al., 1979). Morphine has been reported to potentiate this postictal depression and enhance postictal EEG spiking in kindled rats (Abbott & Melzack, 1978; Caldecott-Hazard et al., 1983; Frenk et al., 1979; Le Gal La Salle et al., 1977; Yitzhaky et al., 1982). Electroconvulsive shock also produces analgesia and catalepsy, both of which are partially blocked by naloxone (Holaday & Belenky, 1980; Nabeshima et al., 1985; Urca, Yitzhaky, & Frenk, 1981). Recently, Tortella and Long (1985) have shown that when cerebrospinal fluid (CSF) is taken from one rat subjected to electroshock-induced seizure, and given to a second, naive animal, the electroshock seizure threshold of the recipient animal is raised. Based on this data, these authors have postulated the exis-tance of an endogenous opioid anticonvulsant. One candidate for this endogenous anticonvul-sant is dynorphin (Przewlocka et al., 1983), a peptide that has been shown to be anticonvul-sant against electroshock and flurothyl seizures (Garant & Gale, 1985; Tortella, Robles, & Holaday, 1985b).

The data concerning naloxone and the kind-led seizure itself are conflicting. Some re-searchers have reported either no change or an anticonvulsant effect of naloxone in kindling (Corcoran & Wada, 1977; Stone, Eggleton, & Berman, 1982). The reason for this discrep-ancy might be different kindling paradigms (Stone et al., 1982). In addition, the experi-ments concerning generalized convulsive sei-zures and kindling do not consider stress which is mediated by nonopiate as well as opiate mechanisms (Lewis, Caldecott-Hazard, Can-non, et al., 1981; Przewlocka et al., 1983). Conceivably, the stress of the seizure rather than the seizure per se could be responsible for the opiate-like affects reported.

Naloxone has also been shown to be procon-vulsant in the mongolian gerbil, a genetic model of epilepsy, possibly by shortening the refrac-tory period via interfering with the postictal state (Bajorek et al., 1984). Conversely, a number of opiate agonists are anticonvulsant in this model (Lee, Bajorek, & Lomax, 1984).

It seems then that there are two contrary data sets, one that supports a proconvulsant and an-other that supports an anticonvulsant role for the opioid peptides. However, the concept of convulsant and anticonvulsant properties of opiate compounds are not mutually exclusive. Experimental and clinical seizure states are ex-ceedingly complex and have no single underly-ing neurochemical mechanism. The electrical and behavioral characteristics of the seizure must therefore be carefully determined prior to extrapolating one group of data to another set of experimental conditions involving different

animal models of epilepsy (Snead, 1983). All the published data regarding anticonvulsant properties of opiate agonists deal with gener-alized seizure phenomena, whether it is the postictal phenomenon associated with these types of seizures in kindled or electroshock sei-zures, or the seizure threshold to exogenously administered generalized convulsants. Those data do not address the question of specific EEG and behavioral effects of intracerebro-ventricularly administered opiate agonists in the context of their similarities and differences. In addition to the different experimental con-siderations alluded to above, it is also conceiv-able that the neurophysiological and neu-rochemical actions responsible for generating one type of seizure (e.g., generalized absence) may be anticonvulsant in another seizure sys-tem (e.g., generalized convulsive).

ACTH AND SEIZURES

ACTH should be considered in any discussion of neuropeptides and seizures because clinical evidence suggests this compound has anticon-vulsant properties, and it is closely related to opiates and opiate peptides.

ACTH-like peptides have been demon-strated to antagonize morphine inhibition of spinal reflex activity (Krivoy, 1970; Zimmer-man & Krivoy, 1973). In addition, ACTH and ACTH fragments show some affinity for the opiate receptor. $ACTH_{4-10}$, a compound nearly devoid of corticotrophic activity, was the shortest sequence to inhibit binding of $\{^3H\}$-naltrexone. Those fragments of ACTH that possess affinity for the opiate receptor also in-hibit morphine-induced analgesia. These ac-tions, together with possible involvement of ACTH in stress analgesia (Lewis, Cannon, & Liebeskind, 1980), the coexistence of ACTH with β-endorphin, and the concomitant secre-tion of ACTH with β-endorphin, all point to a common denominator in the diverse action of ACTH-like peptides and opiates on the central nervous system.

Much of the evidence concerning the action of ACTH on the brain (independent of its endo-crine effect) centers on structure activity relationships of various ACTH peptide fragments in regard to their ability to stimulate the adrenals versus their ability to produce changes in behavior. The observation that ACTH could influence behavior was first made in 1953. These behavioral changes have since been intensively studied and extensively reviewed (de Wied & Gispen, 1979) and will be mentioned only briefly here. ACTH has been found to have various effects. It influences acquisition and extinction of a conditioned avoidance response, facilitates reversal learning, increases resistance to a complex brightness discrimination test, reverses CO_2 retrograde amnesia, and induces excessive grooming followed by stretching and yawning movements.

Several ACTH analogues have been synthesized and tested for behavioral and adrenal activity (de Wied, Witter, & Greven, 1975; Wiegant, Jolles, Colbern, et al., 1979). $ACTH_{4-10}$ and $ACTH_{1-10}$ have no corticotrophic activity. The 4–10 amino acid sequence of ACTH has 10^{-6} times the corticotrophic activity of $ACTH_{1-39}$ and $ACTH_{4-24}$, yet it is behaviorally active. Microinjections of $ACTH_{1-10}$ and $ACTH_{4-10}$ into the posterior thalamus produce behavioral effects while systemic administration produces no behavioral change from control (Steiner, Ruff, & Akert, 1969). The essential elements required for the behavioral effect of ACTH analogs seems to be contained within the 4–7 fragment of ACTH.

ACTH also has an effect on electrical activity of brain. This peptide activates hypothalamic and midbrain cells (Olpe & Jones, 1982; van Delft & Kitay, 1972) and also enhances spinal cord neuron excitability (Krivoy, 1970). Urban and colleagues (Urban & de Wied, 1976; Urban, Lopes da Silva, & Storm van Leeuwen, 1974) have demonstrated that the ACTH fragment 4–10, devoid of corticotrophic activity, has an activating effect on hippocampal theta rhythm in dogs and rats. These fragments also suppress stimulus-induced EEG synchrony in humans, with the $ACTH_{4-10}$ fragment being the most potent (Endroczi, Lissak, & Fekete, 1970).

ACTH has been reported to have anticonvulsant properties against the Mongolian gerbil model of the seizures (Bajorek et al., 1984), amygdaloid kindling (Holmes & Weber, 1985; Rose & Bridger, 1982) and the electroshock seizure model (Honda, White, Chow, et al., 1985).

Corticotrophin Releasing Factor (CRF)

ICV CRF produces a dose related spectrum of effects on EEG and behavior. Doses of 1.5–4 nmol produce long lasting electrographic seizure activity (Ehlers, Henriksen, Wang, et al., 1983). Whether this is due to a direct action on the brain or to release of β-endorphin and ACTH is not clear.

CLINICAL STUDIES

The results obtained from using naloxone in seizure disorders in humans have been disappointing. Montplaisir (Montplaisir, Saint-Hilaire, Walsh, et al., 1981) treated six adult patients with partial seizures with 0.8–2.4 mg naloxone intravenously (iv) and failed to show any change in spontaneous or electrically-induced ictal or interictal EEG discharges or behavior. Engel (Engel, Ackermann, Caldecott-Hazard, et al., 1984) has reported treating adults possessing a variety of generalized seizures with up to 3.6 mg. of naloxone iv with no clear-cut effect except possibly a decrease in interictal spikes. Children with absence seizures or reflex seizures received 0.05 mg/kg iv naloxone without clear cut benefit. These data would suggest that naloxone makes human epilepsy neither better nor worse, in spite of the experimental data reviewed above.

The data concerning ACTH in seizures is a bit more compelling, however. The observation that ACTH and cortisone affected EEGs in humans was first made in the 1940s (McQuarie, Andersson, & Ziegler, 1942). In 1950, Klein and Livingston reported dramatic improvement in the EEG and clinical status of six seizure patients treated with ACTH.

In 1958, Sorel and Dusaucy-Bauloye described remarkable clinical improvement and disappearance of the gross EEG abnormality in children with infantile spasms who were treated with ACTH. This was subsequently confirmed by many authors (for comprehensive review, see Jeavons & Bower, 1964; Lacy & Penry, 1976). Prednisone has also been found to be effective in infantile spasms. There is a single controlled study comparing the efficacy of prednisone to ACTH (Hrachovy, Frost, Kellaway, et al., 1983), which showed that ACTH had no benefit over prednisone. However, an uncontrolled study using much higher doses of ACTH suggests that ACTH is more effective than prednisone, not only against infantile spasms but also against other kinds of intractable, mixed seizures in childhood (Snead, Benton, & Myers, 1983).

The mode of action of ACTH as an anticonvulsant is not known. There are experimental (Torda & Wolff, 1952) and clinical data to support this as an extraadrenal action of ACTH; however, clinical studies utilizing ACTH fragments without adrenal effects have shown little anticonvulsant effect of these fragments (Pentella, Bachman, & Sandman, 1982; Willig & Lagenstein, 1982; Willig, Lagenstein, & Iffland, 1977). Recently, Nalin and colleagues (Nalin, Facchinetti, Galli, et al., 1985) reported reduced ACTH content in cerebrospinal fluid of children suffering from cryptogenic infantile spasms with hypsarrhythmia.

Because of the coexistence of β-endorphin and ACTH, their concomitant secretion by the pituitary, and the neurophysiologic activity of ACTH, these two peptides may form an integrated neuronal system. Given the experimental evidence for the epileptogenic properties of β-endorphin and the clinical evidence for the anticonvulsant effects of ACTH, an imbalance of this system at a specific point in brain development could play a role in certain childhood seizure states, notably, infantile myoclonic seizures.

SUMMARY

There appear to be four lines of evidence for or against a role of neuropeptides in epilepsy:

1. Administration of opiate agonists into the ventricles or the brain of animals produces electrical and behavioral changes, seemingly receptor-specific, that are sensitive to the specific opiate antagonist naloxone as well as to certain anticonvulsant drugs. The primary reservation concerning these data in relation to epilepsy is that the peptides are exogenously administered in relatively high doses. Hence, these data may reflect neurotoxic effects of peptides rather than physiologic function.

2. A number of opiate agonists are anticonvulsant; naloxone shortens the postictal state in some experimental seizure models. One might attempt to reconcile these data with those above by hypothesizing that the spikes and the behavioral changes examined in the latter experimental paradigms represent an isolated model of the postictal state.

3. Naloxone has little effect in clinical epilepsy. These data are not conclusive for two reasons. First, few patients have been studied. Second, because of the issue of opiate receptor heterogeneity and the high doses of naloxone needed experimentally to block non-μ opiate effects, the doses of naloxone used clinically to date are too low to rule out possible opiate mediated effects. The negative clinical data are illustrative of the dangers and difficulties of extrapolating data generated in animal models of seizures to the human condition.

4. ACTH, a peptide that is derived from the same precursor molecule as β-endorphin, is clearly an effective anticonvulsant in certain childhood seizure states. Whether this is due to a direct or indirect (i.e., cortisol) effect on the brain is not clear. Paradoxically, and in contradistinction to other data concerning the pro- and anticonvulsant properties of various opioid peptides, there is no animal model of infantile spasms to help resolve this important question (Snead, 1984).

REFERENCES

Abbott, F.U., & Melzak, K. (1978). Analgesia produced by stimulation of limbic structures and its relation to epileptiform after discharges. *Experimental Neurology, 62,* 720–734.

Abrams, G.M., Nilaver, G., & Hoffman, D., et al. (1980). Immunocytochemical distribution of corticotropin (ACTH) in monkey brain. *Neurology, 30,* 1106–1110.

Adler, M.W. (1980). Minireview: Opioid peptides. *Life Sciences, 26,* 497–510.

Akil, H., Watson, S.J., Young, E., et al. (1984). Endogenous opioids: Biology and function. *Annual Review of Neuroscience, 7,* 223–255.

Augigier, Y., Mazarguil, H., Gout, R., et al. (1980). Structure activity relationships of enkephalin analogs at opiate and enkephalin receptors: Correlation with analgesia. *European Journal of Pharmacology, 63,* 35–46.

Bajorek, J.G., Lee, R.J., & Lomax, P. (1984). Neuropeptides: A role as endogenous mediators or modulators of epileptic phenomena. *Annals of Neurology, 16* (Suppl), S31–38.

Beaumont, A., & Hughes, J. (1979). Biology of opioid peptides. *Annual Review of Pharmacology and Toxicology, 19,* 245–267.

Berman, E.F., & Adler, M.W. (1984). The anticonvulsant effect of opioids and opioid peptides against maximal electroshock seizures in rats. *Neuropharmacology, 23,* 367–371.

Brooks, A., & Bradley, P.B. (1984). Electrophysiological evidence for κ-agonist activity of dynorphin in rat brain. *Neuropharmacology, 23,* 207–210.

Cain, D.P., & Corcoran, M.E. (1984). Intracerebral β-endorphin, met-enkephalin, and morphine: Kindling of seizures and handling-induced potentiation of epileptiform effects. *Life Sciences, 34,* 2535–2542.

Cain, D.P., & Corcoran, M.E. (1985). Epileptiform effects of metenkephalin, β-endorphin, and morphine: Kindling of generalized seizures and potentiation of epileptiform effects by handling. *Brain Research, 338,* 327–336.

Caldecott-Hazard, S., Yamagata, N., Hedlund, J., et al. (1983). Changes in simple and complex behaviors following kindled seizures in rats: Opioid and nonopioid mediation. *Epilepsia, 24,* 539–547.

Chang, K., Cooper, B.R., Hazum, E., et al. (1979). Multiple opiate receptors: Different regional distribution in the brain and differential binding of opiates and opioid peptides. *Molecular Pharmacology, 16,* 91–104.

Chang, K., & Cuatrecasas, P. (1979). Multiple opiate receptors. *Journal of Biological Chemistry, 254,* 2610–2618.

Chavkin, C., James, I.F., & Goldstein, A. (1982). Dynorphin is a specific endogenous ligand of the opioid receptor. *Science, 215,* 413–415.

Coplov, D.L., & Helme, R.D. (1983). Enkephalins and endorphins: Clinical, pharmacological, and therapeutic implications. *Drugs, 26,* 503–519.

Corcoran, M.E., & Wada, J.A. (1977). Naloxone and the kindling of seizures. *Life Sciences, 24,* 791–796.

Cowan, A., Geller, E.B., & Adler, M.W. (1979). Classification of opioids on the basis of change in seizure threshold in rats. *Science, 206,* 465–467.

Crosley, C.J., Richman, R.A., & Thorpy, M.J. (1980).

Evidence for cortisol-independent anticonvulsant activity of adrenocorticotropin hormone in infantile spasms. *Annals of Neurology, 8,* 220.

de Wied, D., & Gispen, W.H. (1979). Behavioral effects of peptides. In H. Gainer (Ed.), *Peptides in neurobiology* (pp. 397–420). New York: Raven Press.

de Wied, D., Witter, A., & Greven, H.M. (1975). Behaviorally active ACTH analogues. *Biochemical Pharmacology, 24,* 1463–1468.

Ehlers, C.L. (1984). Role of selected neuropeptides in the development of epileptiform discharges. In R.G. Fariello, P.L. Morselli, & K.G. Lloyd, et al. (Eds.), *Neurotransmitters, seizures, and epilepsy II* (pp. 295–305). New York: Raven Press.

Ehlers, C.L., Henriksen, S.J., Wang, M., et al. (1983). Corticotropin releasing factor produces increases in brain excitability and convulsive seizures in rats. *Brain Research, 278,* 332–336.

Endroczi, E., Lissak, K., & Fekete, T. (1970). Effect of ACTH fragments on EEG in humans. *Progress in Brain Research, 32,* 254–263.

Engel, J., Ackermann, R.F., Caldecott-Hazard, S., et al. (1984). Do altered opioid mechanisms play a role in human epilepsy? In R.G. Fariello, P.L. Morselli, & K.G. Lloyd, et al. (Eds.), *Neurotransmitters, seizures, and epilepsy II* (pp. 263–272). New York: Raven Press.

Farwell, J., Milstein, J., Opheim, K., et al. (1984). Adrenocorticotrophic hormone controls infantile spasms independently of cortisol stimulation. *Epilepsia, 25,* 605–608.

Foote, F., & Gale, K. (1983). Morphine potentiates seizures induced by GABA-antagonists and attenuates seizures induced by electroshock in the rat. *European Journal of Pharmacology, 95,* 259–264.

Foote, F., & Gale, K. (1984). Proconvulsant effect of morphine on seizures induced by pentylenetetrazole in the rat. *European Journal of Pharmacology, 105,* 179–184.

Frenk, H. (1983). Pro- and anticonvulsant actions of morphine and the endogenous opioids: Involvement and interactions of multiple opiate and non-opiate systems. *Brain Research Reviews, 6,* 197–210.

Frenk, H., Engel, J., Ackermann, R.F., et al. (1979). Endogenous opioid may mediate postictal behavioral depression in amygdaloid kindled rats. *Brain Research, 167,* 435–440.

Frenk, H., McCarty, B.C., & Liebeskind, J.C. (1978). Different brain areas mediate the analgesic and epileptic properties of enkephalin. *Science, 200,* 335–337.

Frenk, H., Urca, G., & Liebeskind, J.C. (1978). Epileptic properties of leucine- and methionine-enkephalin: Comparison with morphine and reversibility by naloxone. *Brain Research, 147,* 327–337.

Frenk, H., Watkins, L.R., Miller, J., et al. (1984). Nonspecific convulsions are induced by morphine but not D-Ala²-methionine-enkephalinamide at cortical sites. *Brain Research, 299,* 51–59.

Garant, D.S., & Gale, K. (1985). Infusion of opiates into substantia nigra protects against maximal electroshock seizures in rats. *Journal of Pharmacology and Experimental Therapeutics, 234,* 45–48.

Gilbert, P.E., & Martin, W.R. (1976). The effects of morphine and nalorphine-like drugs in the nondependent, morphine dependent, and cyclazocine dependent chronic spinal dog. *Journal of Pharmacology and Experimental Therapeutics, 198,* 66–82.

Gispen, W.H., Buitelaar, J., Wiegant, V.M., et al. (1976). Interaction between ACTH fragments, brain opiate receptors, and morphine-induced analgesia. *European Journal of Pharmacology, 39,* 393–397.

Goldstein, A., Fischli, W., Lowney, L.I., et al. (1981). Porcine pituitary dynorphin: Complete amino acid sequence of the biologically active heptadecapeptide. *Proceedings of the National Academy of Sciences of the United States of America, 78,* 7219–7223.

Goldstein, A., Tachibana, S., Lowney, L.I., et al. (1979). Dynorphin (1–13), an extraordinarily potent opioid peptide. *Proceedings of the National Academy of Sciences of the United States of America, 76,* 6666–6670.

Guillemin, R., Vargo, T., Rossier, J., et al. (1977). β-endorphin and adrenocorticotropin are secreted concomitantly by the pituitary gland. *Science, 202,* 1367–1369.

Haffmans, J., & Dzoljic, N.M.R. (1983). Differential epileptogenic potentials of selective mu and delta opiate receptor agonists. *Journal of Neural Transmission, 57,* 1–11.

Harris, D.W., & Sethy, V.H. (1980). High affinity binding of {³H}-ethylketocyclazocine to rat brain homogenate. *European Journal of Pharmacology, 66,* 121–123.

Henriksen, S.J., Bloom, F.E., McCoy, F., et al. (1978). β-endorphin induces non-convulsive limbic seizures. *Proceedings of the National Academy of Sciences of the United States of America, 75,* 5221–5225.

Herman, B.H., & Goldstein, A. (1981). Cataleptic effects of dynorphin (1–13) in rats made tolerant to *mu* opiate receptor agonist. *Neuropeptides, 2,* 13–22.

Holaday, J.W., & Belenky, G.L. (1980). Opiate-like effects of electro-convulsive shock in rats: A differential effect of naloxone on nociceptive measures. *Life Sciences, 27,* 1929–1934.

Hollt, V., Przenlock, R., & Herz, A. (1978). Radioimmunoassay of β-endorphin basal and stimulated levels in extracted rat plasma. *Naunyn Schmiedebergs Archives of Pharmacology, 303,* 171–174.

Holmes, G.L., & Weber, D.A. (1985). Effect of ACTH on seizure susceptibility in the developing brain. *Epilepsia, 26,* 517.

Honda, T., White, H.S., Chow, S.Y., et al. (1985). The effects of ACTH and prednisone on electroshock seizures, development, and brain, water, and electrolyte contents of newborn rats. *Society for Neuroscience Abstracts, 11,* 900.

Houghton, R.A., Johnson, N., & Pasternak, G.W. (1984). {³H}-β-endorphin binding in rat brain. *Journal of Neuroscience, 4,* 2460–2466.

Hrachovy, R.A., Frost, J.D., Kellaway, P., et al. (1983). Double blind study of ACTH vs prednisone therapy in infantile spasms. *Journal of Pediatrics, 103,* 641–645.

Jeavons, P.M. & Bower, B.D. (1964). Infantile spasms: A review of the literature and a study of 112 cases. *Clinics in Developmental Medicine* (No. 15). London: Spastic Society and Heineman.

Joseph, S.A., Pilcher, W.H., & Krigge, K.M. (1985). Anatomy of the corticotropin-releasing factor and opiomelanocortin systems of the brain. *Federation Proceedings, 44,* 100–107.

Katz, R.J. (1980). Behavioral effects of dynorphin: A novel opioid neuropeptide. *Neuropharmacology, 19,* 801–803.

Klein, R., & Livingston, S. (1950). The effect of adrenocorticotrophic hormone in epilepsy. *Journal of Pediatrics, 37,* 733–742.

Kosterlitz, H.W., Lord, J.A.H., Paterson, S.J., et al. (1980). Effects of changes in the structure of enkephalins and of narcotic analgesic drugs on their interactions with μ and δ receptors. *British Journal of Pharmacology, 68,* 333–342.

Krieger, D.T., & Liotta, A.S. (1979). Pituitary hormones in brain: Where, how, and why? *Science, 205,* 366–372.

Krieger, D.T., & Martin, J.B. (1985). Brain peptides. *New England Journal of Medicine, 304,* 876–885.

Krivoy, W.A. (1970). Effects of ACTH and related polypeptides on spinal cord. *Progress in Brain Research, 32,* 108–119.

Lacy, J.R., & Penry, J.K. (1976). *Infantile spasms.* New York: Raven Press.

Le Gal La Salle, G., Calvino, B., & Ben-Ari, Y. (1977). Morphine enhances amygdaloid seizures and increases interictal spike frequency in kindled rats. *Neuroscience Letters, 6,* 255–260.

Law, P., Loh, H.H., & Li, C.H. (1979). Properties and localization of β-endorphin receptor in rat brain. *Proceedings of the National Academy of Sciences of the United States of America, 76,* 5455–5459.

Lee, R.J., Bajorek, L.G., & Lomax, P. (1984). Similar anticonvulsant, but unique, behavioral effects of opioid agonists in the seizure-sensitive mongolian gerbil. *Neuropharmacology, 23,* 517–524.

Lewis, J.W., Caldecott-Hazard, S., Cannon, J.T., et al. (1981). Possible role of opioid peptides in pain inhibition and seizures. *Advances in Biochemical Psychopharmacology, 28,* 213–224.

Lewis, J.W., Cannon, J.T., & Liebeskind, J.C. (1980). Opioid and nonopioid mechanisms of stress analgesia. *Science, 208,* 623–626.

Lord, J.A.H., Waterfield, A.A., Hughes. J., et al. (1977). Endogenous opioid peptides: Multiple agonists and receptors. *Nature, 267,* 495–499.

Mannino, R.A., & Wolf, H.H. (1975). Morphine's proconvulsant action: Importance of endogenous norepinephrine. *Life Sciences, 16,* 1659–1668.

McQuarie, I., Andersson, J.A., Ziegler, M.R. (1942). Observations on antagonistic effects of posterior pituitary and corticoadrenal hormones in the epileptic subject. *Journal of Clinical Endocrinology and Metabolism, 2,* 406–410.

Meldrum, B.S., Menini, C., Stutzmann, J.M., et al. (1979). Effects of opiate-like peptides, morphine, and naloxone in the photosensitive baboon, Papio papio. *Brain Research, 170,* 333–348.

Miller, R.J. (1981). Peptides as neurotransmitters: Focus on the enkephalins, endorphins. *Pharmacology and Therapeutics, 12,* 73–108.

Montplaisir, J., Saint-Hilaire, J.M., Walsh, J.T., et al. (1981). Naloxone and focal epilepsy: A study with depth electrodes. *Neurology, 31,* 350–352.

Nabeshima, T., Matsuno, K., & Kameyama, T. (1985).

Involvement of different opioid receptor subtypes in electrical shock-induced analgesia and motor suppression in the rat. *European Journal of Pharmacology, 114*, 197–207.

Nalin, A., Facchinetti, F., Galli, V., et al. (1985). Reduced ACTH content in cerebrospinal fluid of children affected by cryptogenic infantile spasms with hypsarrhythmia. *Epilepsia, 26*, 446–449.

Nishimura, S.L., Recht, L.D., & Pasternak, G.W. (1984). Biochemical characterization of high affinity {^{3}H}-opioid binding: Further evidence for Mu_1 sites. *Molecular Pharmacology, 25*, 29–37.

Oka, T., Negishi, K., Kajiwara, M., et al. (1982). The choice of opiate receptor subtype by neo-endorphins. *European Journal of Pharmacology, 79*, 301–305.

Olpe, H.R., & Jones, R.S.G. (1982). Excitatory effects of ACTH on noradrenergic neurons of the locus coeruleus in the rat. *Brain Research, 251*, 177–179.

Pasternak, G.W., Childers, S.R., & Snyder, S.H. (1980). Naloxazone, long acting opiate antagonist: Effects in intact animals and on opiate receptor binding in vitro. *Journal of Pharmacology and Experimental Therapeutics, 214*, 455–462.

Pasternak, G.W., Zhany, A., & Tecott, L. (1980). Developmental differences between high and low affinity opiate binding sites: Their relationship to analgesia and respiratory depression. *Life Sciences, 27*, 1185–1190.

Pelletier, G., LeClerc, R., Saveedra, J.M., et al. (1980). Distribution of β-lipotropin (β-LPH), adrenocorticotropin (ACTH), and α-melanocyte stimulating hormone (-MSH) in the rat brain. I. Origin of the extrahypothalamic fibers. *Brain Research, 192*, 433–440.

Pentella, K., Bachman, D.S., & Sandman, C.A. (1982). Trial of an ACTH 4–9 analog (ORG 2766) in children with intractable seizures. *Neuropediatrics, 13*, 59–62.

Pert, C.B., & Snyder, S.H. (1973). Opiate receptor: Demonstration in nervous tissue. *Science, 179*, 1011–1014.

Przewlocka, B., Stala, L., Lason, W., et al. (1983). The effect of various opiate receptor agonists on the seizure threshold in the rat. Is dynorphin an endogenous anticonvulsant? *Life Sciences, 33*(Suppl 1), 595–598.

Quiron, R., & Pert, C.B. (1981). Dynorphins: Similar relative potencies on μ-, δ- and κ-opiate receptors. *European Journal of Pharmacology, 76*, 467–468.

Rose, R., & Bridger, W.H. (1982). Hormonal influences in seizure kindling: the effects of post-stimulation ACTH or cortisone injections. *Brain Research, 231*, 75–84.

Rothman, R.B., & Westfall, T.C. (1981). Allostearic modulation by leucine-enkephalin of {^{3}H}-naloxone binding in rat brain. *European Journal of Pharmacology, 72*, 365–368.

Rothman, R.B., & Westfall, T.C. (1982). Morphine allostearically modulates the binding of {^{3}H}-leucine-enkephalin to a particulate fraction of rat brain. *Molecular Pharmacology, 21*, 538–547.

Rothman, R.B., & Westfall, T.C. (1983). Interaction of leucine-enkephalin with {$3βH$}-naloxone binding in rat brain. *Neurochemical Research, 8*, 913–931.

Shippenberg, T.S., & Altshuller, H.C. (1982). Electroencephalographic effects of alcohol, opiate peptides and tetrahydroisoquinolines. *Federation Proceedings, 41*, 1465.

Shultz, R., Wuster, A., & Herz, A. (1981). Pharmacolog-

ical characterization of the ε-opiate receptor. *Journal of Pharmacology and Experimental Therapeutics, 216*, 604–606.

Snead, O.C. (1983). On the sacred disease: The neurochemistry of epilepsy. *International Reviews of Neurobiology, 24*, 94–180.

Snead, O.C. (1984). Neuropeptides and infantile spasms: Search for an animal model. In R.J. Porter, R.H. Mattson, A.A.Ward, et al. (Eds.), *Advances in epileptology: XVth Epilepsy International Symposium* (pp. 193–196). New York: Raven Press.

Snead, O.C. (1985). Enkephalin-induced seizures: μ or δ? *Society for Neuroscience Abstracts, 11*, 908.

Snead, O.C., & Bearden, L.J. (1980a). Anticonvulsant specific for petit mal antagonize epileptogenic effect of leucine-enkephalin. *Science, 210*, 1031–1033.

Snead, O.C., & Bearden, L.J. (1980b). Naloxone overcomes the dopaminergic, EEG, and behavioral effects of γ-hydroxybutyrate. *Neurology, 30*, 832–838.

Snead, O.C., & Bearden, L.J. (1982). The epileptogenic spectrum of opiate agonists. *Neuropharmacology, 21*, 1137–1144.

Snead, O.C., Benton, J.W., Myers, G.J. (1983). ACTH and prednisone in childhood seizure disorders. *Neurology, 33*, 966–970.

Snyder, S.H., & Innis, R.B. (1979). Peptide neurotransmitters. *Annual Review of Biochemistry, 48*, 755–782.

Sorel, L., Dusaucy-Bauloye, A. (1958). A propos dans d'hypsarhythmia de Gibbs: Son traitement spectaculaire par l'ACTH. *Acta Neurologica Psychiatrica Belgica, 58*, 130–141.

Steiner, F.A., Ruff, A., & Akert, K. (1969). Steroid-sensitive neurones in rat brain: Anatomical localization and responses to neurohumors and ACTH. *Brain Research, 12*, 74–81.

Stone, W.S., Eggleton, C.E., & Berman, R.F. (1982). Opiate modification of amygdaloid-kindled seizures in rats. *Pharmacology, Biochemistry, & Behavior, 16*, 751–756.

Terenius, L., Gispen, W.H., & de Wied, D. (1975). ACTH-like peptides and opiate receptors in rat brain: Structure-activity studies. *European Journal of Pharmacology, 33*, 395–402.

Torda, C., & Wolff, H.G. (1952). Effects of various concentrations of adrenocorticotrophic hormone on electrical activity of brain and on sensitivity to convulsion-inducing agents. *American Journal of Physiology, 168*, 406–415.

Tortella, F.C., Cowan, A., & Adler, M.W. (1981). Comparison of the anticonvulsant effects of opioid peptides and etorphine in rats. *Life Sciences, 29*, 1039–1045.

Tortella, F.C., & Long, I.B. (1985). Endogenous anticonvulsant substance in rat cerebrospinal fluid after a generalized seizure. *Science, 228*, 1106–1108.

Tortella, F.C., Robles, L.E., Holaday, J.W., et al. (1983). A selective role for δ-receptors in the regulation of opioid-induced changes in seizure threshold. *Life Sciences, 33* (Suppl 1), 603–606.

Tortella, F.C., Robles, L., & Holaday, J.W. (1985a). The anticonvulsant effects of DADL are primarily mediated by activation of δ opioid receptor: Interactions between δ and μ receptor antagonists. *Life Sciences, 37*, 497–503.

Tortella, F.C., Robles, L., & Holaday, J.W. (1985b). Seizure threshold studies with dynorphin (1–13) in rats: Possible interactions among κ, μ, and δ opioid binding sites. *Pharmacologist, 27,* 179.

Tulunay, F.C., Jen, M., Chang, J., et al. (1981). Possible regulatory role of dynorphin on morphine and β-endorphin-induced analgesia. *Journal of Pharmacology and Experimental Therapeutics, 219,* 296–298.

Turski, W.A., Czuczuar, S.J., Kleinrok, Z., et al. (1983). Intraamygdaloid morphine produces seizures and brain damage in rats. *Life Sciences, 33,* (Suppl 1), 615–618.

Urban, I., & de Wied, D. (1976). Changes in excitability of the theta generating substrate by ACTH 4–10 in the rat. *Experimental Brain Research, 24,* 325–334.

Urban, I., Lopes da Silva, F.H., Storm van Leeuwen, W., et al. (1974). A frequency shift in the hippocampal theta activity: An electrical correlate of central action of ACTH analogues in the dog? *Brain Research, 69,* 361–365.

Urca, G., & Frenk, H. (1982). Systemic morphine blocks the seizures induced by intracerebroventricular (ICV) injections of opiates and opiate peptides. *Brain Research, 246,* 121–126.

Urca, G., & Frenk, H. (1983). Intracerebral opiates block the epileptic effect of intracerebroventricular (ICV) leucine-enkephalin. *Brain Research, 259,* 103–110.

Urca, G., Frenk, H., Liebeskind, J.C., et al. (1977). Morphine and enkephalin: Analgesic and epileptic properties. *Science, 197,* 83–86.

Urca, G., Yitzhaky, J., & Frenk, H. (1981). Different opioid systems may participate in post-electroconvulsive shock (ECS) analgesia and catalepsy. *Brain Research, 219,* 385–390.

van Delft, A.M.L., Kitay, J.I. (1972). Effect of ACTH on single unit activity in the diencephalon of intact and hypophysectomized rats. *Neuroendocrinology, 9,* 188–196.

Watson, S.J., Richard, C.W., & Barchas, J.D. (1978). Adrenocorticotropin in rat brain: Immunocytochemical localization in cells and axons. *Science, 200,* 1080–1082.

Wiegant, U.M., Jolles, J., Colbern, D.L., et al. (1979). Intracerebroventricular ACTH activates the pituitary-adrenal system: Dissociation from a behavioral response. *Life Sciences, 25,* 1971–1976.

Willig, R.P., & Lagenstein, I. (1982). Use of ACTH fragments in children with infantile spasms. *Neuropediatrics, 13,* 55–58.

Willig, R.P., Lagenstein, I., & Iffland, E. (1977). Cortisoltages profile under ACTH-und Dexamethasontherapie Frühkindlicher Anfälle (BNS-und Lennox Syndrome). *Monatsschr Kinderheilkd, 136,* 191–197.

Wuster, M., Schultz, R., & Herz, A. (1981). Multiple opiate receptors in peripheral tissue preparations. *Biochemical Pharmacology, 30,* 18830–18870.

Yitzhaky, J., Frenk, H., & Urca, G. (1982). Kindling-induced changes in morphine analgesia and catalepsy: Evidence for independent opioid systems. *Brain Research, 237,* 193–201.

Zimmerman, E., & Krivoy, W.A. (1973). Antagonism between morphine and the polypeptides ACTH, $ACTH_{1-24}$, and β- in the nervous system. *Progress in Brain Research, 39,* 383–399.

Zwiers, H., Alogo, V.J., & Gispen, W.H. (1981). Behavior and neurochemical effects of the new opioid peptide dynorphin-(1–13):Comparison with other neuropeptides. *Life Sciences, 28,* 2545–2551.

Chapter 16

Neonatal Seizures

Michael J. Painter

THE DIAGNOSIS OF NEONATAL SEIZURES IS based on clinically observed activity that is stereotyped, repetitive, and usually associated with abnormal eye movements. Five seizure patterns are usually delineated (Volpe, 1977):

1. *Tonic seizures* are characterized by extension of the extremities resembling decerebrate posturing.
2. *Subtle seizures* are characterized by isolated and often brief abnormal eye movements, sucking, rowing, pedaling, or swimming movements.
3. *Multifocal clonic seizures* are characterized by migration of activity from limb to limb in a random pattern.
4. *Focal clonic seizures* are localized to a single limb.
5. *Myoclonic seizures* are repetitive flexion movements of the arms. These seizure pattern types are less developed and less obvious than those observed in older children. The reason for this variance is because of the differing organizations of the immature and mature brains. Glial proliferation, neuronal migration, formation of axonal and dendritic contacts, and myelin deposition are incomplete in the neonatal brain. Additionally, electrical discharges are incompletely spread, tend to remain localized to one hemisphere, and diffuse slowly from their origin (Dreyfus-Brisac, 1964).

Not all repetitive neonatal movements are seizures. Jitteriness, or neonatal clonus, can be distinguished from seizures by being stimulus-provoked, ablated with change in posture or restraint, and unaccompanied by abnormal eye movements.

Observations obtained through video EEG monitoring have cast doubt upon the epileptic nature of some clinical patterns. Tonic "seizures" are usually not associated with cortical electrical discharges, and in many instances are due to a lack of cerebral inhibition (Kellaway & Hrachovy, 1983). Swimming, pedaling, and rowing movements, often called subtle "seizures," may or may not be associated with electrical seizures. Focal clonic activity associated with eye deviation is most often associated with cortical electrical discharge (Kellaway & Hrachovy, 1983; Mizrahi & Kellaway, 1984).

The frequent use of neuromuscular paralyzing agents in the treatment of neonatal cardiorespiratory disorders complicates the task of detecting seizure activity. Electrical seizures occur in a significant number of infants who have been paralyzed in order to facilitate pulmonary ventilation (Tharp & Laboyrie, 1983).

Although some, and perhaps a significant, percentage of neonatal paroxysmal discharges may originate from subcortical gray matter and are not reflected in scalp electrode monitoring, there is little doubt that continuous EEG monitoring will dramatically influence the diagnosis and management of neonatal seizures.

The diagnosis and treatment of neonatal seizures is important. Neonatal seizures are adverse predictors of neurological outcome in asphyxiated newborns (Mulligan et al., 1980), and are predictors of cerebral palsy in high risk populations (Nelson & Broman, 1977; Nelson

& Ellenberg, 1979). Although the underlying etiology and extent of brain injury are obviously crucial, there is experimental evidence to suggest that seizures per se may be damaging to the developing brain. Further, changes in systemic blood pressure and increases in the anterior cerebral blood flow velocity during seizures are harmful to premature neonates, resulting in an increased risk of hemorrhage and elevation of intracranial pressure (Perlman & Volpe, 1983).

Most neonatologists and child neurologists seek the prevention of neonatal seizures, as well as early accurate detection followed by prompt, effective treatment.

ETIOLOGY AND APPROACH

The main diagnostic considerations of neonatal seizures are listed in Table 1. Rational treatment is based on accurate diagnosis. An accurate history is difficult to obtain. The mother is usually remote from the intensive care unit, is often on another floor, and is sometimes located in another hospital. Additionally, infant transportation teams do not always have time to obtain the complete details regarding labor and delivery. It is important for one individual, who is responsible for the infant's care, to review historical details with appropriate individuals. Some causes of neonatal seizures masquerade as hypoxic-ischemic encephalopathy, and are missed without a proper history. Similarly, blood pressure should not be overlooked, because hypertensive encephalopathy may cause seizures in neonates, and the appropriate treatment is the control of blood pressure and not the use of anticonvulsant drugs. Additionally, indirect funduscopy should be carefully performed, as retinal hemorrhages are clues to trauma, and chorioretinitis is a clue to infection. Also, skin lesions can be a clue to infection or to neurocutaneous syndromes. Finally, every infant with neonatal seizures should have a cerebrospinal fluid examination.

Metabolic abnormalities should be considered first in the evaluation of neonates with seizures, as these disorders demand specific therapy. As noted in Table 1, abnormalities of

Table 1. The main diagnostic considerations of neonatal seizures

1. Trauma
   a. Subdural hematoma
   b. Intracortical hemorrhage
   c. Cortical vein thrombosis
2. Hypoxia-ischemia, germinal matrix hemorrhage
3. Cerebral dysgenesis
4. Hypertension
5. Metabolic
   a. Hypocalcemia
      1. Hypomagnesemia
      2. High phosphate load
      3. IDM
      4. Hypoparathyroidism
      5. Maternal hyperparathyroidism
      6. Idiopathic
   b. Hypoglycemia
      1. Galactosemia
      2. IUGR
      3. IDM
      4. Glycogen storage disease
      5. Idiopathic
   c. Electrolyte imbalance
      1. Hypernatremia
      2. Hyponatremia
6. Infections
   a. Bacterial meningitis
   b. Cerebral abscess
   c. Herpes encephalitis
   d. Coxsackie meningoencephalitis
   e. Cytomegalovirus
   f. Toxoplasmosis
   g. Syphilis
7. Drug withdrawal
   a. Methadone
   b. Heroin
   c. Barbiturate
   d. Propoxyphene
8. Pyridoxine dependency
9. Amino acid disturbance
   a. Maple syrup urine disease
   b. Urea cycle abnormalities
   c. Nonketotic hyperglycinemia
   d. Ketotic hyperglycinemia
10. Toxins
    a. Local anesthetics
    b. Isoniazid
    c. Bilirubin
11. Familial seizures
    a. Neurocutaneous syndromes
       1. Tuberous sclerosis
       2. Incontinentia pigmenti
    b. Genetic syndromes
       1. Zellweger
       2. Smith-Lemli-Opitz
       3. Neonatal adrenoleukodystrophy
    c. Benign familial epilepsy

glucose, calcium, amino acid, urea cycle, and organic acid metabolism may cause neonatal seizures as part of their clinical presentation. Pyridoxine dependency must also be considered. The initial laboratory investigation should therefore include tests for blood glucose, calcium, magnesium, electrolytes, blood gases, blood ammonia, a urine screen for amino acids, and, in special circumstances, a urine evaluation of organic acids.

Hypoglycemia, hypocalcemia, and hyponatremia can occur in combination with structural disease such as hypoxia or hemorrhage, and should be treated in the overall approach to these disorders.

Pyridoxine dependency is an autosomal recessive trait characterized by intractable, generalized clonic seizures occurring shortly after birth (Clarke, Saunders, & Feldman, 1979). Infants with pyridoxine dependency are commonly born meconium stained and flaccid. The presence of those symptoms may lead to a misdiagnosis of perinatal hypoxia-ischemia.

The diagnosis of pyridoxine dependency is confirmed when seizures respond after 100 mg. of pyridoxine is given intravenously with EEG monitoring. The seizures cease within minutes, and the EEG, which is characterized by generalized spike, polyspike, and burst suppression patterns, becomes normal in hours. With such patients, pyridoxine supplementation is maintained for life.

Maple syrup urine disease is an autosomal recessive disorder that results when the human body is unable to decarboxylate the amino acids leucine, isoleucine, and valine. Newborns with Maple syrup urine disease usually appear well until protein feeding is instituted. The characteristics of this disorder include vomiting, convulsions, hypertonia, and acidosis.

Seizures in the newborn may be caused by the withdrawal of medications (usually hypnotics or analgesics) taken by the mother during late pregnancy. Seizures usually occur following withdrawal from shorter acting barbiturates such as secobarbital rather than the longer acting agents such as phenobarbital (Desmond, Schwanecke, Wilson, Yasunaga, & Birgdorff,

1972). Maternal heroin addiction frequently results in a neonatal syndrome of jitters, but seizures are uncommon.

The newborn may inadvertently receive substantial amounts of local anesthetic intended for the mother during labor and delivery, and the injection of these procaine substances into the neonate has been described following saddle block, paracervical, and pudendal anesthesia. Local anesthetic toxicity mimics hypoxia ischemia. Meconium staining, flaccidity, and apnea are characteristic findings. The cranial nerve abnormalities and cardiac arrhythmias that are uncommon in asphyxia are also found. Determination of local anesthetic blood levels in the newborn confirms the diagnosis. Testing of levels must be performed shortly after birth, as procaine derivations are rapidly metabolized. Treatment consists of diuresis and acidification of the urine (Hillman, Hillman, & Dodson, 1979). Conventional anticonvulsants may be of some benefit, but measures to promote drug elimination are of greater importance.

Asphyxia and/or intracranial hemorrhage are the most common causes of neonatal seizures in most series (Bergman, Painter, Hirsch, Crumrine, & David, 1983; Volpe, 1977). Neonatal stroke has recently drawn attention as an etiology of neonatal seizures, but its prevalence is unknown.

Seizures due to asphyxia and/or hemorrhage are generalized, clonic, or multifocal in type. The seizures are most severe in the first 72 hours after delivery; seizures then subside, irrespective of therapy. Tonic seizures seen in these disorders may be due to lack of forebrain inhibition.

With improved obstetric delivery techniques, trauma as a cause of neonatal seizures has largely disappeared. Subdural and epidural hematomas, now rarely a cause, are associated with a bulging fontanelle, retinal hemorrhage, and irritability. Large newborns delivered to primigravida mothers with difficult labors, and small newborns delivered precipitously, appear at greatest risk for trauma to the nervous system.

Incontinentia pigmenti and tuberous sclerosis have caused seizures in the newborn. Incontinentia pigmenti is characterized by a vesicular, crusting rash, mimicking herpes simplex. When the vesicular rash heals, it leaves a lightly pigmented, whorled cutaneous lesion. Seizures are usually generalized clonic and respond readily to anticonvulsant therapy. Two neonates with tuberous sclerosis and symptomatic subependymal giant cell tumors have been described. One had patches of unusually pigmented hair and refractory generalized seizures (Painter, Pang, Ahdab-Barmada, & Bergman, 1984).

Neonatal adrenoleukodystrophy, a progressive neurodegenerative disorder, has been found to cause neonatal seizures. Unlike the later childhood variant of this disease, which is transmitted as a sex-linked trait, neonatal adrenoleukodystrophy is transmitted by autosomal recessive inheritance (Jaffe, Crumrine, Hashida, & Moser, 1982).

Benign familial neonatal convulsions have been identified in several families and are characterized by generalized and focal seizures that occur during the first 2 weeks of life (Carton 1978). These seizures are relatively refractory

to anticonvulsant medication, but the outcome is good. The cause is unknown.

ANTICONVULSANT TREATMENT

When a specific metabolic disorder is not found, anticonvulsant drugs are used to treat newborn seizures. There is experimental data suggesting adverse effects of many anticonvulsant drugs on brain growth (Diaz, Schain, & Bailey, 1977; Swaiman, Schrier, Neale, & Nelson, 1980), but most child neurologists and neonatologists agree that neonatal seizures should be effectively treated.

There are no studies demonstrating the superiority of phenobarbital, phenytoin, or the benzodiazepines, but at present, phenobarbital is the initial drug chosen in almost all neonatal units (Boer & Gal, 1982). It is clear that loading doses of at least 20 mg/kg of phenobarbital should be given intravenously to achieve effective but nontoxic levels (Lockman, Kriel, Zaske, Thompson, & Virnis, 1979; Painter et al., 1981) (Figure 1). Seizure control has been reported in 85% of newborns when doses of up to 40 mg/kg are utilized (Gal, Toback, Boer,

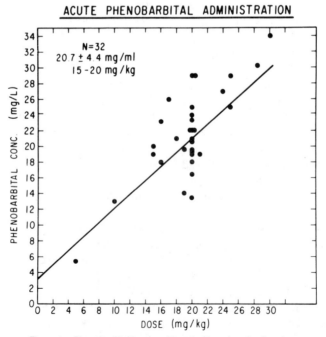

Figure 1.   Phenobarbital levels achieved with various loading doses.

Erkan, & Wells, 1982). As the volume of distribution of phenobarbital in the newborn is 0.9 ± 0.1 L/kg, a significant number of infants will achieve blood levels above 50 mg/l with these high loading doses. At these high blood concentrations, a decrease in heart rate below 100 and decreased heart rate variability have been noted (Svenningsen, Blennow, Lindroth, Gäddlin, & Ahlström, 1982). Data regarding the cardiovascular effects of phenobarbital concentrations above 40 mg/l are limited.

Because the half-life of phenobarbital is relatively long in newborns, maintenance doses of 2–4 mg/kg/day are sufficient. After 2 weeks, metabolism and/or clearance of phenobarbital increases, and plasma concentrations can be expected to decrease. As can be seen in Figure 2, seizure control is unusual below a level of 16 mg/l (Lockman et al., 1979).

Phenytoin is the second agent most often selected when phenobarbital fails. Like phenobarbital, loading doses of 20 mg/kg must be utilized to obtain plasma concentrations of 15–20 mg/l (Figure 3). Intravenous maintenance dosages are within the range of 4–6 mg/kg/

day. Oral doses as high as 12–16 mg/kg/day are necessary to maintain effective plasma concentrations in early infancy. Careful monitoring is necessary, as drug accumulation may be a problem. The brain/plasma ratios of phenobarbital and phenytoin, reflecting distribution of the drug to the brain, are approximately 1.0 and 1.2 (Painter et al., 1981) respectively. These values are comparable to those reported in adults (Sherwin, Wisen, & Sogolowski, 1973; Vajda, Williams, Davidson, Falconer, & Brechenridge, 1974).

Utilizing both phenobarbital and phenytoin at loading doses of 20 mg/k, approximately 70% of neonatal seizures can be controlled (Painter, Pippenger, MacDonald, & Pitlick, 1978).

Primidone may be of value in treating newborns whose seizures are refractory to phenobarbital and phenytoin (Powell, Painter, & Pippenger, 1984). In newborns, primidone is not converted to phenobarbital as it is in older children, but it does impair phenobarbital clearance. This results in a precipitous rise in phenobarbital levels following primidone loading. Primidone loading doses of 15–20 mg/kg

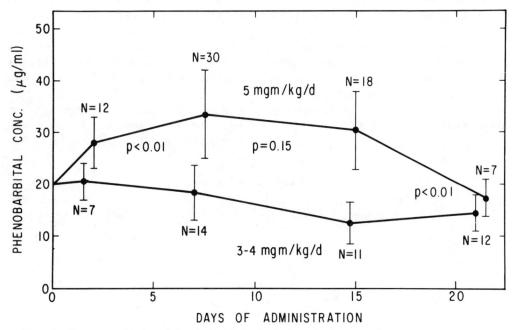

Figure 2.   Plasma concentrations of phenobarbital during the first 3 weeks of therapy utilizing two dosage schedules.

ACUTE DIPHENYLHYDANTOIN ADMINISTRATION

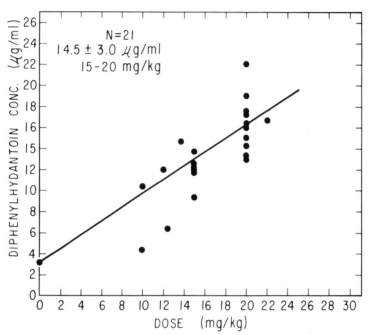

Figure 3.   Phenytoin plasma concentrations at various loading doses.

and maintenance doses of 12–20 mg/kg/day are recommended. The lowest effective primidone level is 6 mg/L.

Similarly, diazepam is an effective anticonvulsant when administered as a continuous intravenous infusion diluted in isotonic saline at a rate of 0.3 mg/kg/hour (Gamstorp & Sedin, 1982). At these doses, the drug causes somnolence in term infants but does not compromise respiration. Effective blood levels are from 35 umol/L to 80.5 umol/L.

Paraldehyde is reported as an effective anticonvulsant in the newborn when administered as a 4% solution intravenously. However, this agent has produced pulmonary edema, pulmonary hemorrhage, and hypotension in older children (Sinal & Crowe, 1976) and should be used with caution in the neonate. Loading doses of 200 mg/kg of paraldehyde followed by infusion of 16–20 mg/kg/hr or 200 mg/kg/hr for 2 hours can be expected to produce effective plasma concentrations (above 10 mg/dl) (Koren, Butt, Rajchgot et al., 1986).

REFERENCES

Bergman, I., Painter, M.J., Hirsch, R.P., Crumrine, P.K., & David, R. (1983). Outcome in neonates with convulsions treated in an intensive care unit. *Annals of Neurology, 14*(6), 642–647.

Boer, H.R., & Gal, P. (1982). Neonatal seizures: A survey of current practice. *Clinical Pediatrics, 21,* 453–457.

Carton, D. (1978). Benign familial neonatal convulsions. *Neuropediatrics, 9*(2), 167–171.

Clarke, T.H., Saunders, B.S., & Feldman, B. (1979). Pyridoxine-dependent seizures requiring high doses of pyridoxine for control. *American Journal of Diseases of Children, 133,* 963–965.

Desmond, M.M., Schwanecke, R.P., Wilson, G.S.,

Yasunaga, S., & Birgdorff, I. (1972). Maternal barbiturate utilization and neonatal withdrawal symptomatology. *Journal of Pediatrics, 80,* 190–197.

Diaz, J., Schain, R. J., & Bailey, B.G. (1977). Phenobarbital-induced brain growth retardation in artificially reared rat pups. *Biology of the Neonate, 32*(1–2), 77–82.

Dreyfus-Brisac, C. (1964). The electroencephalogram of the premature infant and full-term newborn. In P. Kellaway & I. Petersen (Eds.), *Neurological and electroencephalographic correlative studies in infancy* (pp. 186–207). New York: Grune & Stratton.

Gal, P., Toback, J., Boer, H.R., Erkan, M.V., & Wells,

I.J. (1982). Efficacy of phenobarbital monotherapy in treatment of neonatal seizures—relationship to blood levels. *Neurology, 32,* 1401–1404.

Gamstorp, I., & Sedin, G. (1982). Neonatal convulsions treated with continuous intravenous infusion of diazepam. *Upsala Journal of Medical Sciences, 87,* 143–149.

Hillman, L.S., Hillman, R.E., & Dodson, W.E. (1979). Diagnosis, treatment and follow-up of neonatal mepivacine intoxication secondary to paracervical and pudendal blocks during labor. *Journal of Pediatrics, 95,* 472–477.

Jaffe, R., Crumrine, P., Hashida, Y., & Moser, H.W. (1982). Neonatal adrenoleukodystrophy: Clinical, pathologic, and biochemical delineation of a syndrome affecting both males and females. *American Journal of Pathology, 108*(1), 100–111.

Kellaway, P., & Hrachovy, R.H. (1983). Status epilepticus in newborns: A perspective on neonatal seizures. *Annals of Neurology, 34,* 93–99.

Koren, G., Butt, W., Rajchgot, P., et al. (1986). Intravenous paraldehyde for seizure control in newborn infants. *Neurology, 36,* 108–111.

Lockman, L.A., Kriel, R., Zaske, D., Thompson, T., & Virnis, M. (1979). Phenobarbital dosage for control of neonatal seizures. *Neurology, 29*(11), 1445–1449.

Mizrahi, E.M., & Kellaway, P. (1984). Characterization of seizures in neonates and young infants by time-synchronized electroencephalographic/polygraphic/video monitoring. (Abstract). *Annals of Neurology, 16,* 383.

Mulligan, J.C., Painter, M.J., O'Donoghue, P.H., MacDonald, H.M., Hilan, A.C., & Taylor, P.M. (1980). Neonatal asphyxia. II. Neonatal mortality and long-term sequelae. *Journal of Pediatrics, 96*(5), 903–907.

Nelson, K.B., & Broman, S.H. (1977). Perinatal risk factors in children with serious motor and mental handicaps. *Annals of Neurology, 2*(5), 371–377.

Nelson, K.B., & Ellenberg, J.H. (1979). Neonatal signs as predictors of cerebral palsy. *Pediatrics, 64,* 225.

Painter, M.J., Pang, D., Ahdab-Barmada, M., & Bergman, I. (1984). Connatal brain tumors in patients with tuberous sclerosis. *Neurosurgery, 14*(5), 570–573.

Painter, M.J., Pippenger, C., MacDonald, H., & Pitlick, W. (1978). Phenobarbital and diphenylhydantoin levels in neonates with seizures. *Journal of Pediatrics, 92*(2), 315–319.

Painter, M.J., Pippenger, C., Wasterlain, C., Barmada, M., Pitlick, W., Carter, G., & Abern, S. (1981). Phenobarbital and phenytoin in neonatal seizures: Metabolism and tissue distribution. *Neurology, 31*(9), 1107–1112.

Perlman, J.M., & Volpe, J.J. (1983). Seizures in the preterm infant: Effects on cerebral blood flow velocity, intracranial pressure, and arterial blood pressure. *Journal of Pediatrics, 102*(2), 288–293.

Powell, C., Painter, M.J., & Pippenger, C.E. (1984). Primidone therapy in refractory neonatal seizures. *Journal of Pediatrics, 105*(4), 651–654.

Sherwin, A.L., Wisen, A.A., & Sogolowski, C.D. (1973). Anticonvulsant drugs in human epileptogenic brain. Correlation of phenobarbital and diphenylhydantoin levels with plasma. *Archives of Neurology, 29,* 73–77.

Sinal, S.H., & Crowe, J.E. (1976). Cyanosis, cough and hypotension following intravenous administration of paraldehyde. *Pediatrics, 57*(1), 158–159.

Svenningsen, N.W., Blennow, G., Lindroth, M., Gäddlin, P.W., & Ahlström, H. (1982). Brain-oriented intensive care treatment in severe neonatal asphyxia. Effects of phenobarbitone protection. *Archives of Diseases of Childhood, 57*(3), 176–183.

Swaiman, K.F., Schrier, B.K., Neale, E.A., & Nelson, P.G. (1980). Effects of chronic phenytoin and valproic acid exposure on fetal mouse cortical cultures. (Abstract). *Annals of Neurology, 8,* 230.

Tharp, B.R., & Laboyrie, P.M. (1983). The incidence of EEG abnormalities and outcome of infants paralyzed with neuromuscular blocking agents. *Critical Care Medicine, 11*(12), 926–929.

Vajda, F., Williams, F.M., Davidson, S., Falconer, M.H., Brechenridge, H. (1974). Human brain, cerebrospinal fluid, and plasma concentrations of diphenylhydantoin and phenobarbital. *Clinical Pharmacology and Therapeutics, 15*(6), 597–603.

Volpe, J.J. (1977). Management of neonatal seizures. *Critical Care Medicine, 5*(1), 43–49.

Chapter 17

The Epidemiology of Chronic Neurologic Diseases of Children in Sweden

Mårten Kyllerman

AN ADEQUATE KNOWLEDGE OF THE SIZE and composition of the large neuropediatric handicap groups is a necessary prerequisite for the planning of medical diagnostic, therapeutic, and supportive services as well as for everyday clinical work. Exact data can only be derived from well controlled population-based studies; these studies are difficult to perform and consequently there are few of them. Sweden has a well-organized health care community, with a uniform system of health and hospital care and well-developed services for all children with mental and motor handicaps. This system offers good opportunities for population-based epidemiological studies.

CEREBRAL PALSY

Cerebral palsy (CP) is defined as a permanent impairment of movement or posture resulting from a nonprogressive brain disorder. The disorder is caused by hereditary factors or events taking place during pregnancy, delivery, the neonatal period, and the first 2 years of life. The same concept and classification system of CP have been employed in Sweden since 1958 (Hagberg, Hagberg, & Olow, 1975).

Epidemiological Trends

Hagberg and Hagberg (1984) reported on epidemiological trends in CP observed in a population-based series of studies of 773 patients born between 1959 and 1978 in southwest and central Sweden. This series included children with mental retardation. During the first three 4-year periods from 1959–1970, there was a significant decreasing tendency from 1.9 to 1.4 CP cases per 1000 live-born children. This was followed by a significant increase in the last periods, reaching 2.0 CP cases per 1000 children in the period 1975–1978. Preliminary data indicate no decrease from 1979–1980.

The decreases during the 1950s and the 1960s and the increase during the 1970s were mainly referrable to spastic/ataxic diplegia in CP children born preterm and to dyskinetic syndromes in children born at term. Preliminary results indicate an increasing frequency for dyskinetic CP (dystonic and choreo-athetotic) syndromes born at term from the period 1959–1970 to the period 1971–1981 in a separate study by Kyllerman and Hagberg (1984). The syndromes hemiplegia, tetraplegia, and congenital ataxia did not show any significant changes during the period.

Birth Weight and Birth Weight for Gestational Age

In the 681 prenatally and perinatally derived cases of the large Hagberg study, the rate of preterm births (< 37 completed gestational weeks) was 33% compared to 6% in the general Swedish population. Thirteen percent were small-for-gestational-age (SGA, birth weight for gestation age ≤ -2 SD) among term cases and 7% among preterm cases compared to the expected 2.3%. Low birth weight (≤ 2500 g) was present in 36% of CP cases compared to 4.3% of Swedish live births. Weight specific incidences of CP increased steeply by 500 g groups. The factors low birth weight and short gestational age were found to interact in producing increased risks for spastic and dyskinetic CP syndromes.

Leanness, that is, birth weight for birth length, is another important risk factor. This has been shown by Kyllerman (1982) in dyskinetic CP and by Veelken, Hagberg, Hagberg, and Olow (1983) in spastic diplegia. The risk for birth asphyxia was found to increase acutely by increasing leanness in the dyskinetic cases.

Prenatal and Perinatal Risk Factors

Term CP showed a significant increase of defined pre- and perinatal risk factors compared to a non-CP control population (Hagberg & Hagberg, 1984, Kyllerman, 1983). This was true for all syndromes except for simple ataxia. Specifically, the more common risk factors among term cases were maternal disorder, SGA, and twinning. Preterm cases also had significantly more risk factors than preterm controls. The only significantly increased risk factor was being small-for-gestational-age (SGA). In both term and preterm cases untoward interactions between nonoptimal prenatal and perinatal conditions with known brain damaging risk factors have been detected (Kyllerman, 1983; Kyllerman & Hagberg, 1983; Veelken et al., 1983).

Pathogenetic Factors in CP Syndromes

Spastic diplegia is particularly associated with preterm birth, which was found in 55% of the 226 diplegic children, the vast majority (95%) of whom were appropriate for gestational age. Prenatal detrimental events apart from those associated with preterm birth itself seemed to be of little importance. The major determining risk factor was found to be the degree of CNS immaturity. For diplegic cases born at term

(45%), the situation appeared more complex and heterogeneous. Term diplegic cases were more likely to have been affected by factors associated with fetal deprivation of supply and of intrauterine asphyxia.

Altogether, 75% of the brain lesions in term *hemiplegia* of this series were considered to have been prenatally caused or predisposed. Among preterm hemiplegia cases, a similar predisposition for prenatal detrimental events was noted. A prenatal etiology in the majority of spastic hemiplegia was supported by observations in France (Goutières, 1979; Lyon & Robain, 1967) and Germany (Michaelis, Rooschütz, & Dopfer, 1980) but the proportion of cases in which the lesion was caused by direct perinatal brain damage is still a matter of controversy (Kotlarek, Rodewig, Brüll, & Zenner, 1981). The problem is presently being investigated by Dr. Uvebrant (1988) in a special study of CP hemiplegia in children born 1967–1978. Silent prenatal perfusion insufficiency may well result in encephalomalacia and hypoplasia, mainly during the third trimester.

With the Swedish classification, the group with *spastic tetraplegia* turns out to be very small. The prenatal risk factor pattern was more similar to that found in spastic diplegia than in hemiplegia. In a separate study, Tysk (1984) found that 26% of the cases were from prenatal causes such as congenital infections (cytomegalovirus) and CNS malformations, 40% of the cases had prenatal and/or perinatal risk factors, and 20% of the cases had postnatal causes such as meningoencephalitis (Herpes simplex virus) and near miss sudden infant deaths.

Ataxic diplegia was found to have etiological similarities to spastic diplegia. Congenital ataxia differed regarding risk factors from all other syndromes. In a large group, no obvious causes or increased risk factors could be detected. Rather, both in term and preterm cases, there were strong indications of hereditary factors. Gustavson, Hagberg, and Sanner (1969) found ataxia combined with mental retardation in 50% of the cases to be due to hereditary factors in Sweden that are transmitted as autosomal recessive traits. Sanner (1973) and

Sanner and Hagberg (1974) described a dyse-quilibrium syndrome particularly prevalent in northern Swedish populations. The syndrome has since been reported in other populations around the world.

Dyskinetic CP syndromes are the ones most often associated with perinatal brain damaging factors. Hyperbilirubinemia and birth asphyxia are well known causes. In a recent study of 116 dyskinetic cases, Kyllerman (1982) confirmed earlier impressions that choreo-athetosis is the particular syndrome associated with hyper-bilirubinemia and preterm birth. Due to region-alized exchange transfusion routines, hyper-bilirubinemia as a single cause for brain damage disappeared in the early 1960s. The more severely disabled dystonic (tonus chang-ing) syndromes were associated in particular with severe birth asphyxia in babies born at term. Leanness at birth and fetal growth retar-dation correlated with birth asphyxia. All dys-kinetic cases in that series with birth weight for birth length more than 2 SD below the standard mean had had severe asphyxia, and the per-centage decreased successively to zero for those more than 1 SD above the standard mean.

Costs and Benefits
with Modern Neonatal Care

The rate of CP children treated with respirators increased from 1% from 1959–1962 to 18% in 1975–1978 (Hagberg & Hagberg, 1984). In that period, every third preterm CP patient had had respirator treatment. The majority were ap-propriate for gestational age and had birth weights ≥ 1500 g. A neonatal condition neces-sitating respirator treatment seemed to potently prognosticate a later CP syndrome. This was confirmed in a separate study on the outcome of severe asphyxia among all term newborns from 1979–1981 who survived the first month of life (Kyllerman & Hagberg, 1984). Of these full-term newborns who had had an intra-uterine asphyxia, Apgar ≤ 3 by 1 min., ≤5 by 5 minutes, perinatal CNS symptoms, and res-pirator treatment, no less than 83% developed a permanent CNS dysfunction. Although an in-creased perinatal morbidity was recorded, a net gain of healthy babies may be demonstrated as the difference between the decrease in early neonatal mortality and the increase in CP inci-dence (Table 1). Between 1967–1970 and 1975–1978, the perinatal mortality and still-birth rate continuously decreased. From the pe-riod 1967–1970 the CP incidence increased. Compared with the period 1967–1970, 3.2 and 7.2 children per 1000 newborns, respectively, may be calculated to have survived without CP damages, 1971–1974 and 1975–1978, respec-tively. At the same time, compared with the period 1967–1970, 0.1 and 0.5 per 1000 new-borns, respectively, may be calculated to have acquired CP damages. The net gain of surviv-ing healthy newborns is substantial. It should also be observed that ¼ of the population sus-taining permanent brain damage is made up of children who were full-term newborns.

MENTAL RETARDATION

The concept of mental retardation (MR) is in-terpreted differently in different societies. This creates great difficulties when researchers at-tempt to delineate and compare MR in popula-tion based studies. Mild mental retardation (MMR) was defined by the WHO Expert Com-

Table 1.   Calculated "gains" in live births and nonCP survivors, and "losses" in additional CP per 1,000 live born children in Sweden

	1967–70	1971–74	1975–78
Perinatal mortality	17.5	14.3	10.3
Incidence of CP	1.30	1.26	1.66
"Gains" in live births		3.2	7.2
"Losses" in additional CP		0.1	0.5
"Gains" in nonCP survivors		3.1	6.7

140 Kyllerman

mittee on Mental Health in 1968 as being associated with an IQ range of −3.3 to −2.0 SD from the mean IQ of 100 ± 15, that is, an IQ of 50–70. For the range below IQ 50, a simplified grouping into severe mental retardation (SMR) is applied in the following section (Hagberg & Kyllerman, 1983).

Prevalence of MR

Prevalence data are based on five recent epidemiological studies covering various areas of Sweden (Table 2). The Västerbotten studies concern a sparsely populated vast northern county, the Uppsala studies concern a central Swedish county with mixed urban and rural populations, and the Göteborg studies concern the second largest city of Sweden. The prevalence of SMR was 3 per 1000, which was the expected rate. The figure for MMR was surprisingly low, 4 per 1,000, which was only 16% of the expected rate. It was more difficult to be confident about the complete ascertainment of MMR than of SMR. However, a thorough search of all available files of the Board for Provision of Services to the Mentally Retarded, of child habilitation centers, of institutions for the handicapped, and of hospitals caring for sick children was performed. In addition, all school nurses and school psychologists were asked for files concerning children who were suspected of having MR but who were attending ordinary schools. Incomplete ascertainment was thus considered unlikely. An alternative explanation may be the population shifts in general IQ due to developmental

stimulation and altered cultural environment. Considerable IQ gains have been reported in American and in Japanese populations over the last few decades. Old test norms were used in the Swedish studies; a qualified estimation is that currently Göteborg 8–12 year olds have a mean IQ range 112–114 ± 15. This would yield a prevalence of 3 per 1000 in the IQ range 50–70, a figure in agreement with the MMR findings of 4 per 1000.

Causes of MR

Pathological/etiological grouping into pre-, peri-, and postnatal origin in the Göteborg studies revealed a highly probable biological origin in 81% of SMR and in 43% of MMR. Prenatal assignment was based on presumed predominant pathogenetic factors before 28 weeks of gestation, perinatal from that date until the 28th postnatal day, and postnatal after 4 weeks of age. Twenty-three percent of MMR cases and 55% of SMR cases had a prenatal cause. There were indications that no less than 80%–85% of SMR cases were, with great probability, related to negative factors acting before delivery. Perinatal factors accounted for only 15%–20% of cases in both MMR and SMR, even with the applied broad definition of the perinatal period.

Chromosomal Aberrations

Although banding techniques were not regularly applied, 29% of the SMR and 4% of the MMR group had chromosomal aberrations. Down syndrome was the largest single cause of

Table 2. Severe (SMR) and mild mental retardation (MMR) in five Swedish population-based studies, prevalence per 1,000

	Ages (years)	SMR	MMR
Gustavson, Hagberg, Hagberg, and Sars (1977)	11–16	2.8	—
Gustavson, Holmgren, Jonsell, and Blomquist (1977)	5–16	3.5	—
Hagberg, Hagberg, Lewerth, and Lindberg (1981)	8–12	3.0	3.7
Blomquist, Gustavson, and Holmgren (1981)	8–19	—	3.8
Göstasson (1982)	20–60	3.8	5.1

SMR 32%, 33%, and 27%, respectively, in the Uppsala, Västerbotten, and Göteberg studies. In the Västerbotten study fragile X was found in 10% of MMR boys and in 6% of SMR boys. With present knowledge, chromosomal errors are to be expected in at least 40% SMR and 10% MMR cases in Sweden.

Fetal Alcohol Syndrome

The risk for an alcoholic mother of giving birth to a child with a complete fetal alcohol syndrome (FAS) has been estimated to be 20%–50%. A wide range of damage has been shown. Olegård and colleagues (1979) found a complete FAS in 1:600 newborn infants and an incomplete FAS was ascertained in as many infants in the city of Göteborg. Among MMR children, complete FAS accounted for 7% (Hagberg, Hagberg, Lewerth, & Lindberg, 1981). The prevalence of incomplete FAS was far less certain, but at least 10% MMR children in large Swedish city populations may show fetal alcohol effects.

Inborn Errors of Metabolism

The contribution of metabolic disorders in the studied populations was modest, SMR 4%–5%, MMR < 1%. Metabolic disorders occur differently between the Scandinavian countries and within Sweden. Local accumulations are known for Gaucher disease, Norrbottnian type (III) (Eriksson, 1986); Sjögren-Larsson's ichthyosis-spastic diplegia-oligophrenia (Jagell, Gustavson, & Holmgren, 1981); infantile metachromatic leukodystrophy (Gustavson & Hagberg, 1971) and non-Jewish form of GM_2 gangliosidosis. An even geographical distribution has been found for Krabbe's disease, globoid cell leukodystrophy (Hagberg, Kollberg, Sourander, & Åkesson, 1969); phenylketonuria (Alm & Larsson, 1981); the mucopolysacharidoses; methylmalonic aciduria, and glutaric aciduria (Kyllerman, 1980; Kyllerman & Steen, 1977).

The prevalence of Rett's syndrome (Hagberg, 1985) in southwestern Sweden (including the city of Gothenburg) among children and adolescents 6–17 years of age was 0.65/10.000 girls, that is, about twice that of phenylketonuria. In the SMR group of cases caused by progressive metabolic disorders, Rett's syndrome could be considered to be responsible for one-quarter to one-third of such cases.

Intrauterine Infections

In the Västerbotten and Göteborg studies, there were only a few cases of diagnosed congenital toxoplasmosis, rubella, cytomegalovirus, or herpes simplex infections. In a recent prospective study in southern Sweden, Ahlfors (1982) calculated that 0.6/1000 of Swedish newborns, or some 60 infants a year, developed sequelae from congenital cytomegalovirus infections. The majority of these newborns appeared to have isolated sensorineural hearing loss, and a minority had developmental retardation. According to Ahlfors's studies, cytomegalovirus infection as a cause of mental retardation is probably less frequent than was believed only a few years ago.

Perinatal Brain Damage

Perinatal brain damage as a cause for MR has probably also been overestimated. From the Göteborg studies, it may be concluded that perinatal risk factors (from the 28th week of gestation until the 28th postnatal day) are implicated in 15% of SMR cases and in 18% of MMR cases. Only about 10% of the MMR and SMR cases are perinatally derived in a restricted sense (birth and first 7 days of life). In uncomplicated low birth weight appropriate-for-gestational-age children, the risk for MR appears low as a result of present day neonatal Swedish routine care.

HYDROCEPHALUS

In a study in 1963 in the city of Uppsala, Hagberg, Sjögren, Bensch, and Hadenius found a mean birth prevalence of spina bifida cystica of 0.72 per 1000 live births from 1944–1961. The birth prevalence of simple hydrocephalus, not associated with spinal dysraphism, was 0.85/1000 live-born children in central and northern Sweden. In southern Sweden, Kornfält, Lagergren, Börjeson, and Mortensson

(1978), and Lagergren (1981), found birth prevalences of 0.6 per 1000 cases of motor handicaps associated with myelomeningocele among 4–16 year olds born 1968–1972.

The live birth prevalence of infantile expansive hydrocephalus was recently reevaluated in a population-based survey in southwestern Sweden (Fernell, Hagberg, Hagberg, & Wendt, 1986). All live-born infants born from 1967–1982 who developed hydrocephalus in the first year of life and who were unassociated with myelomeningocele, encephalocele, hydranencephaly, or intracranial tumours were included. Of 200 children thus identified, 84% had had a shunting operation. The live-birth prevalence increased from 0.46 per 1000 in 1967–1970 to 0.60 in 1979–1982. The increase was mainly referable to babies born preterm. In this group, the mean birth prevalence increased from 0.16 to 0.29 per 1000. Preliminary observations indicate that the increase noted from 1979–1982 mainly concerned preterm babies with complications necessitating respirator treatment in the neonatal period.

CONCLUDING REMARKS

Completed and ongoing population-based epidemiological studies on cerebral palsy, mental retardation, and infantile hydrocephalus have provided a basis for a better understanding of the size of the problem and the multifaceted handicap profile within the main syndromes. Pathogenetic background mechanisms have been indicated from these studies from which approaches to prevention can be made. There is an urgent need for continuous studies within these fields and on additional neurohandicaps in the pediatric population; these would include: epilepsy (Blom and Heijbel, 1982; Blom, Heijbel, & Bergfors, 1978) hearing deficits (Thiringer, Kankkunen, Lidén, & Niklasson, 1984) and visual failure.

REFERENCES

Ahlfors, K. (1982). *Epidemiologic studies of congenital cytomegalovirus infection.* Thesis, Malmö, University of Lund, Sweden.

Alm, J., & Larsson, A. (1981). Evaluation of a nationwide neonatal metabolic screening programme in Sweden 1965–79. *Acta Paediatrica Scandinavica, 70,* 601–607.

Blom, S., & Heijbel, J. (1982). Benign epilepsy of children with centrotemporal EEG foci. A follow-up study in adulthood of patients initially studied as children. *Epilepsia, 23,* 629–632.

Blom, S., Heijbel, J., & Bergfors, P.G. (1978). Incidence of epilepsy in children: A follow-up study three years after the first seizure. *Epilepsia, 19,* 343–350.

Blomquist, H.K., Gustavson, K.-H., & Holmgren, G. (1981). Mild mental retardation in children in a northern Swedish county. *Journal of Mental Deficiency Research, 25,* 169–186.

Eriksson, A. (1986). *Gaucher disease—Norrbottnian type (III).* Thesis, University of Gothenburg, Sweden.

Fernell, E., Hagberg, B., Hagberg, G., & Wendt, L. (1986). Epidemiology of infantile hydrocephalus in Sweden. I. Birth prevalence and general data. *Acta Paediatrica Scandinavica,* accepted for publication.

Goutières, F. (May, 1979). *Role of circulatory disturbances in the genesis of some prenatal encephalopathies.* Paper presented at the European Federation of Child Neurology Societies, 5th Conference, Brussels.

Göstasson, R. (September, 1982). *Mental retardation and its psychiatric complications. Preliminary report of an epidemiological study in an adult population in Sweden.*

Paper presented at a meeting of the International Association of Scientific Study of Mental Deficiency, Toronto.

Gustavson, K.-H., & Hagberg, B. (1971). The incidence and genetics of metachromatic leucodystrophy in northern Sweden. *Acta Paediatrica Scandinavica, 60,* 585–590.

Gustavson, K.-H., Hagberg, B., Hagberg, G., & Sars, K. (1977). Severe mental retardation in a Swedish county. Epidemiology, gestational age, birth weight and associated CNS handicaps in children born 1959–70. *Acta Paediatrica Scandinavica, 66,* 373–379.

Gustavson, K.-H., Hagberg, B., & Sanner, G. (1969). Identical syndromes of cerebral palsy in the same family. *Acta Paediatrica Scandinavica, 58,* 330–340.

Gustavson. K.-H., Holmgren, G., Jonsell, R., & Blomquist, H.K. (1977). Severe mental retardation in children in a northern Swedish county. *Journal of Mental Deficiency Research, 21,* 161–181.

Hagberg, B. (1985). Rett's syndrome: Prevalence and impact on progressive severe mental retardation in girls. *Acta Paediatrica Scandinavica, 74,* 405–408.

Hagberg, B., & Hagberg, G. (1984). Prenatal and perinatal risk factors in a survey of 681 Swedish cases. In F. Stanley & E. Andermann (Eds.). *The epidemiology of the cerebral palsies* (pp. 116–134). Oxford: SIMP.

Hagberg, B., Hagberg, G., Lewerth, A., & Lindberg, U. (1981). Mild mental retardation in Swedish school children. I. Prevalence. *Acta Paediatrica Scandinavica, 70,* 441–444.

Hagberg, B., Hagberg, G., & Olow, I. (1975). The changing panorama of cerebral palsy in Sweden 1959–70. I. Analysis of the general changes. *Acta Paediatrica Scandinavica, 64*, 187–192.

Hagberg, B., Kollberg, H., Sourander, P., & Åkesson, H.O. (1969). Infantile globoid cell leucodystrophy (Krabbe disease). *Neuropädiatrie, 1*, 74–88.

Hagberg, B., & Kyllerman, M. (1983). Epidemiology of mental retardation—a Swedish survey. *Brain & Development, 5*, 441–449.

Hagberg, B., Sjögren, I.. Bensch, K., & Hadenius, A.-M. (1963). The incidence of infantile hydrocephalus in Sweden. *Acta Paediatrica Scandinavica, 52*, 588–594.

Jagell, S., Gustavson, K.-H., & Holmgren, G. (1981). Sjögren-Larsson's syndrome in Sweden. A clinical genetic and epidemiological study. *Clinical Genetics, 19*, 233–256.

Kornfält, R., Lagergren, J., Börjeson, M.-C., & Mortensson, W. (1978). Barn med ryggmärgsbråck—redovisning av ett 10-årsmaterial (Sw). *Läkartidningen, 75*, 3895–3899.

Kotlarek, F., Rodewig, R., Brüll, D., & Zenner, H. (1981). Computed tomographic findings in congenital hemiparesis in childhood and their relation to etiology and prognosis. *Neuropediatrics, 12*, 101–109.

Kyllerman, M. (1980). Glutaric aciduria. A "common" metabolic disorder. *Archives Françaises de Pediatrie, 37*, 297–281.

Kyllerman, M. (1982). Dyskinetic cerebral palsy II. Pathogenetic risk factors and intrauterine growth. *Acta Paediatrica Scandinavica, 71*, 551–558.

Kyllerman, M. (1983). Reduced optimality in pre- and perinatal conditions in dyskinetic cerebral palsy. Distribution and comparison to controls. *Neuropediatrics, 14*, 29–36.

Kyllerman, M., & Hagberg, G. (1983). Reduced optimality in pre- and peri-natal conditions in a Swedish newborn population. *Neuropediatrics, 14*, 37–42.

Kyllerman, M., & Hagberg, G. (1984). Ökar antalet barn med CP-skador? *Läkaresällskapets Medicinska Riksstämma, Sammanfattningar, PE23*, 250.

Kyllerman, M., & Steen, G. (1977). Intermittently pro-

gressive dyskinetic syndrome in glutaric acid. *Neuropädiattrie, 8*, 397–404.

Lagergren, J. (1981). *Children with motor handicaps. Epidemiology, medical and socio-paediatric aspects of motor handicapped children in a Swedish county.* Thesis, University of Lund, Sweden.

Lyon, G., & Robain, O. (1967). Encéphalopathies circulatoires prénatales et paranatales. *Acta Neuropathologica, 9*, 79–98.

Michaelis, R., Rooschütz, B., & Dopfer, R. (1980). Prenatal origin of congenital spastic hemiparesis. *Early Human Development, 4/3*, 243–55.

Olegård, R., Sabel, K.-G., Aronson, M., Sandin, B., Johansson, P.R., Carlsson, C., Kyllerman, M., Iversen, K., & Hrbek, A. (1979). Effects on the child of alcohol abuse during pregnancy. Retrospective and prospective studies. *Acta Paediatrica Scandinavica (Suppl.), 275*, 112–121.

Sanner, G. (1973). The dysequilibrium syndrome. A genetic study. *Neuropädiatrie, 4*, 403–413.

Sanner, G., & Hagberg, B. (1974). 188 cases of non-progressive ataxic syndromes in childhood. Aspects of aetiology and classification. *Neuropädiatrie, 5*, 224–235.

Thiringer, K., Kankkunen, A.. Lidén, G., & Niklasson, A. (1984). Perinatal risk factors in the aetiology of hearing loss in preschool children. *Developmental Medicine & Child Neurology, 26*, 799–807.

Tysk, K. (September, 1984). Tetraplegic cerebral palsy—a preliminary report. Paper presented at the XIV International Spastic Society Symposium, Cambridge, England.

Uvebrandt, P. (1988). Hemiplegic cerebral palsy: Aetiology and outcome. *Acta Paediatrica Scandinavica*, (Suppl. 345).

Veelken, N., Hagberg, B., Hagberg, G., & Olow, I. (1983). Diplegic cerebral palsy in Swedish term and preterm children. Differences in reduced optimality, relations to neurologic and pathogenetic findings. *Neuropediatrics, 14*, 20–28.

Chapter 18

Biological and Psychological Aspects of Neurodevelopmental Outcome of Very Low Birth Weight Infants

John H. Kennell

OVER THE LAST DECADE MANY CHANGES have been made in the obstetric and neonatal evaluation and treatment of very low birth weight (<1500 gms) and extremely low birth weight (<1000 gms) infants. During this period of increasing skill in the application of intensive care measures in the delivery room and Neonatal Intensive Care Unit (NICU), there has been a progressive increase in the number of both healthy and handicapped preterm infants surviving and graduating from NICUs. (Alberman, Benson, & McDonald, 1982; Fitzhardinge & Ramsey, 1973; Hack, Caron, Rivers, & Fanaroff, 1983; Hack & Fanaroff, 1984; Hack & Fanaroff, 1986; Hack, Fanaroff, & Merkatz, 1979; Hack, Merkatz, Gordon, Jones, & Fanaroff, 1982; Hack, Merkatz, McGrath, Jones, & Fanaroff, 1984; Kitchen, Ryan, & Rickards, 1980; Steward, Reynolds, & Lipscomb, 1981). Table 1 shows that over a 5-year period, almost 81% of very low birth weight children showed normal developmental performance at 33 months.

The premature infant faces two major types of deprivation or pathology: biological and psychological, each with potentially severe, long-term sequelae. Following is a discussion of two biological disturbances—intraventricular hemorrhage and intrauterine growth retardation—which are particularly relevant to preterm infants.

BIOLOGICAL ASPECTS: INTRAVENTRICULAR HEMORRHAGE AND BRAIN GROWTH

For many decades, intraventricular hemorrhage has been recognized as the most common central nervous system lesion identified at autopsy in preterm infants. In the last 10 years, the clinical application of noninvasive imaging techniques has made it possible to identify and follow the progress of germinal-layer and intraventricular hemorrhages in surviving preterm infants (Thorburn et al., 1986). These bleeds can be detected in approximately one-third of surviving very low birth weight infants. The data generated by Papile illustrate the significance of these hemorrhages (Papile, Munsick-Bruno, & Schaefer, 1983). Her classification of intraventricular hemorrhage (IVH) based on CT brain scans defines four grades: Grade 1, isolated germinal matrix hemorrhage; Grade 2, intraventricular hemorrhage with normal ventricular size; Grade 3, intraventricular hemorrhage with ventricular dilation; Grade 4, intraventricular hemorrhage with parenchymal hemorrhage.

Table 1.　Neurodevelopmental outcome: Very low birth
weight children (1975–1979) (N = 463)

	n (%)	Bayley[a] (20 mo.)	Stanford-Binet[a] (33 mo.)
Normal outcome	373 (80.6%)	99 ($\pm$ 11)	99 ($\pm$ 14)

Adapted with permission from Hack, M., Caron, B., Rivers, A., and
Fanaroff, A. A. (1983). The very low birthweight infant: The broader
spectrum of morbidity during infancy and early childhood. *Journal of
Developmental and Behavioral Pediatrics, 4,* 243–249. Copyright © by
Williams & Wilkens, 1983.
　[a]Mean ($\pm$ SD).

In her follow-up study, Papile included only those infants that survived the first 28 days of life. Infants with major congenital malformations, documented congenital TORCH infections, and meningitis were excluded.

The infants with Grades 1 and 2 intraventricular hemorrhage had the same outcome as infants *with no intracranial bleed.*

The outcome for infants with Grades 3 and 4 intraventricular hemorrhage was much poorer. Of those infants with Grades 3 and 4 IVH, 58% had a major handicap, and multiple handicaps were present in 45% of this group. Most Grade 3 and 4 intraventricular hemorrhages are extensive and are usually associated with acute ventricular dilatation. In Grade 4 hemorrhages, there is also the destruction of periventricular white matter.

It is already clear that there can be more optimism for the future of some infants with Grades 3 and 4 IVH than was originally anticipated. In spite of alarming changes on ultrasound and CT scan, some infants have tested normal on developmental and neurologic assessment through early childhood, for example, 4 of 34 in the Papile study (Papile et al., 1983).

Real time ultrasound provides a simple and safe method for scanning the brains of newborn infants. By checking for intraventricular hemorrhages by ultrasound in the first days of life, and by following their resolution and associated brain changes by successive examinations, it should be possible to identify most of the preterm infants who are at high risk for neurodevelopmental handicaps. Also, controlled trials of interventions to prevent intraventricular hemorrhage and neurodevelopmen-

tal handicaps can be carried out with real time ultrasound. In addition, it is already apparent that with the use of PET scans and cerebral blood flow studies, it will be possible to answer more questions about etiology, extent of brain damage, and prevention of intraventricular hemorrhage.

An additional major biologic issue is brain growth. Dobbing and associates (Dobbing, 1974; Dobbing & Smatt, 1973) have carried out studies in rats that simulated human growth failure. They discovered that rats with infantile growth retardation had greater deficits in neurologic maturation, cerebellar cell number, and maximum adult growth than in rats malnourished prenatally. When extrapolated to humans, these studies suggested that proportionately more of the human brain growth spurt occurs after term than *in utero.* Dobbing also suggested that, during the first year of life, an infant may compensate for earlier brain growth failure. If catch-up growth did not occur, there was a high risk of permanent stunting of brain size and of later cognitive impairment. The careful follow-up studies of very low birth weight infants by Maureen Hack (Hack & Fanaroff, 1984; Hack et al., 1982, 1984) in Cleveland appear to confirm Dobbing's data; these studies also provide a physical measurement guide to IQ at 3 years. Specifically, Hack and her colleagues (Hack & Breslau, 1986) recently reported that head circumference at 8 months *corrected age* is the best growth parameter for the prediction of IQ at 3 years of age. Her data show that the first year of life was a crucial period for brain growth. The effects of neonatal growth failure on 3-year IQ could be offset by compensatory growth during the first year. This important information has relevance for the infant with intrauterine growth retardation and also for millions of malnourished infants in developing countries.

PSYCHOLOGICAL ASPECTS: IMPACT OF PRETERM BIRTH ON THE PARENTS AND INFANT

While the potential for biological deprivation or pathology of the premature infant is a major issue, an examination of psychological deprivation or pathology is equally compelling. Early studies in this area were in part stimulated by the disastrous results observed after premature infants were discharged from intensive care units. Some of the infants returned to the hospital because they had been battered or were failing to thrive without organic disease. For example, Figure 1 shows that some infants who

gained weight well in the hospital failed to thrive at home, whereas the opposite was true for another group of preterm infants whose weight gain and progress improved at home. Research centered on the effects of the longer-than-usual period of mother-infant separation caused by the initial hospitalization. As a consequence of these studies, parents were admitted into intensive care nurseries; this benefited both infants and parents. However, many problems remained.

Before the very low birth weight infant—or any high-risk baby—enters the intensive care nursery, certain psychological deprivations may already have occurred. In fact, it is due to these preexisting psychological deprivations that some pregnancies are considered high-risk: for example, the low income, single mother, or the socially unsupported teenage mother. Socioeconomic factors such as these

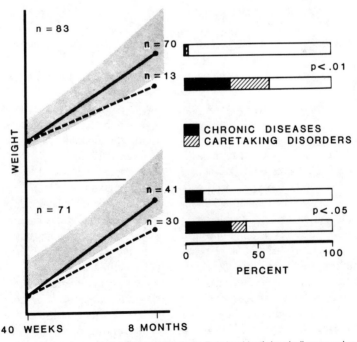

Figure 1. Appropriate for gestational age very low birth weight infants. Relationship of chronic disease and caregiving disorders to weight attainment at 8 months postmenstrual (corrected) age. Stippled area represents the mean ± 2 SD. *Note.* From "The Outcome of Growth Failure Associated with Preterm Birth" by M. Hack and A. A. Fanaroff, 1984, *Clinical Obstetrics and Gynecology, 27*(3),647–663. Copyright © 1984 by J. B. Lippincott. Reprinted by permission.

may result in psychological deprivation of the mother and the infant. While these psychological deprivations do not directly affect the infant, the effects can be both severe and long-reaching as the deprivation takes its toll on the mother-infant relationship from birth onward.

Evidence of psychological deprivation caused by socioeconomic factors can be found in research on the influence of the home environment on cognitive development. Hack and colleagues confirmed the importance of social class on 3-year outcome in very low birth weight infants. Sixty-three percent of the total explained variance in IQ at 3 years could be attributed to social class and race. This is consistent with recent studies that continue to show that prematurely born babies from a disadvantaged population were more at risk for cognitive deficits than were babies from a middle-class population.

Following is an examination of the psychological impact of a preterm birth on the parents and the infant.

There is much evidence available documenting the mutual dependence of the behavior of parent and child. What the parent does influences the behavior of the child, and what the child does influences the parent. These interactions may be present in the unique social and psychological climate of the Neonatal Intensive Care Unit.

The parents are not psychologically prepared at the time of the baby's birth. The mother has not been influenced by the same hormonal changes that are usual with a full-term birth. The parents are often distressed by the apparently abnormal baby they have produced with its scrawny appearance. The mother and father are experiencing a grief reaction, coupled with anger, at the loss of the ideal, healthy full-term baby they had anticipated. In addition, they are frightened and therefore inhibited in their ability to make a commitment or become attached to a baby that they believe may die.

The parents are also handicapped by all the concerns related to a very sick baby and a tense, confusing environment. There are few opportunities for parents to interact with their very small babies or to experience the feelings of confidence that usually come from caring for a full-term infant.

The preterm infant is quite different from a full-term infant. The preterm infant's cry is physiologically more aversive. Preterm babies, because of their immaturity, show neither the same degree of organization in their behavior nor the same ability to enter into "dialogue-like" exchanges as full-term babies. They appear neurologically immature for interaction. This makes it hard for parents to "read" them or to feel close to them. If the mother is unable to settle her baby and to understand her baby's needs, she feels more helpless. Additionally, a large number of different people may provide care for several premature infants, so the nursery staff seldom has time to learn the individual characteristics of each baby. Therefore, it is not possible for them to respond consistently to the infant's signals. What is the effect of this lack of give and take on the infant's later social development?

Clinicians have been aware of the psychological effects of the NICU environment on the parent-infant relationship. Coming from a long period during which the stimulation of premature infants was deliberately restricted, numerous studies in the last 15 years (Barnard, 1975; Hasselmeyer, 1964; Kattwinkel, Nearman, Fanaroff, Katona, & Klaus, 1975; Katz, 1971; Korner, Kraemer, Haffner, & Cosper, 1975; Kramer & Pierpont, 1976; Leib, Benfield, & Guidubaldi, 1980; Scarr-Salapatek & Williams, 1973; Segall, 1972; Solkoff, Yaffe, Weintraub, & Blase, 1969) revealed that if a small premature infant is touched, rocked, fondled, or cuddled daily during the stay in the nursery, he or she may have significantly fewer apneic periods, and may have increased weight gain and fewer stools. In some studies, even an advance in certain areas of higher central nervous system functioning that persisted for a short time after discharge from the hospital was observed in the infants. As a result, parents and caregivers have often begun additional stimulation of the preterm infant after he or she goes home.

As a result of studies by several perceptive

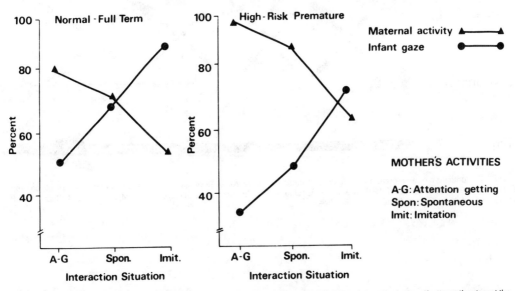

Figure 2.   Relationship between maternal anxiety and infant gaze. Three maternal situations are shown: 1) attempting to get the infant's attention, 2) spontaneous interaction, and 3) mother imitating the baby. *Note.* From "Effects of Early Separation, Interactive Deficits and Experimental Manipulations on Infant-Mother Face-to-Face Interaction" by T. M. Field, 1977, *Child Development, 48,* pp. 763–771. Copyright © 1977 by The Society for Research in Child Development, Inc. By permission.

researchers, our conceptual framework about stimulation after, and possibly before, hospital discharge, may be drastically altered.

Winnicott (1971) noted that in normal mother-infant dyads, the mother was often following or imitating the infant. Trevarthen (1977) confirmed these observations in mothers and infants using fast film technique, and noted that mothers imitate their babies during spontaneous play. Field (1977) noted that the mother and the normal full-term infant are each interacting about 70% of the time in their spontaneous play (Figure 2). In observations of the high-risk premature infant, Field noted that in the spontaneous situation, the mother is interacting up to 90% of the time, whereas the infant is only looking at the mother 30% of the time. If the mother is told to use attention-getting gestures, her activity increases even above the 90% level, and the infant's gaze decreases further. If her interactions are decreased by asking her to imitate the baby's movements, there is then a striking increase in the amount of time the infant gazes at the mother. All these observations suggest that researchers should be careful about simply rec-

ommending increased interaction with the premature infant. Instead, it would appear to be more appropriate to give specific suggestions to the mother on ways she can begin to know her infant and move at her infant's pace.

Easing the Psychological Impact of the Intensive Care Nursery

What can be done about these biological and psychological factors with which the premature infant is faced? With ultrasound, researchers now have a marker to diagnose intraventricular hemorrhages early and to define their long-term effects. The potential of catch-up brain growth in the first year of life has relevance for the management of infants with intrauterine and neonatal growth retardation, as well as for the large number of malnourished infants in developing nations. While those who care for premature infants cannot eliminate the socioeconomic factors that have psychological effects on the infant, they must maintain a sensitivity to the infants in making plans for the care of the child at home. Researchers are limited in their ability to improve the home and cultural environment of the premature infant.

150   Kennell

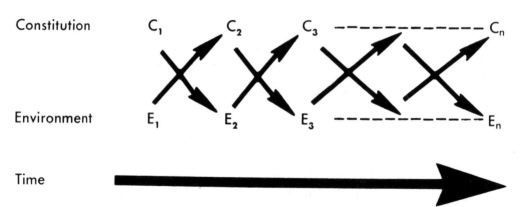

Figure 3.   Continuum of environmental casualty transactional model. *Note.* Reprinted from "Early Influences on Development: Fact or Fancy?" by A. J. Sameroff, 1975, *Merrill Palmer Quarterly of Behavior and Development, 21* (4) pp. 267–294. Reproduced by permission of the Wayne State University Press.

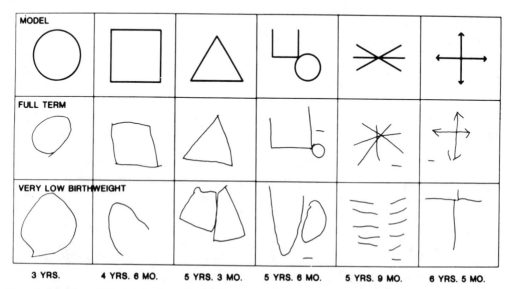

Figure 4.   Developmental test of visual-motor integration. Example indicates difficulty in form copying of child who was very low birth weight infant compared with child born at full term. Both children were 5 years 9 months old at time of study. *Note.* From "Preschool Performance of Children with Normal Intelligence Who Were Very Low Birth Weight Infants" by N. Klein, M. Hack, J. Gallegher, & A. A. Fanaroff, 1985, *Pediatrics, 75,* pp. 531–537. Reproduced by permission of *Pediatrics.*

In contrast, the practices in the intensive care nursery are more accessible to change. When caregivers encouraged mothers to live within their crowded premature nursery and to provide care and breast feed their infants, Tafari and colleagues in Ethiopia (Tafari & Sterky, 1974) were able to care for three times more infants in their unit than in previous years, and the number of surviving infants increased 500%. Baragwaneth in South Africa (Kahn, Wayburne, & Fouche, 1954) provided an earlier successful model for premature infant caregiving. In 1976, a nursery developed by Garrow in High Wycombe, England, to help parents adapt to their premature infants, was opened. No matter how ill they were, preterm babies had their mothers with them from the first hours of life. Improvements in parental care and support, including maternal day care and rooming-in, eased the psychological impact of the neonatal intensive care nursery. A second promising innovation was social support. The studies by investigators such as Minde and colleagues (1980) have demonstrated that when mothers of prematures met in discussion-support groups, their interest in interaction with their infants improved.

Sameroff (1975) has emphasized the transactional model, in which the infant's constitution and environment are continually interacting with each other over time, to explain the massive influence of socioeconomic factors on postnatal development (Figure 3). It is necessary to bear in mind that the high-risk infant is often born to a psychologically high-risk mother. Although the graduates of the intensive care nurseries score well on some developmental tests, these same infants may have more subtle difficulties. Such difficulties include visual-motor integration problems, difficulties with spatial relations, speech and language problems, and passive, withdrawn behavior that may adversely affect school performance (Klein, Hack, Gallagher, & Fanaroff, 1985) (Figure 4). Additional questions that need to be answered are: How many of these problems are attributable in part to the effects of the NICU environment on the parents rather than on the infant? Can they be modified? How?

REFERENCES

Alberman, E., Benson, J., & McDonald, A. (1982). Cerebral palsy and severe educational subnormality in low birthweight children. *Lancet, 1,*606.

Barnard, K. (1975). *A program of stimulation for infants born prematurely.* Seattle: University of Washington Press.

Dobbing, J. (1974). The later development of the brain and its vulnerability. In J.A. Davis & J.W.B. Dobbing (Eds.), *Scientific foundations of pediatrics* (pp. 565–577). Philadelphia: W.B. Saunders.

Dobbing, J., & Smatt, J.I. (1973). Early undernutrition, brain development and behavior. In S.A. Barnett (Ed.), *Clinics in developmental medicine* (No. 47) (pp. 16–36). London: Heineman.

Field, T.M. (1977). Effects of early separation, interactive deficits and experimental manipulations on infant-mother face-to-face interaction. *Child Development, 48,*763–771.

Fitzhardinge, P.M., & Ramsay, M. (1973). The improving outlook for the small prematurely born infant. *Developmental Medicine and Child Neurology, 15,*447–459.

Hack, M., & Breslau, N. (1986). Very low birth weight infants: Effects of brain growth during infancy on intelligence quotient at 3 years of age. *Pediatrics, 77,*196–202.

Hack, M., Caron, B., Rivers, A., & Fanaroff, A.A. (1983). The very low birthweight infant: The broader spectrum of morbidity during infancy and early childhood. *Journal of Developmental and Behavioral Pediatrics, 4,* 243–249.

Hack, M., & Fanaroff, A.A. (1984). The outcome of growth failure associated with preterm birth. *Clinical Obstetrics and Gynecology, 27,*647–663.

Hack, M., & Fanaroff, A.A. (1986). Changes in the delivery room care of the extremely small infant (<750 g): Effects on morbidity and outcome. *New England Journal of Medicine, 314,*660.

Hack, M., Fanaroff, A.A., & Merkatz, I.R. (1979). The low birth weight infant: Evolution of a changing outlook. *New England Journal of Medicine, 301,*1162–1165.

Hack, M., Merkatz, I.R., Gordon, D., Jones, P.K., & Fanaroff, A.A. (1982). The prognostic significance of postnatal growth in very low-birth weight infants. *American Journal of Obstetrics and Gynecology, 143,*693–699.

Hack, M., Merkatz, I.R., McGrath, S.K., Jones, P.K., & Fanaroff, A.A. (1984). Catch-up growth in very-low-birth-weight infants. *American Journal of Diseases of Children, 138,*370–375.

Hasselmeyer, E. (1964). Handling and premature infant behavior: An experimental study of the relationship between handling and selected physiological, pathological, and behavioral indices related to body functioning among a group of prematurely born infants who weighed between 1501 and 2000 grams at birth and were between the ages of seven and twenty-eight days of life. *Dissertation Abstracts, 24,7.*

Kahn, E., Wayburne, S., & Fouche, M. (1954). The Baragwanath premature baby unit—An analysis of the case records of 1000 consecutive admissions. *South African Medical Journal, 28,453–456.*

Kattwinkel, J., Nearman, H., Fanaroff, A.A., Katona, P., & Klaus, M.H. (1975). Apnea of prematurity. *Journal of Pediatrics, 86,588–592.*

Katz, V. (1971). Auditory stimulation and developmental behavior of the premature infant. *Nursing Research, 20,196–201.*

Kitchen, W.H., Ryan, M.M., & Rickards, A., et al. (1980). A longitudinal study of very low birthweight infants: IV. An overview of performance at eight years of age. *Developmental Medicine and Child Neurology, 22,172–187.*

Klein, N., Hack, M., Gallagher, J., & Fanaroff, A.A. (1985). Preschool performance of children with normal intelligence who were very low birth-weight infants. *Pediatrics, 75,531–537.*

Korner, A., Kraemer, H., Haffner, M., & Cosper, L. (1975). Effects of waterbed flotation on premature infants: A pilot study. *Pediatrics, 56,361–367.*

Kramer, L., & Pierpont, M. (1976). Rocking waterbeds and auditory stimuli to enhance growth of preterm infants. *Journal of Pediatrics, 88,297–299.*

Leib, S.A., Benfield, D.G., & Guidubaldi. J. (1980). Effects of early intervention and stimulation on the preterm infant. *Pediatrics 66,83–90.*

Minde, K., Shosenberg, B., Marton, P., Thompson, J., Ripley, J., & Burns, S. (1980). Self-help groups in a premature nursery—a controlled evaluation. *Journal of Pediatrics, 96, 933–940.*

Papile, L.A., Munsick-Bruno, G., & Schaefer, A. (1983). Relationship of cerebral intraventricular hemorrhage and early childhood neurologic handicaps. *Journal of Pediatrics, 103,273–277.*

Sameroff, A.J. (1975). Early influences on development: Fact or fancy? *Merrill-Palmer Quarterly of Behavior and Development, 21,267–294.*

Scarr-Salapatek, S., & Williams, M.L. (1973). The effects of early stimulation on low birth-weight infants. *Child Development, 44,94–101.*

Segall, M. (1972). Cardiac responsibility to auditory stimulation in premature infants. *Nursing Research, 21,15–19.*

Solkoff, N., Yaffe, S., Weintraub, D., & Blase, B. (1969). Effects of handling on subsequent development of premature infants. *Developmental Psychology, 1,765–768.*

Steward, A.L., Reynolds. E.O.R., & Lipscomb, A.P. (1981). Outcome for infants of very low birthweight: Survey of world literature. *Lancet, 2,1038–1941.*

Tafari, N., & Sterky, G. (1974). Early discharge of low birth-weight infants in a developing country. *Journal of Tropical Pediatrics and Environmental Child Health, 20,73–76.*

Thorburn, R.J., Stewart, A.L., Hope, P.L., Lipscomb, A.P., Reynolds, E.O.R., & Pape, K.E. (May 23, 1986). Prediction of death and major handicap in very preterm infants by brain ultrasound. *Lancet,* 1119–1121.

Trevarthen, C. (1977). Descriptive analyses of infant communicative behaviour. In H.R. Schaffer (Ed.), *Studies in mother-infant interaction* (pp. 227–270). New York: Academic Press.

Van den Daele, L.D. (1970). Modification of infant state by treatment in a rockerbox. *Journal of Psychology, 74,161–165.*

Winnicott, D.W. (1971). *Playing and reality.* London: Tavistock Publications, Ltd.

Chapter 19

Pathology of Prenatal Encephalopathies

Philippe Evrard, Philippe de Saint-Georges,
Hazim J. Kadhim, and Jean-François Gadisseux

T HE PRENATAL PERIOD IS DANGEROUS: AN-
tenatal mortality is around 70%. Postnatal
major or minor problems resulting from prenatal disturbances afflict nearly 10% of those
who survive embryonic and fetal life. The nervous system is often a target. Statistical data
suggest that 25% of conceptions are affected by
developmental disturbances of the central nervous system (CNS), and that these embryonic
and fetal neurological disorders account for a
high percentage of fetal deaths (for a review,
see Freeman, 1985; Icenogle & Kaplan, 1981;
Porter & Hook, 1980; Williams & Caviness,
1984). These prenatal disorders often jeopardize postnatal survival and functional perspectives: 40% of infant deaths occurring during the
first year of postnatal life seem to be related in
some way to prenatal malformations of the
CNS, and the subsequent achievement potential for those who survive depends in part on
their prenatal neural development. Furthermore, recent studies demonstrate that postnatal
neurological handicaps result more frequently
from prenatal etiologies than classically re-

ported, and that neonatal problems can often be
provoked or encouraged by prenatal factors
(Freeman, 1985; Nelson & Ellenberg, 1986;
Volpe, 1987).

NEUROPATHOLOGY AND HUMAN PRENATAL DISORDERS

Our understanding of the normal and abnormal
development of the CNS has long remained
poor in comparison with other fields of bio-
medical research. Malformations were considered "vagaries of Nature" so mysterious as to
be unavoidable. Over the last 2 decades, advances in developmental neurobiology (for reviews, see Caviness, Misson, & Gadisseux,
1988; Caviness, Pinto-Lord, & Evrard, 1981;
Caviness & Rakic, 1978; Rakic, 1981) (Figure
1a), especially with regard to mechanisms of
neuronal migration, have revolutionized our
understanding of human brain malformations.
In addition, the analysis of such malformations
(Figure 1b) has raised basic neurobiological
questions about mammalian development and

This chapter owes much to the close collaboration over the last 16 years between Dr. Verne S. Caviness, Jr. (Boston),
Dr. Philippe Evrard, and Dr. Gilles Lyon (UCL, Brussels). We thank Dr. Joëlle Awoust (U.L.B., Brussels), Dr. Georges
Boog (Brest), Dr. Martha Denckla (Baltimore), Dr. A. Henocq (Rouen), Dr. Jeanne-Claudie Larroche, Dr. Bernard Le
Marec (Rennes), Dr. Salvatore Levi (U.L.B., Brussels), Dr. Jean-Paul Misson (Liège), Dr. Dominique Parain (Rouen), Dr.
Cecilia Pinto-Lord (Boston), and Dr. Roger Williams (Billings) for their stimulating discussions. We are especially grateful
to all colleagues who participated in the collaborative study and referred material. Ms. P. Debluts, Ms. C. Defat, Ms. A. M.
Rona, Ms. A. Stefanovic, and Ms. Ch. Vynckier provided valuable help during this work. We also appreciate the generous
support of Mrs. A. Froehlich.

Supported in part by the Action Concertée Gouvernementale, the Fonds de la Recherche Scientifique Médicale, the
Fondation Roi Baudouin, and the Fondation Médicale Reine Elisabeth.

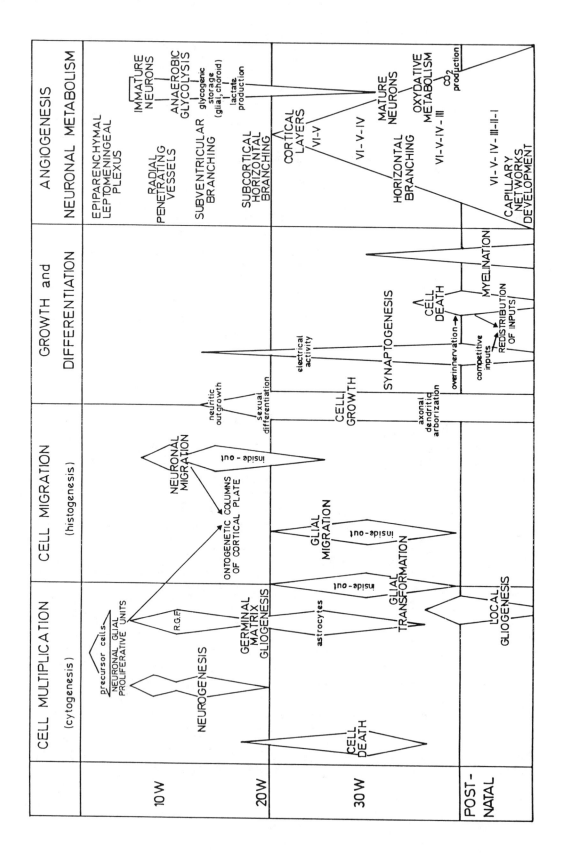

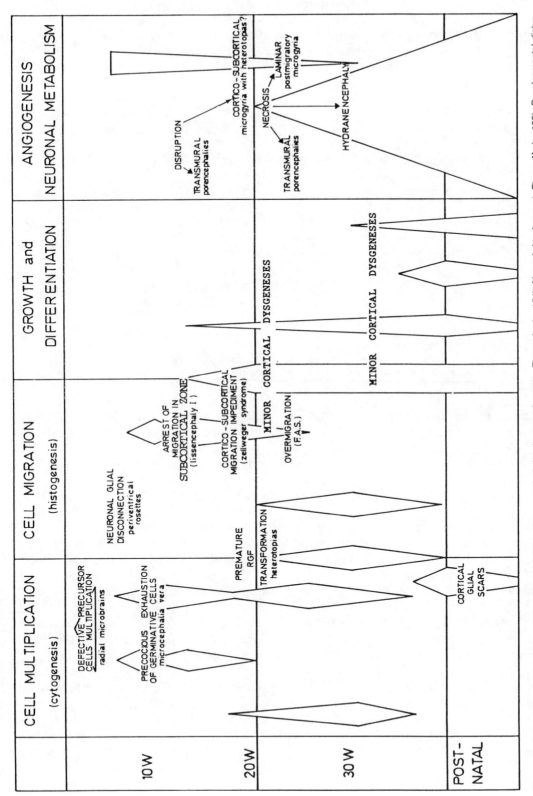

Figure 1. Schematic representation of chronology of the main neocortical developmental events. Figure **1a** (p. 154): Normal development. Figure **1b** (p. 155): Developmental disturbances. This "committed" representation summarizes our reading of the literature, our own data, and our hypotheses.

155

Table 1.   Prenatal developmental steps with examples of abnormal development

A. Cytogenesis and histogenesis : First half of gestation[a]

Main steps	Disturbances in the developmental program[b]
1. Separation of the main embryonic sheets	—Errors of the program
2. Neurulation	—Disturbances in the performance of the program
3. Neuronal multiplication	—Role of aleatory constraints during execution of
4. Neuronal migration	developmental program
5. Regional development of the cerebral vesicles	

B. Growth and differentiation : Second half of gestation[c]

Developmental features	Main lesional mechanisms[d]
—Growth and arborization	1. Disturbances of "residual" histogenesis
—Connections and synaptogenesis	2. CSF hypertension : Prenatal hydrocephalus
—Myelination	3. Perfusion failures—hypoxias[e]
—Gliogenesis	4. Infections[e]
	5. Trauma[e]
	6. "Minor" disturbances
	a. Intrauterine steric hindrance
	b. Minor cortical disturbances during growth and differentiation period

[a]Cyto- and histogenesis not fully completed at mid-gestation.
[b]Growth and differentiation program can be disturbed by same types of mechanisms.
[c]Growth and differentiation continue during postnatal life.
[d]Role of metabolic disturbances not detailed in present table but discussed elsewhere.
[e]These etiological agents can also interfere with cyto- and histogenesis.

has promoted new experimental approaches. Several review papers tried to cover this "swinging motion" between human pathology and basic research approaches. (As examples of such review papers, see Barth, 1987; Caviness et al., 1981; Caviness et al., 1988; Caviness & Williams, 1984; Evrard, Gadisseux, & Lyon, 1982; Evrard, Lyon, & Gadisseux, 1984a, 1984b; Friede, 1975; Larroche, 1977; Williams & Caviness, 1984.) Among the concepts emphasized in most of these reviews is the distinction between two major types of CNS developmental disorders: disturbances interfering with the fundamental program of *cytogenesis and histogenesis* occurring during the first half of gestation, and brain lesions due to destructive processes contemporaneous with CNS *growth and differentiation,* occurring during the second half of gestation (Table 1). Despite its oversimplified character, this distinction provides some useful guidelines for prognosis, genetic counseling, and obstetrical follow-up. It can also be of help in epidemiological and social studies of pre-

natal aspects of child health: the biological and environmental factors interfering with the successive developmental steps seem to be unequally distributed in the various socioeconomic levels. (For a review of some of the social aspects and priorities in prenatal Child Health and Welfare, see Freeman, 1985; Hamburg, 1985.)

The present chapter is focused on conceptual and methodological progress in the study of the neuropathology of human prenatal disorders, and emphasizes clinicopathological correlations in fetal neurology. This chapter considers only a selection of representative examples at different developmental steps. (Cranial hernias are not covered in this chapter [for reviews, see Chapman & Caviness, 1988; Evrard & Caviness, 1974; and Friede, 1975]. Holoprosencephalies were recently extensively reviewed by Leech and Shuman [1986] and will not be dealt with here. Infectious mechanisms will be discussed only in function of their interference with cell multiplication, cytoarchitectonic development, and prenatal brain perfusion.)

METHODOLOGICAL PROGRESS IN THE PATHOLOGICAL APPROACH AND IN CLINICOPATHOLOGICAL CORRELATIONS

Neuropathological Methods

Neuropathological methods exploring developmental disorders were enriched by the collection of normative data and the use of whole brain serial section analysis (see Gilles, Leviton, & Dooling, 1983) and by the application of the Golgi staining process (see Williams & Caviness, 1984). When combined with the concepts of modern developmental neurobiology, these classical tools produced a vast amount of new data about developmental disorders. Furthermore, multicenter collaboration in the collection of pertinent specimens and the emergence of fetal neuropathology expanded this field over the last decade. (Regarding the ethical procedures for the study of human fetal brains: the human brains used for this study have been collected in accordance with the ethical rules of our laboratory. Human fetal brains are obtained for neuropathological and neuroanatomical studies from cases involving miscarriage, abortion, and deceased premature infants. In cases of abortion, we accept specimens only if the obstetrician submitting the specimen formally certifies that the ethical rules applicable in his or her department were respected.)

A major obstacle to the analysis of normal and pathological glial-neuronal relationships and of ontogenesis of the vertical cytoarchitectonic units has been the difficulty in differentiating glial fibers from dendritic and axonal processes in the developing human cortical plate (CP) at the ultrastructural level (Choi & Lapham, 1978). Several new cytological methods were tried for this glial-neuronal differential identification. The rapid Golgi-gold substitution method is difficult to use for such study because of its capriciousness and the limited number of cell impregnations obtained (Pinto-Lord, Evrard, & Caviness, 1982). More recently, immunohistochemical methods using specific antibodies to glial fibrillary acidic pro-

tein and to vimentin in radial glia have been successfully used in rodents (Bignami, Raju, & Dahl, 1982; Bovolenta, Liem, & Mason, 1984; Dupouey, Benjelloun, & Gomes, 1985; Pixley & Vellis, 1984), primates (Rakic, 1984), and human fetuses (Antanitus, Choi, & Lapham, 1976; Choi, 1986). Nevertheless, in the human material, the immunoreactivity discerned in the radial glia by electron microscopic immunoperoxidase methods is a function of tissue preparation, its morphological and other limitations having been pointed out by Choi (1986). The presence of particulate glycogen in glial cells is an essential property that differentiates the glial lineage from most neurons (Brückner & Biesold, 1981; Cataldo & Broadwell, 1986; Gadisseux & Evrard, 1985; Kadhim, Gadisseux, & Evrard, 1988; Peters & Feldman, 1973). On the basis of this property, we recently proposed a modified histochemical method based on Thiéry (1967) and Maxwell (1978) for the preservation and staining of particulate glycogen in the radial glial cell (RGC) population during mammalian and human CNS development (Figures 2 and 3) (Gadisseux & Evrard, 1985; Kadhim et al., 1988). This method has contributed by the following data to our knowledge of the glial-neuronal units in the human fetal brain (Figures 3 and 4): radial glial fibers (RGFs) are grouped in fascicles of five to eight RGFs until around 16 weeks of intrauterine life; RGFs fully *defasciculate* in the neocortical plate by 18 weeks of gestation, paralleling the cortical neuronal saturation. Furthermore, lysosomal proliferation with autophagic resorption, which is one of the cytological mechanisms of transformation of RGCs into astrocytes, displays a grossly centripetal sequence in the human fetus from 21–40 weeks. These data could have several methodological and conceptual implications for developmental neuropathology: they can be used to analyze the vertical cortical units and to study glial disturbances in abnormal neuronal patterns; Potter syndrome with total renal dysplasia (see later discussion) and holoprosencephaly (de Saint-Georges, Della Giustina, Kadhim, & Evrard, 1988) are examples of such

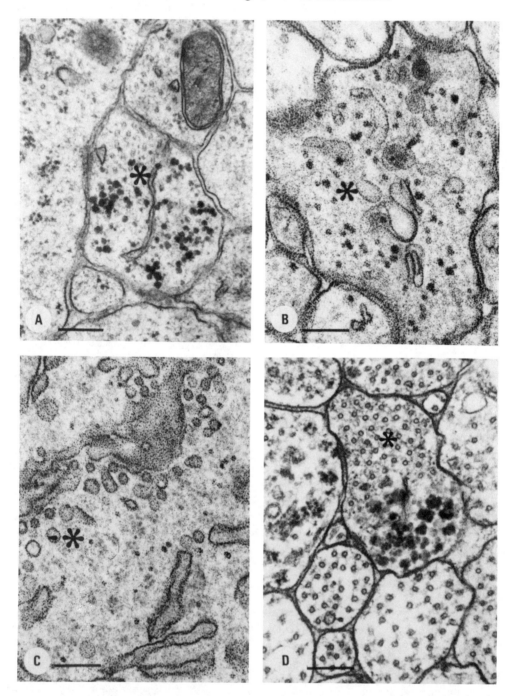

Figure 2.   Ultrastructural features of glycogen in radial glial cells. **a.**   Lower half of the cortical plate, normal mouse, embryonic day 17 (E17), tangential section. Postfixation with reduced osmium and uranyl acetate - lead citrate (U-Pb) staining. **b.**   Spinal cord, cervical region, normal mouse, E14. Postfixation with reduced osmium and modified Thiéry staining method. **c.**   Normal mouse, E14, ventricular zone. Postfixation with reduced osmium and modified Thiéry staining method. **d.**   Human cerebral cortex at 20th fetal week, tangential section. Postfixation with reduced osmium and U-Pb staining. The asterisk indicates a radial glial cell with particulate glycogen. Marker bar=0,5μm. *Note.* From "Glial-neuronal Relationship in the Developing Central Nervous System" by J. F. Gadisseux and Ph. Evrard, 1985, *Developmental Neuroscience, 7,* pp. 12–37. Copyright 1982. Reprinted by permission, S. Karger AG, Basel.

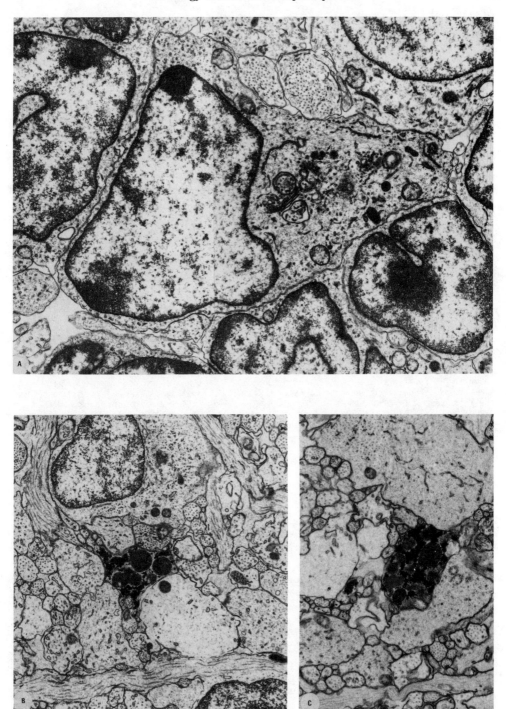

Figure 3.   Identification of RGCs by glycogen labeling in the human fetus. **a.**   Glial cell body in the subventricular zone containing glycogen particles and glial filaments. Normal brain, 18 weeks. Postfixation with reduced osmium and U-Pb staining. **b** and **c.**   Gradual transformation of RGCs into astrocytes during the second half of gestation. Normal brain, 21 weeks, plexiform zone, postfixation with reduced osmium and U-Pb staining. Intense proliferation of the lysosomal apparatus in the peripheral segment of radial glial fibers loaded with glycogen.

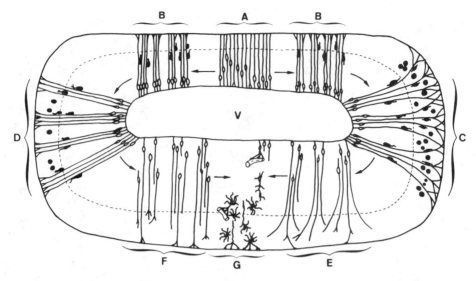

Figure 4. Schematic hypothetical representation of RGC distribution pattern during the different developmental stages in the mammalian neocortex. **a.** Early embryonic stages; RGC regularly aligned. **b.** Migration stage of neurons destined to layers VI to IV. RGC grouped in fascicles throughout the thickness of the neural tube, ventricular zone to pial surface. **c.** RGC distribution in the mammal during migration period of neurons destined for layers III and II. Migrating neurons defasciculate RGFs in the CP via gradual neuronal saturation and glial dilution. **d.** RGC distribution in the Reeler mutant mouse when last waves of migrating neurons reach the cortical plate (**E-17**). There seems to be no intracortical defasciculation of RGC in this mutant. **e.** and **f.** Gradual transformation of RGC into astrocytes after the end of neuronal migration along RGF. In the IZ of the normal human fetus (**e**), normal (**e**) and Reeler mouse (**f**), and in the CP of the Reeler mouse (**f**), glial profiles seem to maintain their fasciculated pattern. In the CP of the human fetus (**e**) and of the normal mouse (**e**), this cytological transformation or "involution" of glial elongated fibers occurs on previously defasciculated RGF. **g.** Stage of full transformation into mature glia. **v:** lumen of neural tube; ● ▮ ; neurons; ⌀ ; glial cell body; dotted line: transition between CP and IZ. *Note.* From "Topographical and Cytological Evolution of the Glial Phase During the Prenatal Development of the Human Brain" by H. J. Kadhim, J. F. Gadisseux, and Ph. Evrard, 1988, *Journal of Neuropathology and Experimental Neurology, 47*, pp. 166–188. Copyright 1988. Reprinted by permission, the American Association of Neuropathologists, Inc.

applications. Presumably, the glycogen staining of the whole glial phase at the electron microscopic (EM) level could be a partial morphological parameter helping to evaluate the glial carbohydrates that might be a critical source of energy during early migration and before neocortical angiogenesis (Kuban & Gilles, 1985; Larrabee, 1985; Norman, 1986).

Clinicopathological Correlations in Fetal Neurology

Most classical neuropathological studies of prenatal disorders have been based on postnatal *a posteriori* reconstructions of developmental events (a necessary but *archeological* method), and prenatal clinical data have been scarce. Since the early 1970s, clinicopathological correlations in this field improved dramatically by the expansion of fetal neuropathology as a dis-

cipline, and by the appearance of precise prenatal clinical data provided by fetal ultrasound methods. The Société Européenne de Neurologie Pédiatrique promoted a multicenter collaborative study in this field (Evrard et al., 1985). At present, 455 observations of prenatal CNS disorders with prenatal ultrasound studies have been collected in this program. To facilitate the clinicopathological analysis of these data, we developed a curve of cranial growth covering prenatal and postnatal life (Figure 5). Recently, we extended the use of this curve to all of the clinical cases in our practice, as this tool has proved useful for the evaluation of the natural history of prenatal disorders. It is also an excellent means of communication between obstetricians, neonatologists, and pediatric neurologists. Some of the data from the European Collaborative Study Program are summarized in Table 2 and in Figure 6.

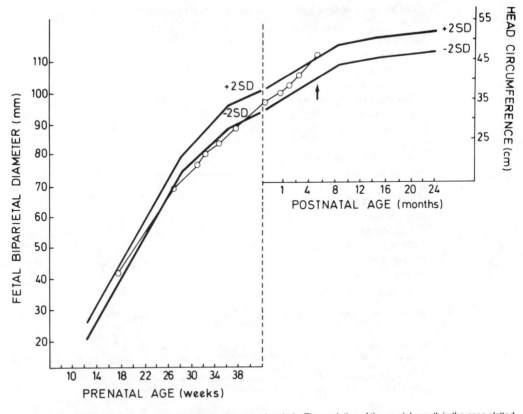

Figure 5. Cranial growth curve covering the pre- and postnatal periods. The evolution of the cranial growth in the case plotted shows the convenience of this composite curve: a maternal severe infectious disease of unknown origin at mid-gestation was followed by relative prenatal microcephaly that ended in postnatal hydrocephalus. *Note.* Modified and adapted from "Les Processus Destructifs Agissant Durant la Seconde Moitié de la Grossesse, Durant la Période de Croissance et de Différenciation du Tissu Nerveux" by Ph. Evrard, G. Lyon, and J. F. Gadisseux, 1984b, *Progrès en Néonatologie, 4,* pp. 71–85.

PATHOGENETIC ANALYSIS OF PRENATAL CNS DISORDERS: REPRESENTATIVE EXAMPLES OF THE PRINCIPAL DEVELOPMENTAL STEPS

Disturbances of Neuronal-Glial Production

Neuronal production and death determine the neuronal complement of the mature brain. While programmed death (estimated at 30%–50% of young neurons) is a normal developmental event, destructive intercurrent processes can result in additional neuronal depletions. Disturbances in cell production, in cell death, or in the balance between them, are the bases for the numerical neuronal deficits pre-

sent in many microcephalies. Impaired differentiation of neuronal processes or their destruction are other factors of reduction of brain size.

On one hand, in *developmental microcephalies,* numerical neuronal deficits and their consequences for the differentiation of neuronal processes are due to insufficient cell multiplication or to excessive programmed cell death. In this section, "radial microbrain" and microcephalia vera will be used as representative examples.

Destructive microcephalies, on the other hand, are secondary to encephaloclastic processes of ischemic, infectious, or toxic origin acting during the pre- or postnatal periods. Examples will be given later in the discussion of brain hypoxias.

Table 2. Multicenter collaborative study of prenatal abnormal brain development[a]

Abnormality	No. Observations (as of 1984)[a]
Anencephaly	130
Hydrocephalus	124
Meningomyelocele	59
Nondestructive microcephaly	34
Encephalocele	23
Holoprosencephaly	11
Hydranencephaly	6
Multicystic encephalomalacia	4
Intracranial tumor	4
Microgyria	3
Porencephaly	3
Megalencephaly	3
Craniostenosis	3
Acardia-acephaly	2
Primary intracerebral hemorrhage	1
TOTAL	410

[a]Collaborative Study Program, Société Européenne de Neurologie Pédiatrique, Branch of the European Federation of Child Neurology Societies. *Note.* From "Diagnostic Anténatal des Affections du Système Nerveux Central: Résultats Prèliminaires d'une Étude Multicentrique Européene" by Ph. Evrard, M. C. Belpaire, G. Boog, N. Elkhazen, J. F. Gadisseux, B. Le Marec, J. P. Misson, J. J. Santini, and M. Van Lierde, 1985, *Journal Français d'Echographie, 2*, pp. 123–126. Copyright 1985 by *Journal Français d'Echographie.* Reprinted by permission. See also "Conclusions d'une Étude Multicentrique Européene sur Les Anomalies du Tube Neural" by M. Van Lierde and Ph. Evrard, 1986, *Journal de Génétique Humain, 34*, pp. 343–365. Copyright 1986 by *Journal de Génétique Humain.* Reprinted by permission.

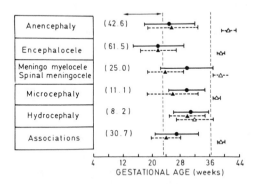

Figure 6. Age of prenatal diagnosis in five groups of prenatal CNS malformations. (Key: (. . .): percentage of diagnosed cases before 24th week of gestation. —●—: age at diagnosis (m+SD). –▲–: age at delivery in cases of interrupted pregnancy (m+SD). –△–: age at delivery in cases of pregnancy to term (m+SD). (m: mean; SD: standard deviation.) *Note.* Modified and adapted from "Diagnostic Anténatal des Affections du Système Nerveux Central: Résultats Preliminaires d'une Étude Multicentrique Européene" by Ph. Evrard, M. C. Belpaire, G. Boog, N. Elkhazen, J. F. Gadisseux, B. Le Marec, J. P. Misson, J. J. Santini, & M. Van Lierde, 1985, *Journal Français d'Echographie, 2*, pp. 123–126.

Distinguishing between these two pathogenic categories of microcephalies has useful clinical and genetic applications, despite the oversimplified character of this distinction. Microcephalies provoked by prenatal viral infections could be caused by mitotic inhibition and/or by destructive neuronal depletion, so they can belong to both categories of microcephalies. The fetal alcohol syndrome (FAS) also offers a classification problem: FAS subnormal brain size can be due to mitotic inhibition, impaired neuronal migration and differentiation, and/or destructive events.

The "Radial Microbrains": Too Few Radial Neuronal-Glial Units? Among the extreme microcephalies in our neuropathological collection, seven cases displayed very homogeneous pathological features (Evrard et al., 1982). The brain size is extremely reduced: postmortem brain weight from 16–50 g. (full-term newborns deceased between birth and day 30). Primary fissures are quite normal, and sec-

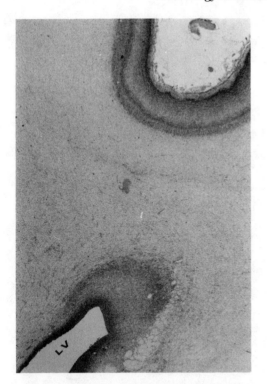

Figure 7. Radial microbrain. Brain of a full-term neonate with the pathological picture of radial microbrain described in the text. Normal cortical lamination and normal residual germinative zone. (**lv**: lateral ventricle.)

ondary and tertiary sulci are developed. There is no evidence of destructive lesions or abnormal gliosis (Figure 7). Neurons are normotopic and display normal microscopical features. The residual germinative zone is appropriate for the age. Cytoarchitectonic analysis studied lamination and striation, and was completed with an estimation of neuronal numbers in the cerebral cortex and per "vertical neocortical column" using a method based on Rockel's (Rockel, Hiorns, & Powel, 1980). The horizontal lamination pattern of cerebral and cerebellar cortex is perfectly normal, the overall number of neocortical neurons seems to be reduced to 30% of normal at a first estimate of the order of magnitude, and the neuronal complement of each "vertical neocortical column" seems normal when evaluated with a method based on Rockel's (1980). On the basis of these data, we suggest that these microbrains result from a severe reduction in the number of adja-

cent vertical neuronal-glial units, each of which contain a neuronal complement seemingly normal in number and organization. We named this abnormal cytoarchitectonic pattern *"radial microbrain."* Cell proliferation in this pattern is grossly defective while neuronal migration remains quite normal, which demonstrates that control mechanisms of multiplication and migration can be independent of each other. The reduction in the number of radial neuronal-glial units could be due to an insufficient number of proliferative neuronal-glial units in the germinative zone. The familial history of radial microbrain cases suggests a genetic basis (our seven cases include two familial observations from two different families). The clinical picture includes inconstant extraneurological signs (acromicria and nephropathy); the maximum postnatal survival was 30 days.

Radial microbrain seems to constitute a distinct clinicopathological entity and a newly recognized model of disturbed neurogenesis.

Microcephalia Vera: Exhaustion of the Germinative Zone? We suggest that the term *microcephalia vera* be used to designate developmental microcephalies other than radial microbrain. (This unusually broad definition perfectly respects the etymology, does not seem contradictory with Giacomini's [Giacomini, 1885], Friede's [Friede, 1975], and Holmes's [Holmes et al., 1972] usage, and is convenient both for clinicians and neuropathologists.) Defined as such, microcephalia vera includes several diseases, among which are autosomal recessive and X-linked conditions.

The clinicopathological picture of autosomal recessive microcephalia vera is rather homogeneous: it presents clinically as moderate mental retardation without sensory or gross motor deficit. A severe neuronal depletion in neocortical layers II and III is the basic cytoarchitectonic finding (Caviness & Williams, 1984; Robain & Lyon, 1972).

Histopathological data from a fetal case of microcephalia vera have contributed to the pathogenetic interpretation of this disorder (Parain, Gadisseux, Henocq, Tayot, & Evrard, 1985). The fetus came from a family with a previously established clinicopathological history of microcephalia vera. In this fetus, sequential ultrasound examinations revealed severe microcephaly with a biparietal diameter at −7 standard deviations. Abortion was induced at the age of 26 fetal weeks. The analysis of neuronal patterns showed that the cerebral neocortex was dominated by neurons of layers V and VI, while neurons of layer II were almost lacking, and those of layer III were scanty. The neuronal complement in the vertical cortical dimension, when compared with normal controls of the same age, was reduced by an order of magnitude compatible with the neuronal shortage in layers II and III. There were no neuronal heterotopias either in the cortex or in the subcortical white matter, and there was no indication of a migration disorder. The germinative zone was depleted of cells in this specimen (Figure 8), while it is at its maximum volume in the normal controls at this age (Jam-

mes & Gilles, 1983). (At this fetal age, the normal germinative zone consists mainly of glial precursors and possibly of residual and/or dying neuronal precursor cells.) These findings suggest that the neuronal shortage in the superficial neocortical layers, the most characteristic cytoarchitectonic feature of most cases of microcephalia vera, was in this case due to early exhaustion of the germinative zone precluding the normal production of last migrating neurons destined for layers III and II.

The following findings on the convolutional pattern, callosal fibers, and the upper cortical appearance support this pathogenetic interpretation of microcephalia vera. The 26th fetal-week brain mentioned above was nonconvoluted and, in our postnatal observations of microcephalia vera, the sulci and gyri were shallow. Such modifications of chronology and wave amplitude in brain folding can be interpreted using the model by Caviness and

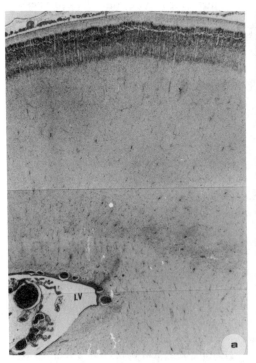 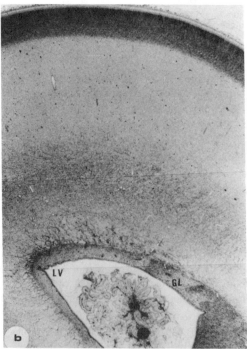

Figure 8.   Premature exhaustion of the germinal layer in microcephalia vera. **a.**   Microcephalia vera, human fetal forebrain, 26 weeks of gestation. **b.**   Normal human fetal forebrain, 26 weeks, same cortical region, for comparison. In microcephalia vera, the germinal layer is exhausted at this age, and the white matter is almost devoid of late migrating glial and neuronal cells. Layers VI to IV are normal while the two superficial layers are almost missing. (**lv:** lateral ventricle; **gl:** germinal layer.)

Pathology of Prenatal Encephalopathies

co-workers for the ontogenesis of brain convolutions (Richman, Stewart, Hutchinson, & Caviness, 1975): they reflect the abnormality in the growth gradient between the upper and lower cortex in microcephalia vera. In most such cases, including our fetal observation, callosal fibers, originating and terminating mainly in the supragranular layers of the normal cortex, are missing or reduced. The presence of a Probst bundle in several microcephalia vera cases could represent neuronal processes originating in deep cortical layers. The excessive and crude vertical columnization and the glomerular aspect in the superficial part of the neocortex are classical cytoarchitectonic features in microcephalia vera. They display similarities with the mouse CP at 17 days of gestation and with the human CP at 16 weeks of pregnancy before neuronal migration for supragranular layers is completed.

In this microcephalia vera group, X-linked microcephaly is a different clinicopathological entity that displays some cytoarchitectonic similarities with the autosomal recessive type. For a review of this condition, see Renier et al. (1982).

Disturbances of Neuronal Migration

Subcortical Arrest of Neuronal Migration Lissencephalies, macroscopically characterized by absent or poor brain sulcation, can be produced by different disorders of neuronal migration. Among these, two clinicopathological entities are well distinguished: the Bielschowsky, or Type I, lissencephaly and the Walker-Warburg, or Type II, lissencephaly. (Macroscopic changes of brain surface are classically used to name and classify malformations. The abnormal appearance of gyration is always the consequence of cytoarchitectonic abnormalities, and different cortical abnormalities may provoke the same abnormal gyral configuration. For this reason, it is crucial to classify cortical malformations on the basis of their abnormal neuronal patterns.)

In the neocortex of *Type I lissencephaly*, the first generated neurons, normally destined for cortical layers VI and V, keep their superficial position after migrating to the interface with

the plexiform zone. Subsequently produced neurons fail to achieve normal migration and settle heterotopically to constitute a diffuse cellular band in the depth of the cerebral mantle. The migratory defect behind this abnormal four-layered pattern of the cerebral mantle seems to occur between 12 and 16 weeks of gestation (Stewart, Richman, & Caviness, 1975). Heterotopic inferior olivary cells are another constant sign of the migratory disorder occurring at the same period. We have collected several cases of Type I lissencephaly for which sequential prenatal ultrasound data are available. In all of these, a defect of cranial growth becomes evident at 16 weeks of gestation (Figure 9). The clinical picture and etiological factors are reviewed by Williams and Caviness (1984), and will not be detailed in this chapter.

In *Type II lissencephaly*, the meninges are thickened and densely adherent to the cortex. The cortex is divided in masses by penetrating vessels and glial septa; the entire cerebral hemispheres and cerebellum are involved. Furthermore, the cerebellar cortex displays a diffuse microgyric aspect. As suggested earlier

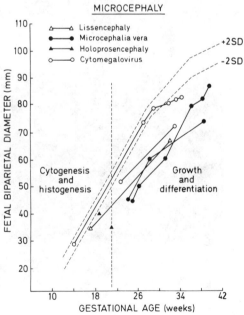

Figure 9. Microcephalies. Prenatal growth of biparietal diameter. The two CMV cases displayed polymicrogyria. (SD = standard deviations.)

(Chan, Egbert, Herrick, & Urich, 1980; Evrard et al., 1982; Williams, Swisher, Jennings, Ambler, & Caviness, 1984), this complex pathological picture, including neuronal heterotopias and a severe prenatal hydrocephalus, suggests a destructive and cicatrizing factor acting over a very protracted period from the second trimester of gestation until at least the age of 24 prenatal weeks. The clinical picture has been reviewed by Lyon & Beaugerie (1988) and will not be discussed in this chapter. A provocative etiological discussion has arisen in the literature to explain the high intrafamilial recurrence rate. In our opinion, the vulnerability to a viral or teratogenic process during successive pregnancies (Williams et al., 1984) explains more features of this clinico-pathological entity than the metabolic or genetic hypothesis (Bordarier, Aicardi, & Goutières, 1984), but there seems to be no way to close this debate with the available data.

Interruption of Neuronal Movement at Midway Along the Migration Trajectory A 16-week brain fetus from our collection introduced this third type of deep subcortical neuronal arrest (Figure 10). A loose neuronal layer containing polymorphic and pyramidal cells, resembling a normal subplate, lies beneath the superficial plexiform zone. The CP was missing. Most neocortical neurons were arrested or slowed down in the intermediate zone (IZ) between the subventricular zone and the thalamocortical projections. An inhibition of neuronal migration or an obstacle along the migratory corridors starting from the 12th week of gestation can explain this neural pattern. Fetal karyotype was normal. The mother had used alcohol and psychotropic drugs.

Cortico-Subcortical Migration Impediments The neocortical cytoarchitectonic disorder always observed in the *Zellweger cerebrohepatorenal syndrome* is characterized by

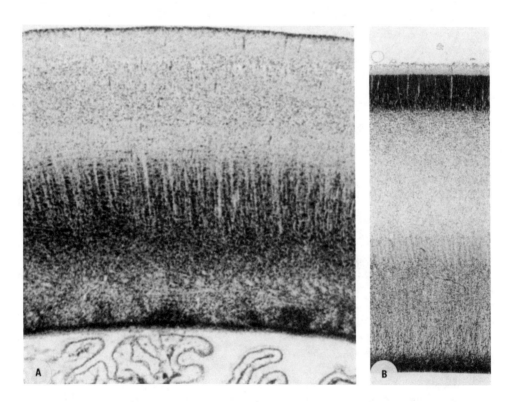

Figure 10. Interruption of neuronal movement in deep intermediate zone. **a.** Diffuse subcortical arrest of neuronal migration in a human fetus at 16 weeks of gestation. **b.** Normal human brain pallium at the same stage for comparison.

many areas of sub- and intracortical hetero-topias consisting of limited numbers of neurons remaining "glued" in the migratory corridors at inappropriately low pallial levels (Evrard, Caviness, Prats-Vinas, & Lyon, 1978). This partial impediment of neuronal migration along RGF results in the following additional abnormal cytoarchitectonic features: large pyr-amidal cells are abnormally superficial and the horizontal lamination is partially inversed, and many radial neuronal columns are too broad. The adjacent radial neuronal columns are somewhat out of register and are displaced up-wards and downwards in relation to each other, giving a somewhat coarse and irregular aspect to the horizontal lamination. Convolutional disturbances (microgyric and pachygyric areas) present in the most affected cortical areas are the macroscopic consequences of the cytoarchitectonic disorders. (See earlier dis-cussion concerning the importance of classify-ing cortical malformations on the basis of their abnormal neuronal patterns.) Golgi impregna-tions (Della Giustina, Goffinet, Landrieu, & Lyon, 1981) showed that all neuronal classes are represented in the heteropias, which per-mits the conclusion that the process hindering the neuronal migration extends over a long pe-riod from the third to the fifth month of intra-uterine life. Moreover, the neocortical abnor-malities are constantly associated with a pachygyric and fragmentory aspect of the in-ferior olivary nuclei, and with neuronal hetero-topias in the cerebellar white matter. The dis-tribution of the olivary discontinuities and of the sheets of cerebellar heterotopias suggest a possible topological relationship between them.

The Zellweger disease is a peroxisomal dis-order associated with some mitochondrial dys-function (for a review, see Vamecq et al., 1986). We still do not know the relationship between the defective peroxisomal function and the migration disturbance. The numerous abnormal astrocytes loaded with sudanophilic material suggest that the causal metabolic de-fect could affect the RGC and disturb gliophilic neuronal migration mechanism. Another

mechanism might be the energy exhaustion of migrating neurons at a time when they could be partially energy-dependent upon peroxisomal function. The deficient plasmalogen biosyn-thesis that is conspicuous in the Zellweger dis-ease could also impair the intercellular rela-tionships during migration.

In the *Potter syndrome with total renal dys-plasia,* migration normally proceeds to the mid-intermediate zone, while migratory im-pediments occur in numerous radial sectors through the external IZ, subplate, and CP; a population of RGFs dispersed through differ-ent glial fascicles display degenerative signs at the EM level (de Saint-Georges et al., un-published data) when using the glycogen stain-ing method described above.

The understanding of migration impedi-ments has been helped by the knowledge de-rived from an *animal model with inversion of the cortical layers: the Reeler mouse* (Cav-iness, 1976; Caviness & Rakic, 1978; Gadis-seux & Evrard, 1985; Goffinet, 1984; Pinto-Lord, Evrard, & Caviness, 1982).

Superficial Ectopias due to Overmigra-tion Abundant colonies of ectopic neurons (sometimes accompanied by glial cells) settled in the plexiform zone or outside the brain in the leptomeningeal space (Figure 11) seem to be constant features in the FAS (Abel, Jacobson, & Sherwin, 1983; Wisniewski, Dambska, Sher, & Qazi, 1983). Additionally, they are encountered in cases of developmental micro-cephaly, mental retardation of unknown ori-gin, and localized injuries to the basal mem-brane or to the surface of the developing brain (Caviness, Evrard, & Lyon, 1978; Choi & Matthias, 1987). It has been reproduced by Lidov and Molliver (1982) using 6 hydroxy-dopamine in the rat (see also Sievers, Pehle-mann, Baumgarten, & Berry, 1985). How-ever, small and isolated ectopias are occasion-ally encountered in normal brains. In our fetal material, these overmigrations or migration re-activations due to derangements in the plex-iform zone, or in the pial-glial membrane, often become conspicuous between 20 and 25 gestational weeks.

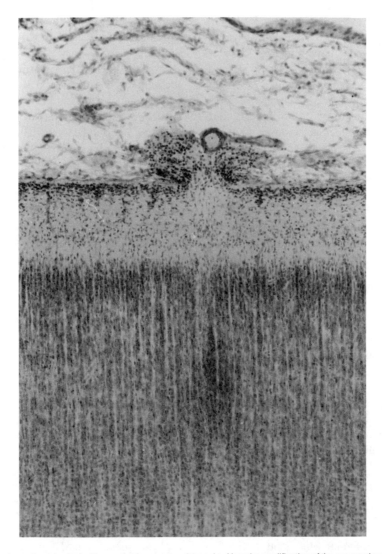

Figure 11.   Leptomeningeal ectopia. Human fetal neocortex, 24 weeks. Note the modification of the neuronal complement in the vertical cortical column beneath the ectopia.

Perfusion Failures and Hypoxias

Perfusion failures and hypoxias are among the frequent causes of viable human brain malformations (Lyon & Robain, 1967; Richman, Stewart, & Caviness, 1974). (For review, see also: Caviness & Williams, 1984; Evrard et al., 1982; Lyon, 1988.) Several etiologies of fetal brain perfusion failure are listed in Table 3. The possible relationship between infections and perfusion failures (Friede & Mikolasek, 1978; Lyon, 1988; Marques-Dias, Harmant-

van Rijckevorsel, Landrieu, & Lyon, 1984) will not be discussed here in detail. Few epidemiological data regarding perfusion failure and hypoxia of the human fetal brain are presently available. Ornoy and co-workers reported that one-third of mothers having newborns with brain abnormalities had experienced genital blood losses during pregnancy, a percentage much higher than in the control population (Ornoy, Benady, & Kohen-Raz, 1976). According to Ornoy and co-workers, this bleeding can be associated with either per-

Table 3. The main known causes of fetal brain perfusion failure

I. Fetal origin
Circulatory disturbances due to an infection (arteritis, systemic hypotension)
Hydrops foetalis, thrombocytopenia
Embolism (placental and others) with arterial occlusion
Multiple monochorial pregnancies with placental vascular anastomoses
Feto-fetal transfusion

II. Placental and cord origin
Premature placental separation
Possibly excessive infarction
See above

III. Maternal origin
Maternal shocks (e.g., toxic, anaphylactic)
Maternal hypoxia (e.g., CO intoxication, butane intoxication)
Extreme maternal stress (?)
Abdominal trauma
Maternal hypo- and hypertension
Maternal thrombophlebitis
Feto-maternal transfusion

The above cited etiologies concern neuropathologically proven fetal brain perfusion failures. Many other causes of fetal brain hypoxia have been reported or suggested. For a review, see Van Lierde (1983).

fusion failures in the fetal brain or fetal malnutrition. These original data are interesting, but their etiological and epidemiological significance needs further support. In our Multicenter Collaborative Study, sequential ultrasound examinations were performed from the time of occurrence of any suspected perfusion failure until birth, and diagnosis was confirmed on the basis of clinical and pathological data; Table 2 gives the occurrence of the different types of prenatal hypoxias in our multicenter study. Data obtained from this program, together with those from our own neuropathological collection, demonstrate the presence of two peaks of perfusion failure at two fetal periods: 20–24 weeks of gestation, and the last 10 weeks of gestation. Ischemia in the second half of gestation can display a vascular territorial distribution, and, in incompletely destroyed cortical areas, it may give rise to a laminar necrosis. Polymicrogyrias, porencephalies, and hydranencephaly are examples of perfu-

sion failures analyzed below. Other hypoxic conditions are listed in Tables 3 and 4.

Microgyrias or Polymicrogyrias Polymicrogyria is a term used to describe an abnormal macroscopic appearance of the brain gyration (see earlier discussion on the classification of malformations on the basis of their abnormal neuronal patterns) that is characterized by too many abnormally small convolutions. The appearance is somewhat variable: small gyri separated by shallow sulci are seen in some cases, while in others, the gyri are wider but with numerous minute indentations (see Figures 12A through 12D). Such abnormalities can often be detected on CT scan and nuclear magnetic resonance.

The basic cytoarchitectonic lesion in polymicrogyria is a mid-cortical ischemic laminar necrosis predominating in layer V (Figure 12A) (Richman et al., 1974). Above this necrotic cortical band, the cortex consists of normal layer IV-, III-, and II-neurons. The cortical laminar necrosis enhances the developmental growth difference between the inner and the outer cortical layers, and this mechanism seems to be at the origin of the polymicrogyric cortical overfolding (Richman et al., 1975). As the late migrating neurons reach their normal positions before the lamilar necrosis takes place, this type of microgyria dates and originates after the 20th fetal week and is considered *postmigratory*.

In some instances, another type of localized pallial disorganization has been described in

Table 4. Examples of perfusion failure—hypoxia

1. During the period of cytogenesis-histogenesis
Lissencephaly type 1 (?)
Onset of rare microgyric variants
Others

2. During the period of growth and differentiation
A. From 6th month on
Microgyria
Porencephaly
Hydranencephaly
B. Last months and perinatal period
Hydranencephaly
Multicystic encephalomalacias
Ulegyria

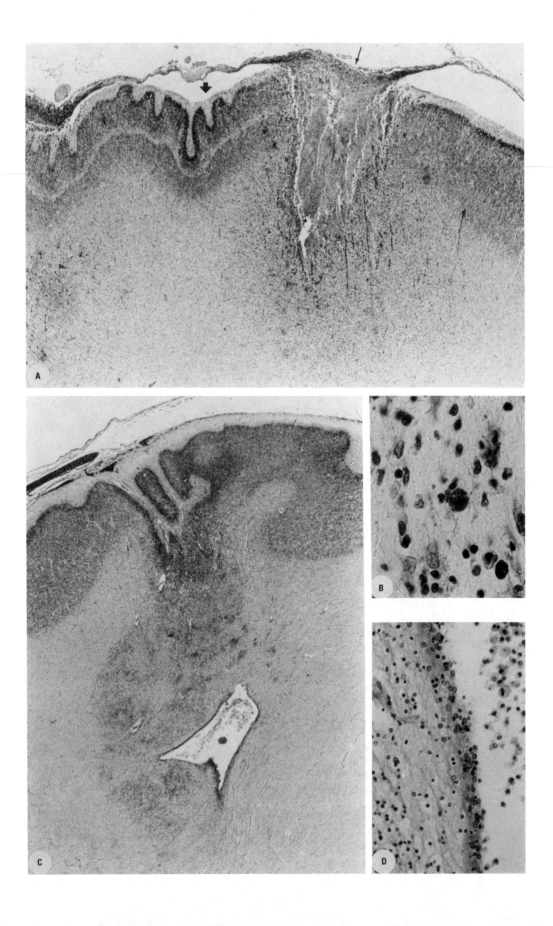

microgyria. Heterotopic neurons are found in the IZ beneath a microgyric cortical area. Ischemia provoking this type of microgyria with heterotopic features originates slightly *before the end of neuronal migration*. A fetal example of this variant is illustrated in Figure 12C. The IZ subjacent to the microgyric cortex contains neuronal heterotopias and displays destructive signs, notably the existence of a porencephalic cavity (Figure 12D) and glial scars.

Variants of microgyria and some other morphogenetic mechanisms have been proposed. For reviews of microgyric variants, see Dvorak and Feit (1977); Ferrer (1984); Lyon (1988); Lyon and Beaugerie (1988); Mac Bride and Kemper (1982); Norman (1980).

Clinicopathological correlations from the Multicenter Study and from our own Neuropathological Collection emphasize two points. First, concerning the etiology of microgyrias, most of the cases were due to perfusion failures provoked by cytomegalovirus (CMV). Other known etiologies were toxoplasmosis (Figures 12A and 12B), syphilis, and maternal shocks. Second, concerning the prenatal clinical evolution, ultrasound followups showed the occurrence of the break in cranial growth curve around 30 weeks in our cases of microgyria due to CMV infection (Figure 8).

Hydranencephaly Hydranencephaly represents an extensive destruction of cerebral territories normally supplied by both carotid arteries (Lyon & Robain, 1967). Nearly the entire cerebral mantle in both hemispheres is destroyed and replaced by a thin membrane of glial tissue covered by meninges. The vertebro-basilar territory is usually preserved with remnants of the temporo-occipital cortex. Some collateral circulation also develops into the basal ganglia. Victims of such accidents are microcephalic or show progressive macrocephaly, depending on whether or not aqueductal stenosis and/or arachnoidal fibrosis by blood or necrotic tissue is present. We have collected six cases of hydranencephaly with combined clinicopathological studies and sequential ultrasound examinations. From these data, the following conclusions were drawn:

1. These cases occurred around 30 weeks of gestation, later than what is often reported in the literature. Most of them were the consequence of either maternal shock (notably of toxic origin) or a sudden fetal accident characterized by a transitory but complete disappearance of fetal movement with no maternal problems.
2. The evolution of the lesions over the last 10 weeks of pregnancy was found to be in either of two patterns: massive hemorrhaging during the days following the initial perfusion failure or a progressive and slow resorption of the hemispheres without hemorrhaging. These two patterns are illustrated by the following examples:
   a. In some cases, fetal movement was reported to have ceased abruptly after 30 weeks of normal gestation. The cortical mantle was then of normal thickness. Subsequent ultrasonic examinations demonstrated progressive resorption of the brain regions irrigated by both internal carotid arteries. Delivery was at term, and the newborns were admitted with hydranencephaly that was confirmed by post mortem examination.
   b. In other cases, after a severe maternal shock around 30 weeks of gestation, the mothers recovered fully and the fetuses were followed up by repeated ultrasound examinations until birth. The day following the maternal shock, the fetal brain was shown to have had a massive hemorrhage.

Porencephalies Porencephalies are focal cerebral defects due to destructive processes (for references, see the beginning of this sec-

---

Figure 12. Microgyrias (see figure at left). **a.** Microgyria of the postmigratory type associated with toxoplasmosis infection. An area of massive cortical destruction (thin arrow) is bordered by a microgyric area (thick arrow) with laminar cortical necrosis (thick arrow). Human fetal brain, 29 weeks of gestation. **b.** Higher magnification of **a**, showing a toxoplasmic cyst. **c.** Microgyria occurring at the end of the migration period. Subjacent to the microgyric cortical area, a porencephalic lesion and glial scar with neuronal heterotopias are observed. Human fetal brain, 29 weeks of gestation. **d.** Higher magnification of the lining of the porencephalic cyst. Numerous macrophages are seen within its cavity.

tion). Most occur during the second half of gestation in areas perfused by major cerebral arteries. A microgyric cortex, caused by a milder ischemia at the border zone, is found adjacent to many porencephalies and helps to date the defect between 20 and 30 gestational weeks. The clinical manifestations may include cerebral palsy and epilepsy. The intellectual function is more often preserved than in many other prenatal perfusion failures. Prenatal porencephalies can continue to expand after birth; several such cases remain treatable during postnatal life (Tardieu, Evrard, & Lyon, 1981). In one of the Multicenter Study observations, sequential ultrasound examinations illustrated the appearance of a porencephaly following perfusion failure at 31 weeks of gestation and its expanding character during prenatal life.

Another type of developmental porencephaly needs to be mentioned. In our fetal neuropathological collection, there are cases in which limited hemorrhagic lesions of the germinative zone, occurring as early as 18 gestational weeks, constituted spherical porencephalic cavities in the deep intermediate zone without initial communication with the ventricule. Germinolytic cysts and rare genetic "porencephalies" were reviewed by Barth (1983); these last cases should not be confused with porencephalies occurring in successive pregnancies of the same mother secondary to nongenetic factors.

After the fetal period, distinction is difficult between the different types of prenatal porencephalies: ischemic accidents through the cerebral mantle in the territories of major cerebral arteries, early hemorrhages of germinative zone within the IZ and, perhaps, deep porencephalic cysts due to nonhemorrhagic lesions of the germinative zone.

"Minor" Cortical Dysgenesis

Many well understood prenatal disorders are disclosed by extensive brain malformations with severe clinical consequences. Identification of minor but unquestionable variations in the cortical pattern correlated with moderate neuropsychological disturbances (Galaburda & Kemper, 1979) opened new hopes but also raised difficult questions in clinicopathological correlations. "Minor" cortical dysgeneses, subtle and quantitative cytoarchitectonic disturbances, and defective neuronal growth and differentiation have been implicated as causative factors or as anatomical witnesses for dyslexia, autism, partial epilepsy, mental deficiency of unknown etiology, and other conditions. The need for careful, systematic, and sometimes serial section studies of a sufficient number of control brains is crucial to the development of this field. The importance of the data reported by Galaburda and Kemper on *dyslexia* has already been cited above. Neuronal ectopias have been discussed in another section. In the *fetal alcohol syndrome,* though constant findings, neuronal ectopias seem to be only a minor accompaniment of more significant disorders of embryogenesis, cell multiplication, growth, and differentiation (Abel et al., 1983; Kennedy, 1984; Rydberg, Alling, & Engel, 1985; Wisniewski et al., 1983). The minor cortical dysgenesis described by Menckee and Janz (1984) regarding *primary generalized epilepsy* has been deeply questioned by Lyon and Gastaut (1985). In our material, in a considerable number of *mentally defective patients* without a precise etiology, significant "minor developmental brain abnormalities" have been detected: abnormal persistance of the subpial cell layer of Ranke-Brun (besides its presence in several minor cortical dysgeneses, a conspicuous persisting Brun layer has also been observed in our material in a case of Neu syndrome). Additional abnormalities include the presence of aggregates of large neurons in the plexiform zone, the fragmentary aspect of the superficial layers, the "rippled" aspect (normally seen in fetal cerebral cortex around 16 weeks of gestation), and the generalized inversion of polarity of neocortical pyramidal neurons and Purkinje cells.

"Minor" dysgenesis and "microdysgenesis" are classically used in the restricted meaning of *minor lesions detected postnatally at the light microscopic level and without Golgi impregnation*. The detection and study of distur-

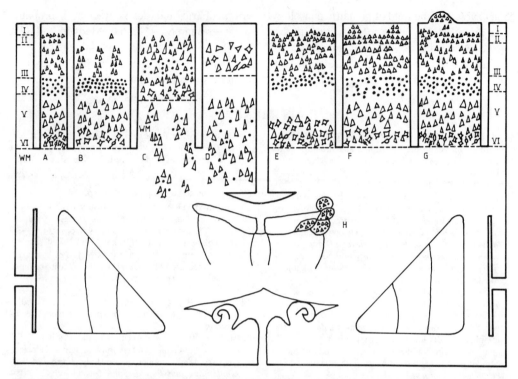

Figure 13.   Composite schematic drawing summarizing cell disposition in various abnormal neocortical neuronal patterns. (Key: **a:** normal cortical pattern in radial microbrain. **b:** microcephalia vera. **c:** Zellweger disease. **d:** Bielschowsky lissencephaly. **e:** microgyria. **f:** atypical microdysgenesis. **g:** neuronal ectopia within the subarachnoid space. **h:** periventricular heterotopias. **I** to **VI:** numerals of neocortical layers in the normal brain. **w m:** white matter. **Dotted lines:** inferior limit of the neocortex. (Figures 13 **a, b, g,** and **h** are derived from Evrard et al., 1982; Figure 13 **c** is derived from Evrard et al., 1978; Figures 13 **d,** and **e** are derived from Richman et al., 1974 and 1975, and from Stewart et al., 1975. The authors of the original papers are not responsible for the geometrical paradoxes of the present caricatural drawing used as a slide at the ICNA meeting.)

bances of neuronal differentiation are often beyond the capacity of Nissl staining. The Golgi method enabled Huttenlocher (1975), Purpura (1975), and others to demonstrate dendritic abnormalities and to suggest a defect in synaptogenesis as an explanation for some cases of mental retardation. EM studies have detected other disturbances of neuronal differentiation. Fetal neuropathology teaches us that "minor" dysgeneses are sometimes the only Nissl detected histological stigmata of major prenatal problems carrying severe consequences.

CONCLUSIONS

In this chapter, we have discussed methodological and conceptual approaches to abnormal neocortical development (Figure 13). Further progress in this field requires a multidisciplinary approach and multicenter coopera-

Table 5.   Neuropathology of human prenatal disorders

Classical limitations	Remedies
1. Collection of relevant material	1. Collaborative programs
2. Archeological approach	2. Use of concepts of developmental neurobiology
3. Difficulties of pathophysiological orientation of the conclusions	3. Use of new dynamic methods (e.g., ultrasound)

tion (Table 5). The field of pediatric neurology is in an optimal position to participate in this effort. A crucial condition is to emphasize again the clinicopathological correlation with more training and research investment in mod-

ern pediatric and developmental neuropathology research, (Gardner-Medwin, 1987), which is one of the tools for dialogue between the fields of clinical pediatric neurology and basic developmental neurobiology.

REFERENCES

Abel, E.L., Jacobson, S., & Sherwin, B.T. (1983). In utero alcohol exposure: functional and structural brain damage. *Neurobehavioral Toxicology and Teratology, 5*, 363–366.

Antanitus, D.S., Choi, B.H., & Lapham, L.W. (1976). The demonstration of glial fibrillary acidic protein in the cerebrum of the human fetus by indirect immunofluorescence. *Brain Research, 103*, 613–616.

Barth, P.G. (1983). Prenatal clastic encephalopathies. In Willemse, J. (Ed.), *Prenatal developmental disturbances. European Federation of Child Neurology Societies Symposium* (pp. 6–13). Noordwijkerhout, Akademisch Ziekenhuis Utrecht.

Barth, P.G. (1987). Disorders of neuronal migration. *Canadian Journal of Neurological Sciences, 14*, 1–16.

Bignami, A., Raju, T., & Dahl, D. (1982). Localization of vimentin, the nonspecific intermediate filament protein, in embryonal glia and in early differentiating neurons. In vivo and in vitro immunofluorescence study of the rat embryo with vimentin and neurofilament antisera. *Developmental Biology, 91*, 286–295.

Bordarier, C., Aicardi, J., & Goutières, F. (1984). Congenital hydrocephalus and eye abnormalities with severe developmental brain defects: Warburg's syndrome. *Annals of Neurology, 16*, 60–65.

Bovolenta, P., Liem, R.K.H., & Mason, C.A. (1984). Development of cerebellar astroglia: Transitions in form and cytoskeletal content. *Developmental Biology, 102*, 248–259.

Brückner, G., & Biesold, D. (1981). Histochemistry of glycogen deposition in perinatal rat brain. Importance of radial glial cells. *Journal of Neurocytology, 10*, 749–757.

Cataldo, A.M., & Broadwell, R.D. (1986). Cytochemical identification of cerebral glycogen and glucose-6-phosphatase activity under normal and experimental conditions: 1. Neurons and glial. *Journal of Electronmicroscopic Technology, 3*, 413–437.

Caviness, V.S. (1976). Patterns of cell and fiber distribution in the neocortex of the reeler mutant mouse. *Journal of Comparative Neurology, 170*, 435–448.

Caviness, V.S., Evrard, Ph., & Lyon, G. (1978). Radial neuronal assemblies ectopia and necrosis of developing cortex. *Acta Neuropathologica, 41*, 67–72.

Caviness, V.S., Misson, J.P., & Gadisseux, J.F. (in press). Abnormal neuronal patterns and disorders of neocortical development. In A.M. Galaburda (Ed.), *From Neuron to Reading: Toward a Neurobiology of Dyslexia*. Cambridge, MA: M.I.T. Press.

Caviness, V.S., Pinto-Lord, M.C., & Evrard, Ph. (1981). The development of laminated pattern in the mammalian neocortex. In T.G. Connely (Ed.), *Morphogenesis and pattern formation* (pp. 102–126). New York: Raven Press.

Caviness, V.S., & Rakic, P. (1978). Mechanism of cortical development: A view from mutations in mice. In M.W. Cowan, Z.W. Hall, & E.R. Kandel (Eds.), *Annual Review of Neuroscience* (pp. 297–326). Palo Alto: Annual Reviews, Inc.

Caviness, V.S., & Williams, R.S. (1984). Cellular patterns in developmental malformations of neocortex: Neuron-glial interactions. In Y. Suzuki, & H. Yabuuchi (Eds.), *The developing brain and its disorders* (pp. 43–67). Tokyo: University of Tokyo Press.

Chan, C.C., Egbert, P.R., Herrick, M.K., & Urich, H. (1980). Oculocerebral malformations. A reappraisal of Walker's "Lissencephaly." *Archives of Neurology, 37*, 104–108.

Chapman, P.H., & Caviness, V.S. (1988). Subtorcular occipital encephaloceles. *Concepts in Pediatric Neurosurgery, 8*, 86–96.

Choi, B.H. (1986). Glial fibrillary acidic protein in radial glia of early human fetal cerebrum: A light and electron microscopic immunoperoxidase study. *Journal of Neuropathology and Experimental Neurology, 45*, 408–414.

Choi, C.H., & Lapham, L.W. (1978). Radial glia in the human fetal cerebrum: A combined Golgi-immunofluorescence and electro-microscopic study. *Brain Research, 148*, 295–311.

Choi, B.H., & Matthias, S.C. (1987). Cortical dysplasia associated with massive ectopia of neurons and glial cells within the subarachnoid space. *Acta Neuropathologica, 73*, 105–109.

Della Giustina, E., Goffinet, A.M., Landrieu, P., & Lyon, G. (1981). A Golgi study of the brain malformation in Zellweger's cerebrohepatorenal disease. *Acta Neuropathologica, 55*, 23–28.

de Saint-Georges, P., Della Giustina, E., Kadhim, H.J., & Evrard, Ph. (in press). Etude du développement fétal du cortex holoprosencéphalique (Study of the fetal development of the holoprosencephalic cortex). (Abstract). *Revue Neurologique.*

de Saint-Georges, P., Kadhim, H.J., Lammens, M., Gosseye, S., Awoust, J., & Evrard, Ph. (1988). Potter syndrome, unpublished raw data.

Dupouey, P., Benjelloun, S., & Gomes, D. (1985). Immunohistochemical demonstration of an organized cytoarchitecture of the radial glia in the CNS of embryonic mouse. *Developmental Neuroscience, 7*, 81–93.

Dvorak, K., & Feit, J. (1977). Migration of neuroblasts through partial necrosis of the cerebral cortex in newborn rats—contribution to the problems of morphological development and developmental period of cerebral microgyria. *Acta Neuropathologica, 38*, 203–212.

Evrard, Ph., Belpaire, M.C., Boog, G., Elkhazen, N., Gadisseux, J.F., Le Marec, B., Misson, J.P., Santini, J.J., & Van Lierde, M. (1985). Diagnostic anténatal des affections du système nerveux central: Résultats préliminaires d'une étude multicentrique européenne. *Journal Français d'Echographie, 2*, 123–126.

Evrard, Ph., & Caviness, V.S. (1974). Extensive developmental defect of the cerebellum associated with posterior fossa ventriculocele. *Journal of Neuropathology and Experimental Neurology, 33*, 385–399.

Evrard, Ph., Caviness, V.S., Prats-Vinas, J., & Lyon, G. (1978). The mechanism of arrest of neuronal migration in the Zellweger malformation: An hypothesis based upon cytoarchitectonic analysis. *Acta Neuropathologica, 41*, 109–117.

Evrard, Ph., Gadisseux, J.F., & Lyon, G. (1982). Les malformations du système nerveux. In P. Royer (Ed.), *Naissance du cerveau (The malformations of the nervous system)*. (pp. 49–74). Paris: Lafayette.

Evrard, Ph., Lyon, G., & Gadisseux, J.F. (1984a). Le développement prénatal du système nerveux et ses perturbations: Mécanismes généraux (The prenatal development of the nervous system and its disturbances: General mechanisms). *Progrès en Néonatologie, 4*, 63–69.

Evrard, Ph., Lyon, G., Gadisseux, J.F. (1984b). Les processus destructifs agissant durant la seconde moitié de la grossesse, durant la période de croissance et de différenciation du tissu nerveux (The destructive processes acting during the second half of gestation and during the period of growth and differentiation of the nervous tissue). *Progrès en Néonatologie, 4*, 71–85.

Ferrer, I. (1984). A Golgi analysis of unlayered polymicrogyria. *Acta Neuropathologica, 65*, 69–76.

Freeman, J.M. (1985). *Prenatal and perinatal factors associated with brain disorders*. (NIH Publication No. 85-1149). Washington, DC: National Institute of Child Health and Development.

Friede, R. (1975). *Developmental Neuropathology*. Heidelberg, New York: Springer-Verlag.

Friede, R., & Mikolasek, J. (1978). Postencephalitic porencephaly, hydranencephaly or polymicrogyria: A review. *Acta Neuropathologica, 43*, 161–168.

Gadisseux, J.F., & Evrard, Ph. (1985). Glial-neuronal relationship in the developing central nervous system: A histochemical-electron microscope study of radial glial cell particulate glycogen in normal and reeler mice and the human fetus. *Developmental Neuroscience, 7*, 12–37.

Galaburda, A.M., & Kemper, T.L. (1979). Cytoarchitectonic abnormalities in developmental dyslexia: A case of study. *Annals of Neurology, 6*, 94–100.

Gardner-Medwin, D. (1987). Pediatric neuropathology. [Editorial]. *Developmental Medicine and Child Neurology, 29*, 143–144.

Giacomini, C. (1885). Contributo allo studio della microcefalia. *Archivi di Psichiatria, 6*, 63–81.

Gilles, F.H., Leviton, A., & Dooling, E.C. (1983). *The developing human brain, growth and epidemiologic neuropathology*. Boston, MA: John Wright.

Goffinet, A.M. (1984). Events governing organization of postmigratory neurons: Studies on brain development in normal and reeler mice. *Brain Research Review, 7*, 261–296.

Hamburg, D.A. (1985). *Reducing the casualties of early life: A preventive orientation*. (Annual report). New York: CarnegieCorporation of New York.

Holmes, M.D., Mosner, H.W., Halldorsson, S., Mack, C., Pant. S.S., & Matzilevich, B. (1972). *Mental retardation, an atlas of diseases with associated physical abnormalities*. New York: Macmillan.

Huttenlocher, P.R. (1975). Synaptic and dendritic development and mental defect. In N.A. Buchwald & M.A.B. Brazier (Eds.), *Brain mechanisms in mental retardation* (p. 123). New York: Academic Press.

Icenogle, D.A., & Kaplan, A.M. (1981). A review of congenital neurologic malformations. *Clinical Pediatrics, 20*, 565–576.

Jammes, J.L., & Gilles, F.H. (1983). Telencephalic development: Matrix volume and isocortex and allocortex surface areas. In F.H. Gilles, A. Leviton, & E.C. Dooling (Eds.), *The developing human brain* (pp. 87–93). Boston, MA: John Wright.

Kadhim, H.J., Gadisseux, J.F., & Evrard, Ph. (1988). Topographical and cytological evolution of the glial phase during the prenatal development of the human brain: A histochemical and electron microscopic study. *Journal of Neuropathology and Experimental Neurology, 47*(2), 166–188.

Kennedy, L.A. (1984). The pathogenesis of brain abnormalities in the fetal alcohol syndrome: An integrating hypothesis. *Teratology, 29*, 363–368.

Kuban, K.C.K., & Gilles, F.H. (1985). Human telencephalic angiogenesis. *Annals of Neurology, 17*, 539–548.

Larrabee, M.G. (1985). Ontogeny of glucose metabolism in sympathetic ganglia of chicken. *Journal of Neurochemistry, 45*, 1193–1200.

Larroche, J.C. (1977). Cytoarchitectonic abnormalities (abnormalities of cell migration). In P.J. Vincken & G.W. Bruyn (Eds.), *Handbook of clinical neurology, congenital malformations of brain and skull, Part I* (Vol. 50, pp. 479–506). New York: Elsevier/North Holland.

Leech, R.W., & Shuman, R.M. (1986). Holoprosencephaly and related midline cerebral anomalies: A review. *Journal of Child Neurology, 1*, 3–18.

Lidov, H.G.W., & Molliver, M.E. (1982). The structure of cerebral cortex in the rat following prenatal administration of 6-hydroxydopamine. *Developmental Brain Research, 3*, 81–108.

Lyon, G. (in press). Neuropathology of prenatal and perinatal ischemic encephalopathies. Physiopathological implications. In *Cerebral ultrasonography* (2nd ed.). New York: Churchill Livingstone.

Lyon, G., & Beaugerie, A. (in press). Developmental abnormalities of the brain. In M.I. Levene (Ed.), *Fetal and neonatal neurology and neurosurgery*. New York: Churchill Livingstone.

Lyon, G., & Gastaut, H. (1985). Considerations on the significance attributed to unusual cerebral histological findings recently described in eight patients with primary generalized epilepsy. *Epilepsia, 26*, 365–367.

Lyon, G., & Robain, O. (1967). Encéphalopathies circulatoires prénatales et périnatales. *Acta Neuropathologica, 9*, 79–98.

Mac Bride, M.C., & Kemper, T.L. (1982). Pathogenesis of four-layered microgyric cortex in man. *Acta Neuropathologica, 57*, 93–98.

Marques Dias, M.J., Harmant-Van Rijckevorsel, G., Landrieu, P., & Lyon, G. (1984). Prenatal cytomegalovirus disease and cerebral microgyria: Evidence for perfusion failure, not disturbance of histogenesis, as the major cause of fetal cytomegalovirus encephalopathy. *Neuropediatrics, 15*, 18.

Maxwell, M.H. (1978). An on-grid method for the specific demonstration of glycogen in electron microscopy. *Medical Laboratory Science, 35*, 201–202.

Meencke, H.J., & Janz, D. (1984). Neuropathological findings in primary generalized epilepsy: A study of eight cases. *Epilepsia, 25*, 8–21.

Nelson, K.B., & Ellenberg, J.H. (1986). Antecedents of cerebral palsy. Multivariate analysis of risk. *The New England Journal of Medicine, 315*, 81–86.

Norman, M.G. (1980). Bilateral encephaloclastic lesions in a 26 week gestation fetus: Effect on neuroblast migration. *Le Journal Canadien des Sciences Neurologiques, 7*, 191–194.

Norman, M.G., & Kusky, J.R. (1986). The growth and development of microvasculature in human cerebral cortex. *Journal of Neuropathology and Experimental Neurology, 45*, 222–232.

Ornoy, A., Benady, S., & Kohen-Raz, A. (1976). Association between maternal bleeding during gestation and congenital anomalies in the offspring. *American Journal of Obstetrics and Gynecology, 124*, 474–478.

Parain, D., Gadisseux, J.F., Henocq, A., Tayot, J., & Evrard, Ph. (1985). Diagnostic prénatal et étude d'une microcephalia vera à 26 semaines de gestation (Prenatal diagnosis and study of a 26 fetal week case of microcephalia vera). In H. Szliwowski & J. Bormans (Eds.), *Progrès en Neurologie Pédiatrique* (pp. 235–236). Bruxelles: Prodim.

Peters, A., & Feldman, M. (1973). The cortical plate and the molecular layer of the late rat fetus. *Zeitschrift für Anatomie Entwicklungs-Geschichte, 141*, 3–37.

Pinto-Lord, M.C., Evrard, Ph., & Caviness, V.S. (1982). Obstructed neuronal migration along radial glial fibers in the neocortex of the reeler mouse: A Golgi-EM analysis. *Developmental Brain Research, 4*, 379–383.

Pixley, S.R., & De Vellis, J. (1984). Transition between immature radial glia and mature astrocytes studied with a monoclonal antibody to vimentin. *Developmental Brain Research, 15*, 201–209.

Porter, I.H., & Hook, E.B. (1980). *Human embryonic and fetal death.* New York: Academic Press.

Purpura, D.P. (1975). Dendritic differentiation in human cerebral cortex: Normal and aberrant developmental patterns. In G.W. Kreutzberg (Ed.), *Advances in neurology* (Vol. 12, pp. 91–116). New York: Raven Press.

Rakic, P. (1981). Developmental events leading to laminar and areal organization of the neocortex. In F.O. Schmitt, F.G. Worden, & S.G. Denis (Eds.), *The organization of cerebral cortex* (pp. 7–28). Cambridge, MA: MIT Press.

Rakic, P. (1984). Emergence of neuronal and glial cell lineages in primate brain. In I.B. Black (Ed.), *Cellular and molecular biology of neuronal development. Proceedings of a symposium on cellular and molecular biology of neuronal development* (pp. 29–50). St. Thomas, U.S. Virgin Islands, March 2–5, 1983. New York: Plenum.

Renier, W.O., Gabreels, F.J.M., Jasper, H.H.J., Hustinx, T.W.I., Geelen, J.A.G., & Van Haelst, U.J.G. (1982). An X-linked syndrome with microcephaly, severe mental retardation, spasticity, epilepsy and deafness. *Journal of Mental Deficiency Research, 26*, 27–40.

Richman, D.P., Stewart, R.M., & Caviness, V.S. (1974). Cerebral microgyria in a 27 weeks fetus: An architectonic and topographic analysis. *Journal of Neuropathology and Experimental Neurology, 33*, 374–384.

Richman, D.P., Stewart, R.M., Hutchinson, J.W., & Caviness, V.S. (1975). Mechanical model of brain convolutional development. *Science, 189*, 18–21.

Robain, O., & Lyon, G. (1972). Les micrencéphalies familiales par malformation cérébrale (The familial microencephalies by cerebral malformation). *Acta Neuropathologica, 20*, 96–109.

Rockel, A.J., Hiorns, R.W., & Powel, T.P.S. (1980). The basic uniformity in structure of the neocortex. *Brain, 103*, 221–244.

Rydberg, U., Alling, C., & Engel. (1985). *Alcohol and the developing brain.* New York: Raven Press.

Sievers, J., Pehlemann, F.W., Baumgarten, H.G., & Berry, M. (1985). Selective destruction of meningeal cells by 6-hydroxydopamine: A tool to study meningeal-neuroepithelial interaction in brain development. *Developmental Biology, 110*, 127–135.

Stewart, R., Richman, D., & Caviness, V.S. (1975). Lissencephaly and pachygyria: An architectonic and topographical analysis. *Acta Neuropathologica, 31*, 1–12.

Tardieu, M., Evrard, Ph., & Lyon, G. (1981). Progressive expanding congenital porencephalies: A treatable cause of progressive encephalopathy. *Pediatrics, 68*, 198–202.

Thiery, J.P. (1967). Mise en évidence des polysaccharides sur coupes fines en microscopie électronique (The discernment of polysaccharides on thin sections on electron microscopy). *Journal de Microscopie, 6*, 987–1018.

Vamecq, J., Draye, J.P., Van Hoof, F., Misson, J.P., Evrard, Ph., Verellen, G., Eyssen, H., Van Eldere, J., Schutgens, R., Wanders, R., Roels, F., & Goldfischer, S. (1986). Multiple peroxisomal enzymatic deficiency disorders. A comparative biochemical and morphologic study of Zellweger cerebrohepatorenal syndrome and neonatal adrenoleukodystrophy. *American Journal of Pathology, 125*, 82–93.

Van Lierde, M. (1983). Attitude obstetricale devant le retard de croissance foetale. *L'Enfant, 3*, 10–22.

Van Lierde, M., & Evrard, Ph. (1986). Conclusions d'une étude multicentrique européenne sur les anomalies du tube neural (Conclusions of a European multicenter study about the anomalies of the neural tube). *Journal de Génétique Humaine, 34*, 343–365.

Volpe, J.J. (1987). *Neurology of the newborn* (2nd ed.). Philadelphia: W.B. Saunders.

Williams, R.S., & Caviness, V.S. (1984). Normal and abnormal development of the brain. In R.E. Tarter & G. Goldstein (Eds.), *Advances in clinical neuropsychology* (Vol. 2, pp. 1–62). New York: Plenum.

Williams, R.S., Swisher, C.N., Jennings, M., Ambler, M., & Caviness, V.S. (1984). Cerebroocular dysgenesis "Walker-Warburg" syndrome: Neuropathologic and etiologic analysis. *Neurology, 34*, 1531–1541.

Wisniewski, K., Dambska, M., Sher, J.H., & Qazi, Q. (1983). A clinical neuropathological study of the fetal alcohol syndrome. *Neuropediatrics, 14*, 197–201.

Chapter 20

Sonographic Anatomy of the Neonatal Head

Thomas P. Naidich, David K. Yousefzadeh, and Debra A. Gusnard

NEW ULTRASOUND EQUIPMENT NOW DIS-plays many anatomic structures far more clearly than was possible previously. This paper discusses the "new" sonographic anatomy.

SONOGRAPHY OF THE NEONATAL HEAD

Previous works have provided initial descriptions of neonatal ultrasonic brain anatomy (see Supplementary Resources at end of chapter). This communication illustrates the fine anatomy depicted by the Acuson 128 Computed Sonography Unit using 3.5 and 5.0 MHz sector and linear array transducers.

Coronal ultrasound sections through the anterior fontanelle display the neonatal calvarium as thin, hyperechoic plates of bone that taper medially toward the fontanelle (Figure 1). The walls of the superior sagittal sinus appear as an echogenic triangle. The lumen is normally hypoechoic. The falx may be resolved as a hyperechoic line that descends from the inferior point of the sinus into the interhemispheric fissure.

The brain surface appears as an echogenic line where the sound beam intersects the crown of a gyrus, and as a hyperechoic scallop where the beam cuts through a sulcus to expose the full face of the gyrus. The cortical gray matter forms a thin, relatively hypoechoic ribbon deep to the hyperechoic brain surface. The white matter cores of each gyrus manifest as hyperechoic central echoes. These echoes probably reflect vessels within the white matter rather than the substance of the white matter itself. The gray-white matter junction is easily discerned.

Narrow sulci and fissures appear hyperechoic because the film of anechoic cerebrospinal fluid (CSF) within them cannot be resolved separate from the apposing brain surfaces. Wide sulci and fissures appear anechoic or hypoechoic, because the contained anechoic CSF can be resolved separately. Cisterns that contain multiple pulsing vessels may still appear hyperechoic even when wide.

In the midline, ultrasound demonstrates the vertical interhemispheric fissure, the nearly horizontal callosal and cingulate sulci, and the intervening cingulate gyrus (Figure 1). Inferiorly, the gyrus rectus lies between the interhemispheric fissure and the olfactory sulcus on each side. The basal (suprasellar) cistern appears as a three-pointed crown: the middle point extends upward toward the interhemispheric fissure. The two lateral points pass toward the cisterns of the insulae. The sella turcica and cavernous sinuses lie inferiorly. The temporal lobes delimit the inferolateral borders of the basal cistern. The middle cerebral arteries can usually be discerned as horizontal tubes, with echogenic walls and hypoechoic lumina. These course laterally from the basal cistern to the cistern of the insula on each side.

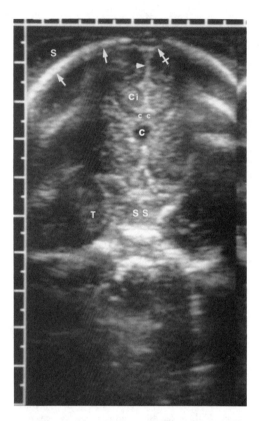

Figure 1. Coronal 5.0 MHz sonogram. Sonography demonstrates the scalp (S), hyperechoic bone plates of the calvarium (white arrows), superior sagittal sinus (crossed white arrow), echogenic interhemispheric fissure (white arrowhead), the hypoechoic gray matter and hyperechoic white matter of the cingulate gyrus (Ci), thin, hypoechoic trapezoidal corpus callosum (cc), cavum septi pellucidi (C), crown-shaped suprasellar cistern (SS), and temporal lobe (T).

The medial-most surface of the temporal lobe is formed by the parahippocampal gyrus. This is delimited laterally by the collateral sulcus. Anteriorly, the parahippocampal gyrus hooks medially to form the uncus. Just posterior to the uncus, the medial surface of the temporal lobe appears to be rolled into the inferomedial temporal horn as the hippocampal formation (Figure 2). The hippocampal formation lies just below the choroidal fissure and surrounds the deep hippocampal fissure. The dentate gyrus lies just superior to the hippocampal fissure. The subiculum lies just inferior to the hippocampal fissure. The hippocampus surrounds the lateral end of the hippocampal fissure forming a ''C'' (or reverse C) of gray matter that is open medially. The lateral arc of

the C bulges into the temporal horn. The upper portion of the hippocampus recurves medially above the dentate gyrus. The alveus and fimbria of the fornix form the superior lateral border of the hippocampus and the dentate gyrus. Along the temporal lobe, the fornix is separated from the thalamus by the perimesencephalic cistern and the choroidal fissure.

The neonatal corpus callosum appears as a thin sonolucent band that forms the roof of the cavum septi pellucidi. The left and right leaves of the septum pellucidum form the lateral walls of the cavum. The frontal horns appear as hypoechoic spaces situated lateral to the cavum septi pellucidi. Prominent hyperechoic zones that flare outward from the lateral angles of the frontal horns are believed to represent prominent periventricular vasculature, especially in premature infants. The subependymal germinal matrix and the caudate nuclei are modes-

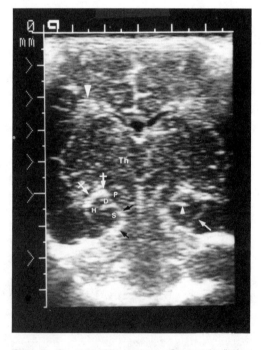

Figure 2. Coronal 5.0 MHz sonogram. Sonography displays the flaring echogenicity of periventricular vessels (large white arrowhead), the ovoid thalami (Th), the hypoechoic cerebral peduncle (P), the echogenic perimesencephalic cistern (black arrows) that continues laterally through the choroidal fissure to the temporal horn (crossed white arrows), the echogenic collateral sulcus (white arrow) and hippocampal fissure (small white arrowhead), the subiculum (S), the dentate gyrus (D), and the hippocampus (H).

tly echoic structures that form the lateral borders of the frontal horns.

The major portions of the internal capsule are readily identified by ultrasound. The anterior limbs of the internal capsules appear as thin, hyperechoic, obliquely oriented lines situated between the caudate nuclei and the putamina. The genus of the internal capsules appear as isoechoic curves that are concave inferolaterally where they pass over the lentiform nuclei. The posterior limbs of the internal capsules appear as hypoechoic curves that are concave medially where they arc around the lateral borders of the thalami. The hypoechoic posterior limbs lead directly inferiorly into the hypoechoic cerebral peduncles.

Ultrasonic sections through the genu of the internal capsule display the lentiform nucleus, external capsule, claustrum, extreme capsule, and insula as a series of crescentic bands of alternating hyperechoic white matter and hypoechoic gray matter (Naidich, Gusnard, & Yousefzadeh, 1985). The heights of these crescents decrease progressively from lateral to medial forming a "striated lateral wedge" (Figure 3). The most lateral, the tallest, and the

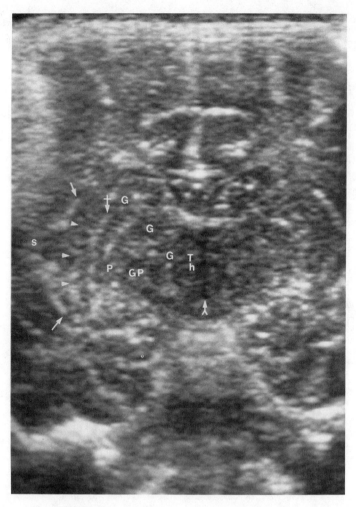

Figure 3.   Coronal 5.0 MHz sonogram. Sonography displays the wide, anechoic sylvian fissure (S) that leads to the cistern of the insula, the top and bottom of the circular sulcus (white arrows) of the insula, the echogenic surface of the insula (white arrowheads), the echogenic external capsule (crossed white arrow), the putamen (P), the globus pallidus (GP), the curving isoechoic genu (G) of the internal capsule, and the thalamus (Th) that flanks the anechoic third ventricle (fishtail white arrow). *Note:* From "Sonography of the Internal Capsule and Basal Ganglia in Infants" by T.P. Naidich, D.A. Gusnard, & D.K. Yousefzadeh, 1985, *American Journal of Neuroradiology, 6*, pp. 909–917. Reprinted by permission.

brightest hyperechoic crescent is the surface of the insula. The top and bottom of that crescent is the circular sulcus. The next brightest and shorter echo situated further medially is the external capsule that separates the putamen from the claustrum laterally. The putamen is often slightly more echoic than the globus pallidus medial to it. On occasion, the lateral and medial nuclei of the globus pallidus may be discerned separately. The claustrum and extreme capsule are rarely depicted clearly.

The thalami manifest as two large ovoids of slightly inhomogeneous echogenicity that correspond to the diverse nuclear groups of the thalamus. The posterior limbs of the internal capsules separate the thalami from the posterior portions of the lenticular nuclei. These posterior portions are composed of the *lateral* nuclei of the globi pallidi and the putamina.

Midsagittal ultrasound sections display the relationships among the medial gyri, corpus callosum, midline cava, and third ventricle (Figure 4). The thin curvilinear hypoechoic corpus callosum is delimited superiorly by the hyperechoic callosal sulcus and the vessels it contains. It is delimited inferiorly by a hyperechoic line that probably corresponds to the interface between the corpus callosum and CSF. The hypoechoic gray and the hyperechoic white matter of the cingulate gyrus form arcs just superficial to the callosal sulcus.

The CSF space deep to the corpus callosum is the cavum septi pellucidi and, if present, the cavum vergae. The fornices arc anteriorly just

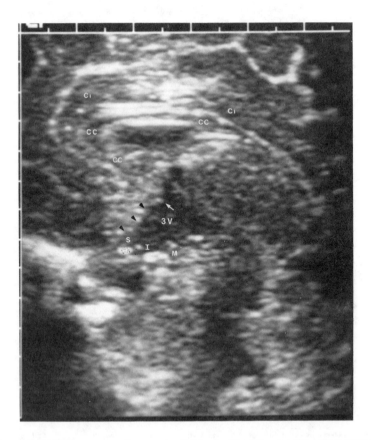

Figure 4.   Midline sagittal 5.0 MHz sonogram. Sonography displays the cingulate gyrus (Ci), corpus callosum (CC), anterior commissure (white arrow) indenting the anterior wall of the triangular third ventricle (3V) just inferior to the foramen of Monro, the lamina terminalis (black arrowheads), supraoptic (S) and infundibular (I) recesses of the third ventricle enclosing the chiasm, and the mamillary body (M).

below the corpus callosum and then curve downward over the foramina of Monro to form columns of the fornices along the anteromedial borders of the foramina of Monro. The thalami lie below the fornices but are separated from them by the transverse fissure. The fissure contains the velum interpositum, the cistern of the velum interpositum, the choroidal vessels, and the internal cerebral veins.

The third ventricle appears as a vaguely triangular hypoechoic zone. The lamina terminalis angles anteroinferiorly from the foramen of Monro to form the straight anterior wall of the third ventricle. It is notched superiorly by the anterior commissure. The supraoptic and infundibular recesses of the third ventricle appear as hypoechoic outpouchings that enclose the optic chiasm. The chiasm protrudes inferiorly into the basal (suprasellar) cistern, where it is outlined by suprasellar CSF. The mammillary bodies form hypoechoic "nodules" at their expected positions along the floor of the third ventricle. The massa intermedia that crosses the third ventricle is highly variable in size. It usually appears as a hyperechoic ovoid with a hypoechoic center.

More lateral sagittal sonograms display the lateral ventricle, portions of the basal ganglia, the thalamus, and the temporal lobe. Two distinct angulations produce different, equally valuable images. When the transducer is angled far laterally, sonographic sections display the full contour of the lateral ventricle and nearly the full contour of the choroid plexus. The choroid glomus forms a hyperechoic nodule that projects posteriorly into the atrium.

When the transducer is angled less far laterally, the sonographic section displays the body of the lateral ventricle but only a small portion of the medialmost temporal horn. Variable amounts of choroid plexus will be seen to extend around the thalamus from the caudothalamic notch anteriorly toward the temporal horn inferiorly. In this section, the roof of the lateral ventricle is corpus callosum. The floor of the lateral ventricle is formed by the caudate nucleus anteriorly, the thalamus posteriorly, and the intervening caudothalamic groove (or notch). The caudate nucleus, lenticular nu-

cleus, and thalamus take the shape of a "gangliothalamic ovoid" (Figure 5) (Naidich, Yousefzadeh, Gusnard, 1986a; 1986b).

The upper border of the ovoid has a double hump formed by the caudate anteriorly, the thalamus posteriorly, and the intervening caudothalamic groove (Bowie, Kirks, Rosenberg, & Clair, 1983). The anterior pole of the ovoid is the head of caudate nucleus. This is delimited anteriorly by the radiations of the corpus callosum. The posterior pole of the ovoid is the pulvinar. This is delimited by the glomus of the choroid plexus and the atrium. The inferior contour of the ovoid exhibits three arcs that are convex inferiorly (Naidich, Yousefzadeh, & Gusnard, 1986; Naidich, Yousefzadeh, Gusnard, & Naidich, 1986). The anterior arc is formed by the caudate and lenticular nuclei. This is the ganglial arc. The middle arc is formed by the cerebral peduncle and is the peduncular arc. The posterior arc is formed by the thalamus and is the thalamic arc. The entire inferior surface of the ovoid is delimited by the perimesencephalic cistern and choroidal fissure. Beneath the ovoid lies the temporal lobe, specifically the hippocampal formation. The anterior limb, genu, and posterior limb of internal capsule subdivide the gangliothalamic ovoid into an anterior ganglial portion and a posterior thalamic portion.

The senotexture of the gangliothalamic ovoid typically exhibits four obliquely oriented parallel zones of increased and decreased echogenicity (Figure 5) (Naidich, Yousefzadeh, & Gusnard, 1986; Naidich, Yousefzadeh, Gusnard, & Naidich, 1986). The most anterior band, band 1, is hyperechoic. Band 2 is hypoechoic. Band 3 is hyperechoic. The posterior band 4 is hypoechoic. Hyperechoic band 1 is composed predominantly of caudate nucleus with small, variable components of putamen and globus pallidus.

Hypoechoic band 2 is formed by two different structures. The posterior portion of band 2 corresponds to the internal capsule and has the shape of a γ. The anterior arm of the γ is the anterior limb of internal capsule. The stem of the γ is the genu of internal capsule that leads inferiorly to the peduncular arc of the ovoid.

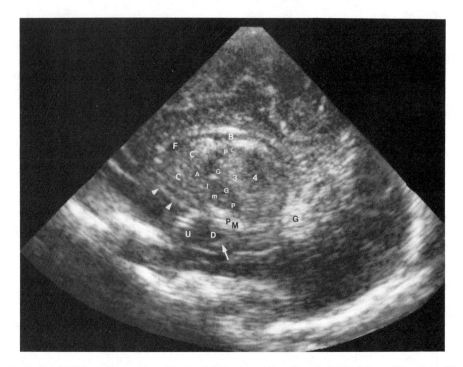

Figure 5.   Sagittal 3.5 MHz sector sonogram. The gangliothalamic ovoid is outlined by the frontal horn (F) and body (B) of the lateral ventricle, the radiations of the corpus callosum (white arrowheads), the perimesencephalic cistern (PM), and the glomus (G) of the choroid plexus behind the pulvinar. The anterior limb (A), genu (G), and posterior limb (PL) of the internal capsule and the cerebral penduncle (P) form a hypoechoic, ν-shape that subdivides the ovoid into an anterior, ganglio-capsular portion and a posterior thalamic portion. The anterior portion contains the caudate nucleus (C) and the medial (m) and lateral (l) nuclei of globus pallidus. The posterior portion contains the ventral and lateral nuclei of thalamus (3) and the pulvinar (4). The dentate gyrus (D) lies anteroinferior to the peduncle (P) across the perimesencephalic cistern. (U = uncus; white arrow = hippocampal fissure.) *Note.* From "Sonography of the Internal Capsule and Basal Ganglia in Infants" by T.P. Naidich, D.K. Yousefzadeh, D.A. Gusnard, and J.B. Naidich, 1986, *Radiology, 161,* pp. 615–621. Reprinted by permission.

The posterior arm of the γ is part of the posterior limb of the internal capsule. The anterior portion of hypoechoic band 2 lies anterior to the internal capsule within the arch formed by the anterior limb and stem of the γ-shaped internal capsule. This anterior portion of band 2 corresponds to the lenticular nucleus, particularly the globus pallidus.

Hyperechoic band 3 consistently starts immediately behind the caudothalamic groove and angles posteroinferiorly to the ganglial arc of the inferior border of the ovoid. Hyperechoic band 3 appears to correspond to the lateral and the ventral groups of thalamic nuclei (exclusive of the pulvinar). Hypoechoic band 4 appears to correspond to the pulvinaric nuclei of the thalamus.

Inferior to the gangliothalamic ovoid is the temporal lobe (Figure 6). The long parahip-

pocampal gyrus sweeps anteroinferiorly to the anterior temporal fossa and then recurves posterosuperiorly to form the uncus. The hippocampal formation lies between the parahippocampal gyrus and the gangliothalamic ovoid. The choroidal fissure, perimesencephalic cistern, and hippocampal fissure form a distinct hyperechoic zone between the gangliothalamic ovoid and the hippocampal formation. The dentate gyrus lies between the perimesencephalic cistern and the hippocampal fissure anterior and inferior to the cerebral peduncle. The subiculum appears as a stripe of hypoechoic gray matter that parallels the perimesencephalic cistern. The fornix curves upward posteriorly and is separated from the pulvinar by the choroidal fissure.

Far lateral sagittal sonograms display the sylvian fissure as an oblique hyperechoic line

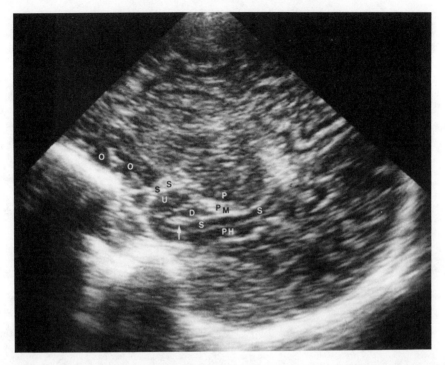

Figure 6.   Sagittal 3.5 MHz sector sonogram. Sonography displays the orbital gyri (O) at the base of the frontal lobe, the sylvian fissure (black S), the long parahippocampal gyrus (PH) that sweeps forward and recurves to form the uncus (U), the dentate gyrus (D) above the hippocampal fissure (white arrow), the subiculum (white S) below the fissure, and the perimesencephalic cistern (PM) that separates the hippocampal formation from the gangliothalamic ovoid. (P = cerebral peduncle.) *Note.* From "Sonography of the Normal Neonatal Head" by T.P. Naidich, D.K. Yousefzadeh, & D.A. Gusnard,1986,*Neuroradiology, 28,* pp. 408–427. Reprinted by permission.

that rises posterosuperiorly. The superior and middle temporal gyri each appears as *two layers* of hypoechoic gray matter surrounding a thin hyperechoic white core. The superior and inferior temporal sulci are readily identified as oblique hyperechoic stripes that course parallel to the sulvian fissure and that are usually thicker and more intensely echoic than the white matter cores of the gyri. The Island of Reil appears as a triangular zone of cortical surface, delimited by the circular sulcus and containing the hypoechoic crowns of the short and long gyri of the insula.

CONCLUSION

Recent improvements in ultrasound equipment have permitted the physician to display anatomic features more clearly than was previously possible. With further application of current and future technology, sonography is expected to display most of the significant anatomic features of the infant brain. Proper use of this new technology and exploitation of its full potential will then require that the physicians who interpret these studies increase their knowledge of neuroanatomy commensurately.

REFERENCES

Naidich, T.P., Gusnard, D.A., & Yousefzadeh, D.K. (1985). Sonography of the internal capsule and basal ganglia in infants, Part 1: Coronal sections. *American Journal of Neuroradiology, 6,* 909–917.

Naidich, T.P., Yousefzadeh, D.K., & Gusnard, D.A. (1986). Sonography of the normal neonatal head. Supra-

tentorial structures: State-of-the-art imaging. *Neuroradiology, 28,* 408–427.

Naidich, T.P., Yousefzadeh, D.K., Gusnard, D.A., & Naidich, J.B. (1986). Sonography of the internal capsule and basal ganglia in infants, Part II: Localization of pathologic processes in the sagittal section through the caudothalamic groove. *Radiology, 161,* 615–621.

184   Naidich, Yousefzadeh, and Gusnard

SUPPLEMENTARY RESOURCES

Atlas, S.W., Shkolnik, A., & Naidich, T.P. (1985). Sonographic recognition of agenesis of the corpus callosum. *American Journal of Neuroradiology, 6*, 369–375.

Babcock, D.S., & Han, B.K. (1981). The accuracy of high resolution, real-time ultrasonography of the head in infancy. *Radiology, 139*, 665–676.

Babcock, D.S., & Han, B.K. (1981). Cranial ultrasonography of infants. Baltimore: Williams & Wilkins.

Babcock, D.S., Han, B.K., & LeQuesne, G.W. (1980). B-mode gray scale ultrasound of the head in the newborn and young infant. *American Journal of Roentgenology, 134*, 457–468.

Birnholz, J.C. (1982). Newborn cerebellar size. *Pediatrics, 70*, 284–287.

Bowie, J., Kirks, D., Rosenberg, E., Clair, M. (1983). Caudothalamic groove: Value in identification of germinal matrix hemorrhage by sonography in preterm neonates. *American Journal of Roentgenology, 141*, 1317–1320.

Corrales, M., del Villar, S., Hevia, R., & Saez, M. (1983). Sonography of the posterior fossa. *American Journal of Neuroradiology, 4*, 665–667.

Couture, A., & Cadier, L. (1983). *Echographie cerebrale par voie transfontanellaire [Transfontanelle cerebral echography]*. Paris: Vigot.

Cremin, B.J., Chilton, S.J., Peacock, W.J. (1983). Anatomical landmarks in anterior fontanelle ultrasonography. *British Journal of Radiology, 56*, 517–566.

de Vlieger, M. (1980). Evaluation of echoencephalography. *Journal of Clinical Ultrasound, 8*, 39–47.

DiPetro, M.A., Brody, B.A., & Teele, R.L. (1985). The calcar avis: Demonstration with cranial US. *Radiology, 156*, 363–364.

Edwards, M.K., Brown, D.L., Muller, J., Grossman, C.B., & Chua, G.T. (1980). Cribside neurosonography: Real-time sonography for intracranial investigation of the neonate. *American Journal of Neuroradiology, 1*, 501–505.

Goodwin, L., & Quisling, R.G. (1983). The neonatal cisterna magna: Ultrasonic evaluation. *Radiology, 149*, 691–695.

Grant, E.G., Schellinger, D., Borts, F., McCullough, D.C., Friedman, G.R., Sivasubramanian, K.N., &

Smith, Y. (1980). Real-time sonography of the neonatal and infant head. *American Journal of Neuroradiology, 1*, 487–492.

Heimburger, R.F., Fry, F.J., Franklin, T.D., et al. (1979). Two-dimensional ultrasound scanning of excised brains: I. Normal anatomy. *Ultrasound in Medicine and Biology, 2*, 279–285.

Johnson, M., Mack, L., Rumack, C., Frost, M., & Rashbaum, C. (1979). B-mode echoencephalography in the normal and high-risk infant. *American Journal of Roentgenology, 133*, 375–381.

Kossoff, G., Garrett, W.J., & Radavanovich, G. (1974). Ultrasonic atlas of normal brain of infant. *Ultrasound in Medicine and Biology, 1*, 259–266.

Pigadas, A., Thompson, J.R., Grube, G.L. (1981). Normal infant brain anatomy: Correlated real-time sonograms and brain specimens. *American Journal of Neuroradiology, 2*, 339–344.

Rumack, C.M., & Johnson, M.L. (1984). Perinatal & infant brain imaging. Role of ultrasound & computed tomography. Chicago: Yearbook Medical Publishers.

Sauerbrei, E.E., & Cooperberg, P.L. (1981). Neonatal brain: Sonography of congenital abnormalities. *American Journal of Neuroradiology, 2*, 125–128.

Shuman, W.P., Rogers, J.V., Mack, L.A., Alvord, E.C., Jr, & Christie, D.P. (1981). Real-time sonographic sector scanning of the neonatal cranium: Technique and normal anatomy. *American Journal of Neuroradiology, 2*, 349–356.

Siedler, D.E., Mahony, B.S., Hoddick, W.K., & Callen, P.W. (1985). A specular reflection raising from the ventricular wall: A potential pitfall in the diagnosis of germinal matrix hemorrhage. *Journal of Ultrasound in Medicine, 4*, 109–112.

Slovis, T.L., & Kuhns, L.R. (1981). Real-time sonography of the brain through the anterior fontanelle. *American Journal of Roentgenology, 136*, 277–286.

Stannard, M.W., Binet, E.F., & Jimenez, J.F. (1984). Cranial sonography: Anatomic and pathological correlation. *CRC Critical Reviews in Diagnostic Imaging, 22(3)*, 163–268.

Yousefzadeh, D.K., & Naidich, T.P. (1985). US anatomy of the posterior fossa in children: Correlation with brain sections. *Radiology, 156*, 353–361.

Chapter 21

Neuropathological Validation of Cranial Ultrasound Diagnosis in Low Birth Weight Infants

Some Preliminary Observations

Jennifer Pinto, Nigel Paneth, Ram Kairam, and Raoul Rudelli

THE FIRST PUBLISHED COMMUNICATION DE-scribing the ultrasonographic (USG) iden-tification of neonatal brain hemorrhage dates from 1979 (Pape, Blackwell, Cusick, et al., 1979). Since then, only a few studies have sys-tematically compared ultrasonographic diag-nosis of brain hemorrhage with its ultimate val-idator, neuropathological findings. Leaving aside reports that have dealt with only a handful of cases, just six published studies, with sam-ple sizes of 24 to 57 infants, have attempted this comparison (Gould, Hamilton, Costello, et al., 1986; Nwasei, Pape, Martin, et al., 1984; Pape, Bennett-Britton, Szymonowicz, et al., 1983; Szymonowicz, Schafler, Cussen, & Yu, 1984; Thorburn, Lipscomb, Reynolds, et al., 1982; Trounce, Fagan, & Levene, 1987).

Our ongoing, population based study of brain hemorrhage in infants weighing 501–2,000g has further explored the relationship between cranial USG and neuropathology. Un-like previous studies of ultrasonographic and autopsy correlation, the authors have utilized whole brain microscopic sections for valida-tion analysis. This study takes place in three Level III neonatal intensive care units in New Jersey: Jersey Shore Medical Center, Mon-mouth Medical Center, and St. Peter's Medical Center. These three units are the only Level III

services for the central New Jersey counties of Middlesex, Monmouth, and Ocean.

In the first year of this 3-year study, which began in September 1984, 85% of all 3-county births weighing 501–2,000g, and 91% of those weighing 501–1,500g, were enrolled as sub-jects. Selection bias should therefore be mini-mal in this research project. The study is both an investigation of etiology of hemorrhage, and a study of its consequences for develop-mental outcome. In the study of etiology, the dependent variables are periventricular hemor-rhage and other USG associated or recognized abnormalities diagnosed according to a pro-tocol described below. The independent vari-ables are events in pregnancy, delivery, and the neonatal period, ascertained both through chart abstraction and maternal interview. Develop-mental outcome is based on the findings of a 24-month (gestational age-corrected) examina-tion of survivors that includes tests of neu-rological, psychometric, behavioral, visual, and auditory functioning.

METHODS

Ultrasound Protocol

In the first week of the infant's life, specially trained ultrasound technologists perform cranial USG examinations of the infant at 4 hours, 24 hours, and 7 days. Later ultrasounds are also obtained, but these will not be discussed in this preliminary report. Diasonics DRF 20 scanners equipped with 5 or 7.5 mH$_z$ transducers are used at each hospital to scan through the anterior fontanelle as follows: *A midline coronal view* is obtained through the Foramen of Monro; *oblique coronal views* are obtained at the anterior limits of the frontal horns and the posterior limits of the occipital horns of the lateral ventricles; *a midline sagittal view* and *angled parasagittal views* through the bodies of the lateral ventricles after identification of the sylvian fissure are also obtained. A minimum of six views are printed in duplicate. Films are read by one of five study radiologists based at the three hospitals who are blind to the clinical state of the infant. Our study calls for a second independent reading of all films by an observer not affiliated with a study hospital, but these duplicate readings are not considered in this report.

Neuropathology Protocol

Following fixation in Perfix (TM), brains are initially sectioned in angled coronal planes corresponding to the ultrasound beams for macroscopic examination, and then whole brain sections (celloidin-paraffin) at 10–20 micron intervals are prepared. Pathologic interpretations are conducted blind to both ultrasound diagnosis and to the clinical state of the infant.

In the first 16 months of the study, 95 deaths occurred in 557 subjects, and 49 autopsy consents were obtained. Five infants with autopsies died before the first ultrasound, leaving 44 infants with both ultrasound and autopsy. Mean birth weight was 969 g; mean gestational age was 27.9 weeks. Median age at death was 32.5 hours.

RESULTS

Correspondence between ultrasound and autopsy varied with age at death and with number of ultrasounds. Thus, analysis of the relationship between ultrasound and pathology was evaluated separately for: 1) *18 infants* with one 4-hour ultrasound whose median age at death was 12.5 hours, 2) *13 infants* with two ultrasounds whose median age at death was 47 hours, and 3) *13 infants* with three ultrasounds whose median age at death was 13.7 days. Analysis of the concordance was by hemisphere, with two possible sites of agreement or disagreement for each type of hemorrhage in each infant. All germinal matrix and ventricular hemorrhages were counted as hemorrhage, regardless of their size.

The time interval between the final ultrasound and death was variable and ranged from 30 minutes to many weeks. A postmortem ultrasound was available in only one infant. For this reason, the emphasis in this analysis is on the validity of *positive* ultrasound findings, rather than on the validity of *negative* findings. A low sensitivity may simply reflect the fact that new lesions had arisen between the last ultrasound and death. This is especially true in our study, in which 41% of deaths occurred in the first 24 hours of life, a time when new lesions would evolve.

Germinal Matrix Hemorrhage (GMH)

The autopsy prevalence of GMH was similar in all three groups of infants, but USG diagnosis of hemorrhage increased steadily with increasing age at death. Among infants who died with only a single 4-hour film, most GMH noted at autopsy were *not* seen on ultrasound. Sensitivity was only 3 of 25 despite the short time interval between ultrasound and autopsy for these cases, averaging 8½ hours.

However, for infants who survived long enough to have three films (7 days), sensitivity increased with the increasing age at last ultrasound, reaching just under 90% (16 of 18).

At all ages, specificity of USG diagnosis was high, with virtually all GMH diagnosed on ultrasound later confirmed at autopsy. For the entire series, among 34 GMH diagnosed on ultrasound, 31 (92%) were pathologically confirmed.

Intraventricular Hemorrhage (IVH)

The pattern for IVH was similar to that for GMH; the first 4-hour film rarely imaged the ventricular hemorrhages later found at autopsy, but the sensitivity increased with increasing age at last ultrasound. However, even at seven days, presence of ventricular bleeding was missed on USG in 35% of cases (8 of 23). In most of these instances, the amount of ventricular blood was small. Specificity of USG diagnosis of IVH was, however, perfect: all 29 ultrasound diagnosed ventricular hemorrhages were confirmed at necropsy.

White Matter Lesions

Our most interesting finding relates to the neuropathological diagnosis corresponding to echodensity in parenchymal areas other than the germinal matrix. These lesions are often interpreted as "Grade IV" or "parenchymal" (hemispherical) hemorrhages, but we will refer to them here simply as intraparenchymal echodensity (IPE).

Sixteen IPE in 10 infants were seen on ultrasound. Virtually all of these echodense lesions were interpreted by our study radiologists as parenchymal hemorrhages. For the purpose of correlation, however, ultrasonographic parenchymal echodensities were counted as a correct match to autopsy findings when *either* hemorrhage or infarction in the corresponding hemisphere was found at autopsy.

Table 1. Neuropathological findings in infants with parenchymal echodensities

Case no.	Birth weight (G)	Nature of echodensities	Age at death	White matter lesion	Other
1. S622[a]	590	Left only, 4 hrs.	9 hrs.	Edema (B)	GMH(B), IVH, Brain stem infarct, cerebellar hemorrhage
2. H747	1080	Bilateral, 24 hrs.	42 hrs.	Edema, congestion (B)	GMH(B), CPH, IVH
3. F316[a]	830	Bilateral, 24 hrs.	47 hrs.	Edema, perivascular hemorrhage (B)	GMH(B), Asymmetric hemocephalus
4. B604	785	Left only, 3 days	3d 16 hrs.	Edema, perivascular hemorrhages (B)	GMH(B), Asymmetric hemocephalus, cortex and basal ganglia infarct, cerebellar hemorrhage
5. S535	630	Bilateral, 4,24 hrs.	4d 4 hrs.	Hemorrhage infarct (U) Edema (U)	GMH(B), Asymmetric hemocephalus, basal ganglia infarct, bilateral
6. S105	730	Bilateral, 7 days	7 days	Edema, perivascular hemorrhages (B)	GMH(B), Asymmetric hemocephalus, cortex infarcts, cerebellar hemorrhage
7. E601	555	Right only, 4 hrs, 24 hrs, 7 days	7d 22 hrs.	Ischemic infarct (B)	GMH(B), Asymmetric hemocephalus, cortex, basal ganglia infarcts
8. W620	1035	Left only, 7 days	38d 16 hrs.	Periventricular leukomalacia (B)	GMH(B), IVH
9. R314[a]	570	Bilateral, 8 weeks	58 days	Ischemic infarct (B)	GMH(B), CPH, Asymmetric hemocephalus, cortex, basal ganglia, brain stem infarcts, cerebellar hemorrhage
10. C529	650	Right only, 24 hrs; bilateral 7 days	59 days	Periventricular leukomalacia (B)	GMH(B), CPH, IVH, Cortex, brain stem, and cerebellar infarcts

[a]2nd of twins; all others singletons.
(B): Bilateral.
(U): Unilateral.
CPH: Choroid Plexus Hemorrhage.

Hemispherical white matter lesions at autopsy were rare in infants dying early. Only one hemispheric white matter infarct was diagnosed among 32 infants dying in the first week of life. However, eight IPE were seen in five infants with only early ultrasounds. The positive predictive value of ultrasound for white matter infarcts was thus very poor in the first days of life (1 of 8). Among infants who died at 7 days or later, parenchymal echodensity did generally represent a specific parenchymal lesion. The positive predictive value of ultrasound for this group of five infants was 71% (5 of 7). Sensitivity to parenchymal lesions was fairly good. Seven of the 10 autopsy documented parenchymal infarctions were noted on ultrasound as IPE. Age at last ultrasound was a significant predictor, then, of the likelihood of IPE representing a white matter infarct.

What kinds of lesions were present when IPE was seen? Details of the findings in the 10 infants in whom IPE was noted are given in Table I. In cases where white matter infarcts and hemorrhage were absent, the white matter abnormalities present when echodensities were seen on ultrasound consisted of edema, vascular congestion, and small ("sleeve") perivascular hemorrhages.

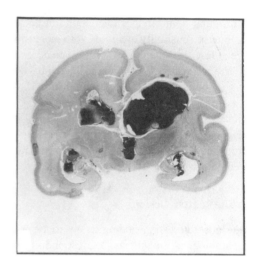

Figure 2.   Massive asymmetrical enlargement of ventricle: tissue section.

A frequent finding in the infants both with and without infarctions was a massive asymmetrical enlargement of one blood filled ventricle (see Figures 1 and 2; figures are not of the same infant) which we have termed *hemocephalus*. The asymmetric USG echodensity seen in these cases has mistakenly suggested to several sonologists the presence of intraparenchymal hemorrhage.

The most common definite hemispheric (corona radiata) lesion represented by IPE in our series *was not* an extension of a ventricular hemorrhage. Instead, the most common hemispherical pathologic lesions found in infants with IPE were, in order of frequency: infarcts, edema of the centrum semiovale, and perivascular hemorrhages. Massive asymmetrical hemocephalus often accompanied these lesions.

DeVries et al. have also noted that an asymmetrical hemocephalus can simulate a lesion in the white matter on ultrasound (DeVries, Dubowitz, Dubowitz, et al., 1985). Careful evaluation by experienced ultrasound readers failed to discern any observable features of the IPE lesions that would assist in the discrimination between those with and those without a discrete white matter infarct. The only distinct discriminating variable present in this series was the age at which the final ultrasound was taken.

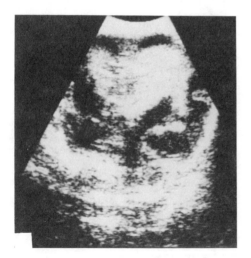

Figure 1.   Massive asymmetrical enlargement of ventricle: ultrasound.

Lesions seen early were *most likely not* to represent white matter infarcts. Lesions seen at 7 days or later were *most likely* associated with white matter infarcts. One important implication of our findings is that early ultrasounds should not be used for prognostication, as for example, in very ill, very low birth weight infants in whom the advisability of aggressive medical management is frequently questioned.

DISCUSSION

The validity of cranial USG diagnosis of hemorrhage in the first day of life is uncertain. Although almost all USG diagnosis of GMH and IVH are confirmed at autopsy, many autopsy-proven lesions had not been imaged in those infants who died early. This could represent a limitation of early USG, or could perhaps be an indication of the rapidity with which lesions evolve in the first day, and their proximity to time of death. Seven day films proved reasonably sensitive and specific in the diagnosis of GMH and IVH.

For parenchymal lesions, however, our results suggest the need to revise prevalent concepts of pathogenesis.

The literature on brain hemorrhage in low birth weight infants commonly makes three assumptions:

1. That a complication of severe germinal matrix and intraventricular hemorrhage is an extension of the hemorrhage, presumably through an ependymal rupture, into hemispherical white matter surrounding the ventricles
2. That this intraparenchymal or "Grade IV" hemorrhage represents the most severe gradation of a single pathological continuum that has its origin in the germinal matrix bleeding. Milder manifestations of this disorder are hierarchically graded from I to III
3. That the intraparenchymal hemorrhage is diagnostically visualized on ultrasound as a homogeneously echodense lesion in the periventricular region, or more extensively in the white matter

Both the use of the term "periventricular" hemorrhage and the current classification system tend to reinforce the putative pathophysiologic mechanism expressed in the first two assumptions listed above.

The demonstration by Volpe et al. (1983), using positron emission tomography, that IPE lesions were often associated with marked hemispherical white matter ischemia was probably the first evidence that simple extension of hemorrhage into the white matter was not the entire explanation for the lesion being imaged. Nwaesei et al. (1984) showed that IPEs generally corresponded to infarcts that were not necessarily hemorrhagic. In fact, in Nwasei's series, most of the white matter infarcts were nonhemorrhagic, with USG appearances indistinguishable from those of hemorrhagic infarctions. Similar findings were reported by Rushton et al. (Rushton, Preston, & Durbin, 1985) who advocated abandoning the term "periventricular hemorrhage." These data reinforce the separation between ischemic and hemorrhagic lesions described by Pape and Wigglesworth prior to the ultrasound era (Pape & Wigglesworth, 1979). Their careful pathological work contains no description of a parenchymal extension of IVH; rather, it describes white matter lesions of a predominantly ischemic nature.

A review of earlier literature on the pathology of the GMH-IVH complex reveals scant evidence for direct extension of ventricular blood into the hemispheres. Large series, such as those of Gruenwald (1951) and Ross and Dimmette (1965) did not describe intraparenchymal extensions of blood. Hemsath (1934) and Grontoft (1953) each saw only one instance of associated hemispherical bleeding in their respective series, and each suggested a possible ischemic origin for these hemorrhages. Unique among early pathological studies, Claireaux's work (1959) pointed to the possibility of "bursting of the blood outwards from the subendymal region of the ventricles." Thus, the pathological evidence for the existence of such a lesion, let alone its correspondence with ultrasonographic findings, is sparse indeed.

Our own preliminary data represent one of the largest series of infants so far published in which cranial ultrasound and neuropathological correlation have been obtained. It is also the only such series in which whole brain microscopic examinations were used to define the nature of the pathological process.

In this series, which covers 44 autopsies derived from a population of over 500 low birth weight infants, no instance of an intraparenchymal extension of intraventricular hemorrhage into *normal hemispheric white matter* was seen. Thus, if this pathophysiologic process occurs at all, it must be rare. In only two instances was ependymal rupture suspected, and in both of these cases, the hemorrhagic lesion neighboring the ventricle was characterized by extensively infarcted white matter.

Our data, taken together with the work cited, suggest a need for reevaluation of the utility of ultrasound in the diagnosis of hemorrhage/ischemia in the neonatal brain. Infarction of white matter may or may not have similar determinants to those of the germinal matrix-intraventricular hemorrhage. Of these two pathophysiologic processes, it is likely that white matter infarction is the more pertinent to the eventual neurologic outcome. Whether manifested as infarction or as periventricular leukomalacia, it is likely to be an antecedent of cyst formation, asymmetrical loss of paraventricular tissue and cortical atrophy, and lesions which have recently been recognized to correlate very closely with the development of cerebral palsy (Graham, Levene, Trounce, & Rutter, 1987; Graziani, Pasto, Stanley, et al., 1986; Guzzetta, Schackelford, Volpe, et al., 1986). It is to be hoped that future investigations will lead to a better understanding of the evolution and characteristics of parenchymal echodense lesions in ultrasound and of their prognosis in surviving infants.

REFERENCES

Claireaux, A.E. (1959). Cerebral pathology in the newborn. *Guy's Hospital Report, 108,* 2–20.

DeVries, L.S., Dubowitz, L.M.S., Dubowitz, V., et al. (1985). Predictive value of cranial ultrasound in the newborn baby: A reappraisal. *Lancet, ii,* 137–140.

Gould, S.J., Hamilton, P.A., Costello, A.M., et al. (1986). Sensitivity of detection of brain lesions in very pre-term infants by ultrasound. Abstract, *Pediatric Research, 20,* 1054.

Graham, M., Levene, M.I., Trounce, J.Q., & Rutter, N. (1987). Prediction of cerebal palsy in very low birthweight infants: Prospective ultrasound study. *Lancet, ii,* 593–596.

Graziani, L.J., Pasto, M., Stanley, C., et al. (1986). Neonatal neurosonographic correlates of cerebral palsy in preterm infants. *Pediatrics, 78,* 88–95.

Grontoft, O. (1953). Intracerebral and meningeal hemorrhages in perinatally deceased infants. *Acta Obstetricia et Gynecologica Scandinavica, 32,* 308–334.

Gruenwald, P. (1951). Subependymal cerebral hemorrhage in premature infants and its relation to various injurious influences at birth. *American Journal of Obstetrics and Gynecology, 61,* 1285–1292.

Guzzetta, F., Schackelford, G.D., Volpe, S., et al. (1986). Periventricular intraparenchymal echodensities in the premature newborn: Critical determinant of neurologic outcome. *Pediatrics, 78,* 995–1006.

Hemsath, F.A. (1934). Ventricular cerebral hemorrhage in the newborn infant. *American Journal of Obstetrics and Gynecology, 28,* 343–354.

Nwaesei, C.G., Pape, K.E., Martin, D.J., et al. (1984). Periventricular infarction diagnosed by ultrasound: A postmortem correlation. *Journal of Pediatrics, 105,* 106–110.

Pape, K.E., Bennett-Britton, S., Szymonowicz, W., et al. (1983). Diagnostic accuracy of neonatal brain imaging: A postmortem correlation of computed tomography and ultrasound scans. *Journal of Pediatrics, 102,* 275–280.

Pape, K.E., Blackwell, R.J., Cusick, G., et al. (1979). Ultrasound detection of brain damage in preterm infants. *Lancet,* June 16, 1261–1264.

Pape, K.E., & Wigglesworth, J.S. (1979). *Hemorrhage, ischemia and the perinatal brain.* Philadelphia: J.B. Lippincott.

Ross, J.J., & Dimmette, R.M. (1965). Subependymal cerebral hemorrhage in infancy. *American Journal of Disease in Children, 110,* 531–542.

Rushton, D.I., Preston, P.R., & Durbin, G.M. (1985). Structure and evolution of echodense lesions in the neonatal brain. *Archives of Disease in Childhood, 60,* 798–808.

Szymonowicz, W., Schafler, K., Cussen, L.V., & Yu, V.Y.H. (1984). Ultrasound and necropsy study of periventricular hemorrhage in preterm infants. *Archives of Disease in Childhood, 59,* 637–642.

Thorburn, R.J., Lipscomb, A.P., Reynolds, E.O.R., et al. (1982). Accuracy of imaging of the brains of newborn infants by linear-array real-time ultrasound. *Early Human Development, 6,* 31–46.

Trounce, J.Q., Fagan, D., & Levene, M.I. (1987). Intraventricular hemorrhage and periventricular leukomalacia: Ultrasound and autopsy correlation. *Archives of Disease in Childhood, 61,* 1203–1207.

Volpe, J.J., Herscovitch, P., Perlman, J.M., et al. (1983). Positron emission tomography in the newborn: Extensive impairment of regional cerebral blood flow with intraventricular hemorrhage and hemorrhagic intracerebral involvement. *Pediatrics, 72,* 589–601.

Chapter 22

Vascular Flow and Metabolic Study of the Neonatal Brain

Hans C. Lou, Gorm Greisen, and Arnold Tweed

IN RECENT YEARS THERE HAS BEEN A GROW-ing awareness of the significance of hemodynamic factors in the pathogenesis of perinatal neurologic disorders. In particular, the "lost autoregulation hypothesis" has received attention as a key to the understanding of the development of hypoxic-ischemic encephalopathy and periventricular hemorrhage. According to this hypothesis, in normal conditions, the adult as well as the unstressed newborn is capable of regulating vascular resistance in order to obtain a constant cerebral perfusion during wide changes of perfusion pressure. This autoregulation of cerebral blood flow (CBF) is lost in the stressed newborn, and exposes the brain to ischemia, in even moderate hypotension, and to increased pressure gradient across the capillary wall in even moderate hypertension; the result is increased risk of intracranial hemorrhage (Lou, 1980; Lou, Lassen, & Friis-Hansen, 1979a; 1979b). These data have stimulated efforts by researchers to define the factors that regulate cerebral perfusion *in utero,* and to identify the stresses surrounding the birth process.

AUTOREGULATION OF CBF

Using an animal model, the chronically prepared near term fetal lamb, the authors have examined, with Dr. Arnold Tweed, London, Ontario, the autoregulation of CBF *in utero* in normoxic and hypoxic conditions (Tweed, Coté, Pash, & Lou, 1983). CBF was measured

using an isotope labelled 15 um microspheres 24–48 hours after surgical preparation. Seventeen animals were studied. Eight were considered to be normoxic; ascending aortic O_2 saturation (SaO_2) was 50% or higher, and nine were considered to be spontaneously hypoxic (SaO_2 less than 57%); the fetal hemoglobin averaged 11.5 g/100 ml. CBF autoregulation was assessed in four regions: telencephalon, right and left (grey and white matter), diencephalon, cerebellum, and brain stem. Autoregulation was found to be functionally active in all regions of the normoxic fetuses, but was absent in the mildly hypoxic fetuses.

The demonstrated 50%–60% threshold of SaO_2 for impairment of autoregulation corresponds to an arterial O_2 concentration of about 3 millimoles/1; this is very similar to the threshold for impairment of autoregulation in newborn lambs (Tweed, Coté, Lou, Gregory, & Wade, 1986) and adult dogs (Häggendal & Johansson, 1965). This threshold is a little higher than the level required for fetal hypoxic hyperemia (Johnsson, Palahniuk, Tweed, Jones, & Wade, 1979) in which a hyperbolic relationship between CBF and arterial O_2 concentration has been reported (Jones, Sheldon, Peeters, Makowski, & Meschia, 1981).

It may be concluded from these observations that the regulation of fetal CBF is fragile, apparently due to the relatively hypoxic conditions in utero: a minor additional hypoxic insult is sufficient to abolish this protective mechanism. The normal birth process may constitute

191

such an insult, and this may explain why a number of investigators find that vaginally born premature infants are more prone to develop periventricular hemorrhages than prematures born by cesarean section (Dolfin et al., 1982; Lou, Phibbs, Wilson, & Gregory, 1982).

Mild periventricular hemorrhage probably indicates good prognosis. However, if the hemorrhage penetrates into the ventricular system, there is a substantial risk hydrocephalus will develop due to impaired CSF outflow (Papile, Munsick, Weaver, & Pecha, 1979). But the most serious turn of events will develop if the hemorrhage spreads into the brain parenchyma. Should this occur, the clinical conditions of the infant are likely to deteriorate abruptly, with death as a result in many cases.

ISCHEMIC LESIONS OF THE BRAIN

There is some evidence that ischemic lesions of the brain parenchyma precede this development. In our original series of 19 patients, in whom CBF had been measured a few hours after birth, four of the patients died with clinical signs of hemorrhage verified at autopsy at the ages of 2–37 days. In all four, very low values of CBF had been measured immediately after birth. In a subsequent study, we found a low flow state prior to detectable intracranial hemorrhage, accompanied by electrophysiologic signs of ischemic brain dysfunction. In this study, fifteen infants of 32 weeks of gestation or less, were studied using continuous recording of amplitude integrated electroencephalogram (aEEG) and repeated Doppler ultrasound determination of mean blood flow velocity in the internal carotid artery (cMFV). The recording was started after initiation of mechanical ventilation for respiratory distress, if no signs of germinal layer hemorrhage (GLH) were found by ultrasound scanning. Seven of the 15 infants had cMFV increases of 100% or more associated with blood pressure increases following volume expansion (group I), thus indicating absence of autoregulation. Initial minimum blood pressure and minimum

cMFV were lower in these infants compared with the remaining eight infants in whom the cMFV was stable (group II). Six of the infants in group I, all with low Apgar scores at birth, later developed GLH, whereas only two infants in group II bled ($p = 0.039$). In all infants, the aEEG showed suppression burst activity, whereas no period of sustained electrical silence was seen in any infant. In group II, the burst rate increased over the first 6 hours to 150 bursts/h. In group I, the burst rate increased less and seemed unaffected by the increased blood flow, thus indicating an abnormal function of neural tissue that was not readily reversed with improved energy supply. Timing of eventual GLH by repeated ultrasound scanning showed this abnormality to be present before any hemorrhage in most of the infants, indicating that the hemorrhage occurs in brains that have already been damaged by ischemia (Figure 1).

The hemorrhage itself may, in its turn, aggravate ischemia. Volpe and co-workers have shown with PET scanning that intraparenchymal hemorrhage is surrounded by a zone of severe ischemia (1983). In order to obtain a better understanding of the mechanism of this regional ischemia, we have examined the effect of blood admixture to mock spinal fluid on its ion composition *in vitro* (Edvinsson, Lou, & Tvede, 1986). It was found that during the first 2 to 3 days, the K^+ concentration increased dramatically up to about tenfold, depending upon the concentration of blood in the mixture with mock spinal fluid. This level was maintained for at least 2 weeks. Such a K^+ concentration of about 20–50 meq had a marked vasoconstrictor effect which very well could have been responsible for the perihemorrhagic ischemia. Likewise, it should be mentioned that a similar K^+ concentration is capable of inducing neuronal depolarization and spreading depression. Spreading depression is known to be accompanied by a considerable *increase* in glucose utilization (Shinohara, Pollinger, Brown, Rapoport, & Soholoff, 1979). Hence, not only does the hemorrhage induce, or aggravate, ischemia in surrounding tissue, it may also greatly increase its energy demand.

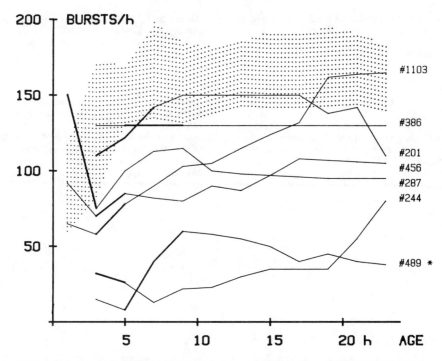

Figure 1.   EEG bursts per hour in premature infant (Gestational age <32 wks) prior to eventual intracranial hemorrhage. Shaded area represents eight infants with stable mean flow in carotid artery. Seven infants with unstable carotid flow (increase >100%) are depicted individually. Heavy lines indicate the periods of flow increase. (*died suddenly.)

SUMMARY

In summary, the following sequence of events may be hypothesized:

1. Hypoxemia impairs autoregulation
2. Lack of autoregulation and initial hypotension induce ischemic infarction
3. Subsequent blood pressure increase leads to periventricular hemorrhage
4. Hemorrhage may then spread in infarcted tissue
5. Perihemorrhagic ischemia is induced
6. Ischemia is then aggravated by increased energy demand due to spreading depression

REFERENCES

Dolfin, T., Skidmore, M.B., Fong, K.W., Hoskins, E.M., Milligan, J.E., Moore, D.C., & Shennan, A.T. (1982, December). *Perinatal factors that influence the incidence of subependymal and intraventricular hemorrhage in low birthweight infants*. Second Special Ross Laboratories Conference on Perinatal Intracranial Hemorrhage, Washington, DC.

Edvinsson, L., Lou, H.C., & Tvede, K. (1986). On the pathogenesis of regional cerebral ischemia in intracranial hemorrhage. A causal role of K^+? *Pediatric Research, 20,* 478–480.

Häggendal, E., & Johansson, B. (1965). Effects of arterial carbon dioxide tension and oxygen saturation on CBF autoregulation in dogs. *Acta Physiologica Scandinavica Supplement, 258,* 27–53.

Johnsson, G.N., Palahniuk, R.J., Tweed, W.A., Jones,

M.V., & Wade, J. (1979). Regional cerebral blood flow changes during severe fetal asphyxia produced by slow partial umbilical cord compression. *American Journal of Obstetrics and Gynecology, 135,* 48–52.

Jones, P.M., Sheldon, R.E., Peeters, L.L., Makowski, E.L., & Meschia, G. (1981). Regulation of cerebral blood flow in the ovine foetus. *American Journal of Physiology, 235,* H162–H166.

Lou, H.C. (1980). Perinatal hypoxic-ischemic brain damage and intraventricular hemorrhage. A pathogenetic model. *Archives of Neurology, 41,* 825–829.

Lou, H.C., Lassen, N.A., & Friis-Hansen, B. (1979a). Impaired autoregulation of cerebral blood flow in the distressed newborn infant. *Journal of Pediatrics, 94,* 118–121.

Lou, H.C., Lassen, N.A., & Friis-Hansen, B. (1979b). Is

arterial hypertension crucial for the development of intraventricular haemorrhage in the neonate? *Lancet, i,* 1215–1217.

Lou, H.C., Phibbs, R.H., Wilson, S.L., & Gregory, G.A. (1982). hyperventilation at birth may present early periventricular hemorrhage. *Lancet, i,* 1407.

Lou, H.C., Skov, H., & Pedersen, H. (1979). Low cerebral blood flow: A risk factor in the neonate. *Journal of Pediatrics, 95,* 606–609.

Papile, L.A., Munsick, G., Weaver, N., & Pecha, S. (1979). Cerebral intraventricular hemorrhage in infants <1500 g. Developmental follow-up at one year. *Pediatric Research, 13,* 528.

Shinohara, M., Pollinger, B., Brown, G., Rapoport, S., & Soholoff, L. (1979). Cerebral glucose utilization: Local changes during and after recovery from spreading cortical depression. *Science, 203,* 188–190.

Tweed, W.A., Coté, J., Lou, H.C., Gregory, G.A., & Wade, J. (1986). Impairment and recovery of autoregulation of cerebral blood flow in the newborn lamb. *Pediatric Research, 20,* 516–519.

Tweed, W.A., Coté, J., Pash, M., & Lou, H.C. (1983). Arterial oxygenation determines autoregulation of cerebral blood flow in fetal lamb. *Pediatric Research, 17,* 246–249.

Volpe, I.I., Herscovitch, P., Perlman, J.M., & Raichle, M.E. (1983). Position emission tomography in the newborn: Extensive impairment of regional cerebral blood flow with intraventricular hemorrhage and hemorrhagic intracerebral involvement. *Pediatrics, 72,* 589–601.

Chapter 23

11C-Glucose Positron Emission Tomography of Intracerebral Hemorrhage in Infancy

Mikio Hiraiwa,
Chizuru Nonaka, Toshiaki Abe, Ryochi Fujii, and Masaaki Iio

IN INFANCY, INTRACEREBRAL HEMORRHAGE (IH) may have various causes, and tends to result in a severe sequelae. However, the exact pathophysiology and mechanism of IH and its sequelae have not yet been determined. Positron emission tomography (PET) is a new technique that has been useful in the evaluation of the morphological, physiological, circulatory, and metabolic conditions *in vivo*. We applied PET for two infants with IH using 11C-glucose.

PET STUDY

All PET studies were performed with orally administered 11C-glucose; this was obtained by photosynthesis of green spinach using 11C-carbon dioxide which was produced with a cyclotron BC-105. The dosage of orally administered 11C-glucose was between 5 and 15 mCi. PET images were visualized with Head-tome II. The spatial resolution of the apparatus was 10mm full width at half maximum in the center of view (Kanno, Uemura, Miura, Miura, et al., 1981). For the measurement of regional distribution of radioactive concentration in the brain, the profile procedure and ROI (region of interest) were utilized. For a comparison to the PET study, x-ray CT (computed tomography) was employed with CT scanner CT/T-8800.

Case Studies

Case 1 Case #1 involved a 1 year, 3-month-old Japanese boy. He had been healthy until 3 months of age, when he fell into unconsciousness and status epilepticus. An immediate x-ray CT scan of the brain revealed a high density area at the right front temporal lobe, cerebrospinal fluid (CSF) was bloody and the CSF pressure was high. Blood hemoglobin was 6.0 g/dL. Under the temporary diagnosis of IH, the boy was treated with mannitol and anticonvulsants, and received a blood transfusion. Further examination disclosed a marked decrease in the boy's factor 8 (13.0%) with mild decrease in the mother's factor 8.

The boy was diagnosed as having hemophilia A, and was accepted for replacement therapy. After the boy recovered from unconsciousness, we noted left hemiparesis and developmental retardation. Four months later, convulsions involving head nodding and twitching limbs began. A record of electroencephalogram (EEG) disclosed typical hypsarrhythmia. Administration of pyridoxal phosphate brought cessation of the seizures and an improvement in the EEG. At 1 year and 3 months, he was retarded in motor, mental, and emotional development. Both PET and x-ray CT scans were performed during this period. X-ray CT showed the area-limited right front-

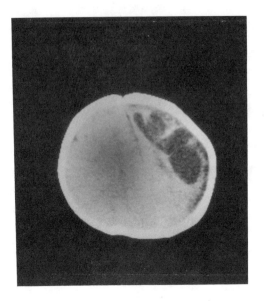

Figure 1.   Case 1. X-ray CT: cystic low density area is noted at the right front-temporal lobe (CM 50mm).

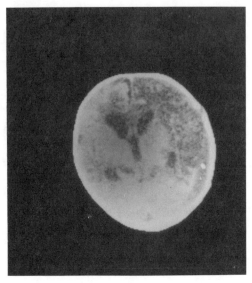

Figure 3.   Case 2. X-ray CT: low density area without obvious cystic formation in the right front-temporal area.

temporal cystic low density area with mild enlargement of the right lateral ventricle (Figure 1). PET scanning revealed widespread low radioactive accumulation in the right hemisphere (Figure 2). The damaged area on the PET scan was larger than that of x-ray CT scan, and the ratio of damaged area of x-ray CT to PET was 1 and 1.5, respectively.

Case 2   Case #2 involved a 3-month-old Japanese boy. His health had been uneventful and he had been breast-fed until 1 month of life; at 1 month, his consciousness was disturbed. The laboratory data disclosed decreased hemoglobin (8.3g/dL), hematocrit (24.3%), RBC (235×10^4/cmm), and hemorrhagic tendency. The hemorrhagic tendency was improved im-

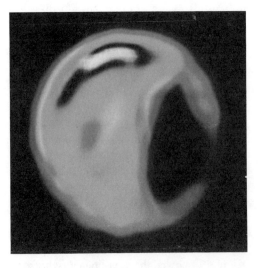

Figure 2.   Case 1. PET with 11C-glucose: low radioactive concentration in the similar area in x-ray CT, but larger.

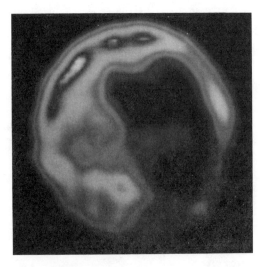

Figure 4.   Case 2. PET with 11C-glucose: large low radioactive concentration as compared to x-ray CT.

mediately after the boy was injected with vitamin K. X-ray CT revealed a left temporal high density area with edema of the right hemisphere and enlargement of the left lateral ventricle. Then the boy received a surgical decompression. At 3 months of life, he showed retarded motor development and was accepted for PET and x-ray CT. X-ray CT revealed the right front-temporal low density area without an obvious cystic formation and a mild enlargement of bilateral lateral ventricles (Figure 3). PET showed significant low radioactive accumulation in the whole right hemisphere (Figure 4); similar to case #1, the damaged area was larger in PET scan, and the ratio of the damaged area of x-ray CT to PET was 1 and 1.6, respectively.

DISCUSSION

It is well known that intracerebral hemorrhage in infancy often induces severe developmental sequelae. In the adult, focal intracranial lesions are usually combined to only focal symptoms after the recovery from acute illness. It is problematic why IH in infancy causes not only related focal symptoms, but developmental deficit. To detect a metabolic and circulatory aspect of the pathological conditions *in vivo*, PET is an excellent technique. The use of 11C-glucose study in PET is conventional and minimally invasive even in the examination of infants and children, as previously reported (Hiraiwa, Nonaka, Abe, & Iio, 1983; Hiraiwa, Nonaka, Ushijima, Abe, & Iio, 1984). The rationale for using 11C-glucose study is that it provides a visual image of the circulation and metabolism of glucose. Radioactive isotope accumulation may indicate the presence of

glucose and its metabolites (mainly glutamic acid) in the brain transported by the blood stream (Hara & Nozaki, 1982). A regional low radioactive accumulation can suggest a regional disturbance of the blood stream and/or hypometabolism. Upon examination by x-ray CT, severe damage in regional blood stream usually presents regional loss of density. In our study, low density areas on x-ray CT were not so large and could not explain the developmental deficit from the size and localization. In the acute stage of illness, brain edema might bring some influence in circulation and metabolism of surrounding area. But our PET study was performed in the late stage, after the recovery from brain edema. Then the largely damaged areas revealed by PET are thought to be mainly based on the regional hypometabolism and are not a simple result of the affected blood stream. This hypometabolism might be responsible for the severe developmental sequelae of IH in infancy.

SUMMARY

Intracerebral hemorrhage (IH) is a severe neurological disorder in the clinical course and sequelae, especially in infancy. For an evaluation of IH in infancy, two infants with IH (hemophilia A and hypovitaminosis K) were studied using positron emission tomography (PET) with 11C-glucose. Compared to the low density area and cystic lesion on x-ray CT, the area of low radioactive accumulation was large in PET, even after the patient's recovery from acute illness. A discrepancy in x-ray CT and PET can be specific in IH of infancy, and the widely damaged area revealed by PET suggests severe neurological sequelae.

REFERENCES

Hara, T., & Nozaki, H. (1982, June). *Radioactivity labeling of C-1 position of glucose and mannose—synthetic methods, metabolism, and application of the compounds for* in vitro *determination of regional glucose utilization rate in the brain and for detection of tumors in the body.* Paper presented at the Fourth International Symposium on Radiopharmaceutical Chemistry, Tokyo, Japan. Abstract p. 355.

Hiraiwa, M., Nonaka, C., Abe, T., & Iio, M. (1983). Positron emission tomography in systemic lupus erythematosus: Relation of cerebral vasculitis to PET

findings. *American Journal of Neuroradiology, 4*, 541–543.

Hiraiwa, M., Nonaka, C., Ushijima, H., Abe, T., & Iio, M. (1984). Positron computed tomography in West syndrome (infantile spasms): 11C-labelled glucose ingestion study. *Annales Universtat Turkuensis D, 17*, 283–287.

Kanno, I., Uemura, K., Miura, Y., Miura, H., et al. (1981). Headtome: A hybrid emission tomograph for single photon and positron emission imaging of the brain. *Journal of Computer Assisted Tomography, 5*, 216–226.

Chapter 24

The High-Risk Infant: A Clinical Model for Prevention, Identification, Assessment, and Treatment of Children at Risk for Developmental Disabilities

A Plan for Interaction of Community and Medical Center Resources

Shaul Harel, Abraham Tomer, and Galya Rabinovitz

I N RECENT YEARS, THERE HAS BEEN IN-
creasing concern for early identification of
young children at risk for developmental problems. Children at risk for later sensory, motor,
mental, and social handicaps may never be able
to achieve their full potentials as productive
citizens without appropriate interventions. Differences between social groups within a society, the so-called "ethnic" or "social" gap
that exists in many countries, may have significant effects upon individual and group levels of
cultural, social, and economic achievement.
Detection and assessment of infantile developmental defects need to be carried out at the
earliest possible age. The prevention and treatment of developmental problems, as well as the
closing of these "social" gaps, are foremost
for all professions caring for the child.

There is widespread agreement supporting
the investigation of developmental disabilities
in children prior to their onset rather than after
their occurrences. Our present knowledge of
human development, neurology, biochemical

genetics, immunology, obstetrical care, and
environmental effects should enable us to establish preventive practices. If followed, the
emotional and financial impact accompanying
the birth and long-term management of a handicapped child could be minimized for the family, as well as for the community. Combined
with early detection, via screening of an "at
risk" population, there should also be a program for a more careful follow-up of these children, as well as for the early implementation of
remedial steps to ameliorate the various handicapping conditions.

In previous years, the major focus of concern was on the development of preschool or
school-age children. Many remedial programs
yielded disappointing results because of their
failure to recognize that children may have
reached a "point of no return" for effective
intervention. It is now apparent that biological
and environmental events in that early period
of human development may have a unique and
profound impact on the course of subsequent

development. Our current knowledge of human brain development has shifted the major focus of concern to intrauterine brain growth and to the first 2 or 3 years of life, a so-called "critical period" (Dobbing, 1973). During this highly critical period of development, the fetus is especially sensitive and vulnerable to both ante-perinatal insults and to neglect. It is also crucial to begin early rehabilitation at this stage, provided the brain is protected from further injuries.

According to Dobbing (Dobbing, 1973, 1980), the human brain growth spurt begins about the middle of gestation and ends between the second and third year of life. The adult number of neurons is already present in the brain before the brain-growth spurt begins. The late dividing granular neurons of the cerebellum are the only neurons which continue to divide after the growth spurt period. After division and differentiation, there follows a long period of neuronal development resulting in the growth and development of the dendritic tree and its synaptic connections. Fetal and infant malnutrition may indeed affect these vital developing structures. Current experimental studies using animal models show that malnutrition or ischemic conditions during the growth spurt period can reduce the number of synapses per neuron by up to 40% (Dobbing, 1980).

However, if rehabilitation is started during the above period, the brain is still able to compensate (Winick, 1969). Some regions in the brain are more permanently affected than others; the most vulnerable of these is the cerebellum. The selective effect on the cerebellum seems related to its accelerated growth rate within the growth-spurt period (Dobbing, 1980). It is for this reason that the cerebellum (and its functional correlates) is by far the most sensitive index of the effects of malnutrition or ischemia on the growing brain (Dobbing, 1980). This may have important consequences for future motor coordination. It may also be responsible for the "clumsy child" and some of the manifestations related to the syndrome of "minimal cerebral dysfunction." For the un-

derprivileged world, malnutrition is only one of the many adversities with which the infant is constantly surrounded (Dobbing, 1980).

The recognition of a "critical period" in brain development led to the concept of "high-risk" pregnancy and "high-risk" infancy. The theoretical background for these definitions derived from the concept of "a continuum of reproductive casualty" which was first introduced by Knoblock and Pasamanick (Knoblock & Pasamanick, 1959; Knoblock & Pasamanick, 1960). This means that in some instances, events that take place in the prenatal period are not independent of insults that occur perinatally. Knoblock and Pasamanick's hypothesis consists of two components described as lethal and sublethal manifestations. The lethal component consists of abortions, stillbirths, and neonatal deaths, while the sublethal manifestations include sensory, motor, and mental disabilities. To be "at risk" means that individuals with certain characteristics are more likely to later develop detrimental conditions than are individuals without these characteristics (Finkelstein & Ramey, 1980). High-risk infants generally fall within three categories: 1) those with environmental deprivation contributing to deficiencies in cognitive and emotional development, 2) those with genetic malformations, and 3) those exposed to biologic stress, such as hypoxia and trauma leading to a variety of developmental disabilities (cerebral palsy, mental retardation, and epilepsy, and communication, behaviour, and learning problems) (Denhoff, 1980; Legum, 1983).

In western countries, between 3% and 5% of all live-born infants are affected with major structural anomalies, chromosomal aberrations, or with serious single gene hereditary diseases. Such disorders account for more than 20% of infant mortality in the United States, and are major etiologic factors in the causation of mental retardation and chronic disabling conditions in childhood (Kaback, 1980). Among other chief biological factors are maternal-fetal vascular insufficiency, low birth weight, asphyxia, jaundice, intracranial hemorrhage, and neonatal seizures.

INFLUENCE OF
SOCIOECONOMIC ENVIRONMENT

As early as 1862, Little postulated that brain damage (in the form of cerebral palsy) is caused by perinatal events (Buck, Gregg, Stavraky, et al., 1960). However, prospective studies have failed to show a significant correlation between most single perinatal or postnatal events and later disabling outcomes (Buck et al., 1960; Finer, Robertson, Richards, Pinnell, & Peters, 1981; Hack & Breslau, 1986; Kohler, Svenningsen, & Lindquist, 1979; Parmelee & Haber, 1973; Stern, 1980; Westwood, Kramer, Munz et al., 1983). It has been shown that long-term outcomes are strongly influenced by the socioeconomic circumstances of the children's environment. These influences, it would appear, are often stronger than those of earlier potentially damaging biological events (Broman, Nichols, & Kennedy, 1975; Drillen, 1964; Furstenberg, 1976; Knoblock & Pasamanick, 1960; Parmelee, Sigman, Kopp, & Haber, 1974; Sameroff & Chandler, 1975; Werner, Simonia, Bierman, & French, 1968; Wiener, Rider, Opel, & Harper, 1968). However, there is also evidence that early biological problems lead children to be more vulnerable to adverse environments. Some health problems during pregnancy and early infancy are related to socioeconomic status; the two variables must be considered as inextricably interwoven (Parmelee et al., 1974). These findings are in concordance with data from the National Institutes of Health Collaborative Project, with its prospective follow-up of 40,000 pregnancies (Broman, 1980; Broman, Nichols, & Kennedy, 1975; Nelson & Ellenberg, 1986; Smith, Flick, & Ferris, 1972). Analysis of data from this study showed no significant correlation between most single abnormal ante-perinatal events and academic performance at the age of 7. Low birth weight, regardless of gestational age, maternal level of education, and the socioeconomic status of the children's parents, were far more significant factors in determining intelligence scores than were most single perinatal events (Njiokiktjien & Kurver, 1980; Siegel, 1983). It seems that at least in cases of mild dysfunction, the environment may be relatively more important than the initial damage in terms of prognosis (Njiokiktjien & Kurver, 1980).

In the context of the influence of the socioeconomic environment on the child, the major role parents can play in causing a child to be at risk became increasingly apparent (Njiokiktjien & Kurver, 1980). It is well known that the infant is totally dependent on his or her parents, especially on the mother. This period has been called "second" or "extra-abdominal pregnancy." This link is crucial for the critical transition period from reflex to perceptive and cognitive life. The more competent the parents, the greater the chance for the child to achieve a better social maturation and adaptability. It is also a known factor that parents who are deprived of proper management during their childhood may be inadequately equipped to provide appropriate care and education for their own children. Based on this knowledge, the concept of the "at-risk" parent was derived. Therefore, malfunctioning parents who were themselves "at-risk" infants will usually have an "at-risk" child. Not only is it likely that the child "at risk" is born to a mother "at risk," but both mother and infant usually reside in an environment that is less than adequate to meet either the infant's or the parents' needs. Factors found to be detrimental to parental functioning are: poverty, low level of education, single parenthood, inexperience, as in the case of teen-age parents, severe marital conflicts, drug use, and mental illness. Thus, the infant and the environment transact in a mutually reciprocal manner to either deepen the "at-risk" factors or to overcome them (Anastasiow, 1980). Many day care centers were planned and opened to counteract some of these risky factors that can occur in parent-infant interactions.

The complexity of the interrelationship between the various biological and environmental factors affecting brain development has brought many investigators to look upon the clusters of pregnancy, neonatal, and environmental events and factors that may interact cumulatively. When these additive factors are combined with repeated assessment, they can be significant predictors of later developmental disabilities. On this basis, the concept of a "cumulative risk score system" as a method for early identification of infants at risk was defined (Parmelee et al., 1974; Werner et al., 1968).

As previously stated, the validity of the linear model correlating single perinatal events with dysfunction later in life has been strongly questioned (Sameroff & Chandler, 1975). It seems that the interactional or transactional model of development may better relate to the "cumulative risk" approach and may more clearly account for the complexities of the developmental process. This model stresses the importance of both the infant's status and the environment as sources of variance in predicting future functioning. Development is viewed as an ongoing interactive process between the status of the organism and the environment in which it develops. The researcher attempting to assess and predict later development (Fox, 1980; Hack & Breslau, 1986) must regard the infant's environment at successive ages during the early years of life as an equal partner to infant status variables.

Recognition of the complex interactions of biological and environmental factors and of their influence on early development has inspired the growth of a broad spectrum of approaches and resources aimed at constructive interventions for "at-risk" infants. Collectively. the concepts guiding these developments span the total ecology of the developing infant—from the macro level, involving society's attitudes and beliefs—to the micro level of diadic interventions (Hack & Breslau, 1986; Harel, 1980).

It is the purpose of this review to propose a simple practical model for early identification and intervention for children with disabilities. The model is designed to effectively and economically integrate community and medical center services. Among the prime goals of such a program are the following:

1. To prevent, or diagnose and treat, as early as possible, any cause of developmental handicaps
2. To provide every child with the kind of environment that will enable the child to reach his or her full innate potential

We are aiming at a health care model rather than a "sickness-cure" model. We hope to develop a health care system based upon an understanding of prevention at all levels of action. While such general aims are common to all health services for children, the more detailed objectives will vary from country to country. The general state of child care, the staff and materials available. and the socioeconomic conditions in the country concerned will, in turn, influence the priority in which the objectives are approached (Mackenzee, 1977).

Trained professionals and paraprofessionals will constitute the core of the program at the medical center, as well as at the community level. The approach is multidisciplinary: many of the concerns are related to biological, social, economic, cultural, and environmental factors, and must be considered from different points of view.

In the past, many programs yielded disappointing results because their approaches were narrow and limited, and they tended to focus inordinate amounts of time on isolated issues that reflected only the special interests of the program designers. Evidence suggests that in order to prevent, detect, and treat developmental disabilities as early as possible, there is no acceptable alternative to comprehensive health surveillance. This investigation must be a part of a general health service program for all children. The program should include among its procedures the collection of questionnaires concerning high-risk patients, repeated screening and clinical examinations of patients, and implementation of early intervention steps by well-trained personnel. It is interesting to note that policies concerning screening procedures and perinatal services, and the operations of intensive neonatal care units and assessment centers for handicapped children are usually attacked on the grounds that their value has not been established. What these critics overlook is that a health service is a very complex human activity and not an isolated entity to be judged as always being scientifically effective or ineffective (Mackenzee, 1977).

The proposed project, unlike other prospective studies, is rather clinical and service-oriented, although its special computerized design should enable recorded data to be equally applicable to clinical research. We have tried to avoid an elaborate collection of unimportant and irrelevant material, and have focused instead on known factors associated with brain dysfunction and environmental deprivation.

In 1968, Prechtl (1980) introduced a fruitful "optimality concept" as a method of risk scoring that has since proven its practicability and efficiency. Prechtl pointed out the following facts: prenatal and perinatal complications are often poorly defined, a clear distinction between the normal child and the at-risk child is often difficult to determine, complications from case to case may vary from mild to severe, and complications rarely occur alone, because they are often associated with other risk factors. Therefore, it is difficult to define a certain condition as being either positively pathological or abnormal. It seems easier to define an optimal range for a specific condition. This concept is also useful since it takes into account the cumulative effect of several coincidental, unfavorable factors. The more nonoptimal conditions are present, the more at risk is the infant. It should be noted that the optimal score concept has to be modified according to the rapidly changing aspects of neonatology and obstetrics in order to maintain the sensitivity and specificity of this system (Hobel, 1980; Ohrt & Flehmig, 1980; Stern, 1980). The use of a normal/abnormal dichotomy rating system and the lack of flexibility in changing the weighing of risk factors with time, have caused the failure of some previous high risk registers (Forfar, 1968; Oppe, 1967; Rogers, 1968).

In the following model, screening procedures have been selected not only for their own reliability and validity. but also for their practicality and convenient application. This will ensure long-term participation by families and cooperation from health care personnel.

In order for the program to be most effective and economical, specific intervention programs will be aimed at specific high-risk populations of children and families. These include: overt handicapping conditions, potential handicapping conditions, emotional or physical neglect or abuse, and culturally disadvantaged families.

Another major need that must be met for the successful implementation of such a program is purposeful public and professional education in the field of child development and general public health care.

To summarize, the design of our "at risk" project is based on the following concepts:

1. The transactional ecological model of development
2. A continuum of reproductive casualty
3. The cumulative risk score system
4. The optimality concept

PROJECT FLOW PLAN

The design of the project (a detailed protocol is available upon request) as illustrated in the flow chart plan (Figure 1 and Figure 2), consists of the following stages: preconception. pregnancy, newborn, infants—9 months, infants—2 years, and school-age. At each stage, high-risk factors (HRF) that are potentially harmful in regard to later developmental problems will divide the general population of parents, newborns, and infants into low- and high-risk groups. High-risk factors for each stage are defined according to their lethal and sublethal manifestations.

The optimal and nonoptimal scoring rate of each condition will be based on data from the literature and on the author's professional experience regarding factors associated with potential brain dysfunction. Special emphasis is placed on biological stress events and nonbiological factors, such as low socioeconomic status and poor environment.

A pilot study is then conducted for each stage to determine the range and distribution of

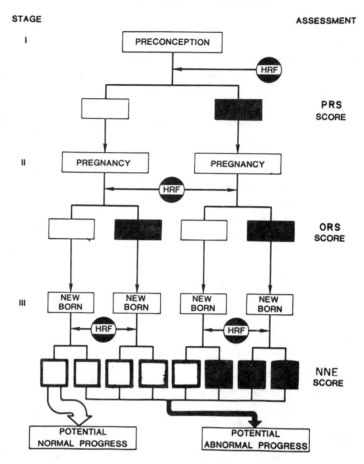

Figure 1.   Cumulative risk assessment: Preconception, pregnancy, and newborn. (HRF = high risk factors; PRS = Parental Risk Scale; ORS = Obstetrical Risk Scale; NNE = Newborn Neurobehavioral Examination.)

scores. The spread of scores, from optimal to nonoptimal, is established for each step, and the raw scores are converted to standardized scores. In this way, the individual scores for each stage are treated equally in the summation of the cumulative risk assessment.

According to the range of scores for each stage, a critical cutoff point is arbitrarily determined in order to define the terms "low risk" and "high risk." Any newborn who is found to be "at risk" at stages I, II, or III is assigned for follow-up in the "high-risk" infant group. From the flow chart plan (Figure 1), it can be seen that at the end of Stage III, a heterogeneous population of newborns is obtained. At one extreme are newborns (white block)

with no harmful influence from high-risk factors at any stage; at the other extreme are newborns affected at each step (black block). In between are groups of potentially high-risk newborns possessing all possible combinations of risk factors (fading black blocks, Figure 1).

In order to allow interaction with the environment and possible compensation for transient insults, the "high-risk" newborn group still without obvious neurodevelopmental disabilities is fully assessed at the age of 9 months. A cumulative risk score (CRS) based on the summation of previous assessments at 9 months (Parental Risk Scale (PRS), Obstetrical Risk Scale (ORS), Newborn Risk Scale (NRS), Newborn Neurobehavioral Examina-

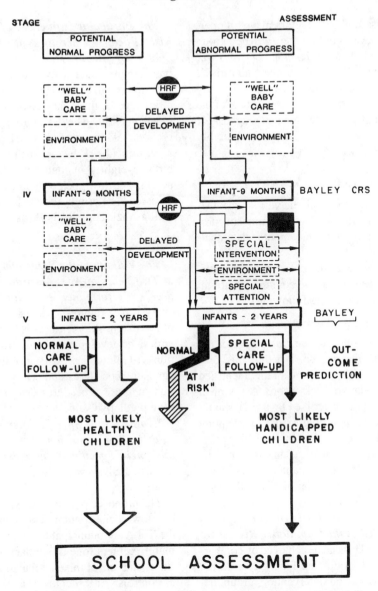

Figure 2.   Cumulative risk assessment: 9 months–2 years. (HRF = high risk factors; Bayley = Bayley Scales of Infant Development; CRS = Cumulative Risk Score.)

tion (NNE), and the Bayley Scales of Infant Development) is used to identify those infants who are high "high risk" (black block) and for whom a special intervention program will be provided (Figure 2). At the age of 2 years, the whole group of "high-risk" infants will be re-assessed (using Bayley Scales). Infants who apparently "catch-up" and show normal de-

velopment (normal–"at risk") will continue to receive special follow-up services.

The infants who still have low scores at the age of 2 years, who show no obvious "catch-up," will "most likely" end up in the group of handicapped children. Some of these children will probably continue to improve with time, provided that they get special care and attention. Because high-risk factors may still operate in the first years of life, there will be a group of infants with delayed development who will switch from the "normal" to the "high-risk" group. It should be clear that specific early interventions can be applied at any stage of the project, and that the detection and diagnosis of any obvious neurodevelopmental disability will be treated accordingly.

RESEARCH AND DATA ANALYSIS

Clinical information from the various risk factor scales and from selected diagnostic procedures are recorded for computer data analysis.

Concomitant with the delivery of appropriate medical services to the community, it will be possible to assess the following:

At the Age of Two Years

The Effectiveness of the Early Special Intervention Program To expedite this process, the high-risk group of infants identified by the Cumulative Risk Score Assessment (CRS) at 9 months of age (see Figure 2), should be divided into a high "high-risk" intervention group (black block) and a "high-risk" nonintervention group. Statistical analysis of variance using tests for significant differences will be needed to determine the validity of the early intervention program.

The Validity of the Early Diagnostic Measures Included in the Cumulative Risk Score Assessment This can be achieved by comparing the normal group (see Figure 2) with the low "high-risk" nonintervention group derived from the CRS assessment at 9 months. Analysis using tests of correlation will be needed to determine which of the diagnostic measures are most predictive of 2-year status.

The Particular Influences of the Various Risk Factors Operating at the Different Stages of Brain Development Statistical breakdown of data analysis using correlational techniques will be needed to determine the specific value of these factors when they operate independently, whether at a specific stage of brain development or in combinations. In this way, critical risk factors such as anoxia, low birth weight, malnutrition, hyperbilirubinemia, and low socioeconomic status can be assessed to determine their individual effects as well as their combined effects.

At School Age

The Validity of the "Outcome Prediction" at Two Years of Age, According to the Children's Performance at School Age This analysis (see Figure 2) will also indicate which of the diagnostic measures is better correlated with later development. This crucial information will allow reassessment of the various diagnostic procedures and will permit elimination of those procedures determined to have little predictive value.

Evaluation of Specific Intervention Strategies in Regard to their Target Populations and their Specific Achievements (specific detailed analysis will be decided at appropriate time).

The proposed pilot project will be applied in one low socioeconomic community center in the Tel Aviv municipal area. Two other community centers (one of similar socioeconomic status and one of mixed population) will serve as controls. At 9 months of age, 2 years, and school age (6 years), all children from the three family health care stations will be evaluated and compared for levels of neuropsychological development and school achievement.

REFERENCES

Anastasiow, N. (1980). Introduction to Workshop I: Prospective parents. In S. Harel (Ed.), *The at risk infant* (pp. 15–18). Princeton: Excerpta Medica.

Broman, S.H. (1980). Outcome of adolescent pregnancy: A report from the collaborative perinatal project. In S. Harel (Ed.), *The at risk infant* (pp. 45–49). Princeton: Excerpta Medica.

Broman, S., Nichols, P.L., & Kennedy, W.A. (1975). *Pre-school IQ: Prenatal and early developmental correlates*. Hillsdale, NJ: Lawrence Erlbaum Associates.

Buck, C., Gregg, R., Stavraky, K., et al. (1960). The effect of single prenatal and natal complications upon the development of children of mature birthweight. *Pediatrics, 43*, 942–955.

Denhoff, E. (1980). Assessment of "at risk" infant and early stimulation. In S. Harel (Ed.), *The at risk infant* (pp. 138–142). Princeton: Excerpta Medica.

Dobbing, J. (1973). The later development of the central nervous system and its vulnerability. In J. A. Davis & J. Dobbing (Eds.), *Scientific Foundation of Pediatrics* (pp. 565–577). London: William Heinemann Medical Books.

Dobbing, J. (1980). Nutrition and brain development: In S. Harel (Ed.), *The at risk infant* (pp. 124–128). Princeton: Excerpta Medica.

Drillen, C.M. (1964). *The growth and development of the prematurely born infant.* Baltimore: Williams & Wilkins.

Finer, N.N., Robertson, C.M., Richards, R.T., Pinnell, I.E., & Peters, K.L. (1981). Hypoxic-ischemic encephalopathy in term neonates: Perinatal factors and outcome. *Journal of Pediatrics, 98,* 112–117.

Finkelstein, N.W., & Ramey, C.T. (1980). Information from birth certificates as a risk index for educational handicap. *American Journal of Mental Deficiency, 84,* 546–552.

Forfar, J.O. (1968). "At risk" registers. *Developmental Medicine and Child Neurology, 10,* 384–395.

Fox, N. (1980). Assessment of the mother-infant interaction: A research design for clinical evaluation and intervention. In S. Harel (Ed.), *The at risk infant* (pp. 80–84). Princeton: Excerpta Medica.

Furstenberg, F.F. (1976). The social consequences of teenage pregnancy. *Family Planning Perspectives, 8,* 148–164.

Hack, M., & Breslau, N. (1986). Very low birth infants: Effect of brain browth during infancy on intelligence quotient at three years of age. *Pediatrics, 77,* 196–202.

Harel, S. (Ed.). (1980). *The at risk infant.* Princeton: Excerpta Medica.

Hobel, C.J. (1980). A dynamic maternal risk factor scale. In S. Harel (Ed.), *The at risk infant* (pp. 143–147). Princeton: Excerpta Medica.

Kaback, M.M. (1980). Prospective identification of parents at risk for hereditary diseases or congenital defects in their offspring. In S. Harel (Ed.), *The at risk infant* (pp. 90–95). Princeton: Excerpta Medica.

Knoblock, H., & Pasamanick, B. (1959). The syndrome of minimal brain damage in infancy. *Journal of the American Medical Association, 70,* 1384–1387.

Knoblock, H., & Pasamanick, B. (1960). Environmental factors affecting human development before and after birth. *Pediatrics, 26,* 210–218.

Kohler, L., Svenningsen, N.W., & Lindquist, B. (1979). Early detection of preschool health problems—Role of perinatal risk factors. *Acta Paediatric Scandinavia, 68,* 229–237.

Legum, C. (1983). Antenatal screening for fetal malformations and genetic disorders. In S. Harel & N. Anastasiow (Eds.), *The at-risk infant: Psycho/socio/medical aspects* (pp. 115–119). Baltimore: Paul H. Brooks Publishing Co.

Mackenzee, J. (April, 1977). Health for children, the 1977 Donald Peterson Memorial Lecture. In G.D. Robinson (Ed.), *Redesigning the child care.* The proceedings of a pediatric symposium held in Vancouver, British Columbia.

Njiokiktjien, C., & Kurver, P. (1980). Predictive value of neonatal neurological examination for cerebral function in infancy. *Developmental Medicine and Child Neurology, 22,* 736–747.

Ohrt, B., & Flehmig, I. (1980). The neurological evaluation of the newborn. In S. Harel (Ed.), *The at risk infant.* Princeton: Excerpta Medica.

Oppe, T.E. (1967). Risk registers for babies. *Developmental Medicine and Child Neurology, 9,* 13–21.

Parmelee, A.H., & Haber, A. (1973). Who is the "risk infant?" *Clinical Obstetrics and Gynaecology, 16,* 376–387.

Parmelee, A.H., Sigman, M., Kopp, C.B., & Haber, A. (1974, March). *The concept of a cumulative risk score for infants.* Paper presented at the Symposium on Aberrant Development in Infancy P.I., Gatlinburg, Tennessee.

Prechtl, H.F.R. (1980). The optimality concept [Editorial]. *Early Human Development, 4/3,* 201–205.

Rogers, M.G.H. (1968). "At risk" registers. *Developmental Medicine and Child Neurology, 10,* 813–814.

Sameroff, A., & Chandler, M.J. (1975). Reproductive risk and the continuum of caretaking casualty. In F.D. Horowitz, M. Hetherington, S. Scarr-Salpatek, & G. Siegal (Eds.), *Review of child development research* (Vol. 4). Illinois: University of Chicago Press.

Siegel, S.L. (1983). Biological and environmental variables as predictors of intellectual functioning at six years of age. In S. Harel & N. Anastasiow (Eds.), *The at-risk infant: Psycho/socio/medical aspects* (pp. 65–73). Baltimore: Paul H. Brookes Publishing Co.

Stern, L. (1980). Evaluation of the efficacy of neonatal care. In S. Harel (Ed.), *The at risk infant* (pp. 202–209). Princeton: Excerpta Medica.

Werner, E., Simonia, K., Bierman, J.M., & French, J.E. (1968). Cumulative effect of perinatal complications and deprived environment on physical, intellectual and social development of pre-school children. *Pediatrics, 39,* 490–505.

Westwood, M., Kramer, N.S., Munz, D., et al. (1983). Growth and development of full term nonasphyxiated small for gestational age newborns: Follow-up through adolescence. *Pediatrics, 71,* 376–382.

Wiener, C., Rider, R.V., Opel, W.C., & Harper, P.A. (1968). Correlates of low birth weight. Psychological status at eight to ten years. *Pediatric Research, 2,* 110–118.

Winick, M. (1969). Malnutrition and brain development. *The Journal of Pediatrics, 74,* 667–679.

Chapter 25

Pediatric Identification of Learning Disabilities

Murray M. Kappelman

THERE ARE MANY REASONS WHY CHILDREN fail in school. The school failure is merely a signal; it is the message of what has caused it that is of most importance to the pediatrician, parent, and teacher. Zuckerman and Chase (1984) indicated that there were four major areas that served as etiologic bases for school failure. The first area was the neurologically based sensory and motor disturbances, including hearing, visual, and motor impairment. Another was environmental interference, including school environment, bilinguality, school absence, and a dysfunctional family. Emotional disorders, including lack of motivation, depression, and psychosis made up a third category. The fourth category was one of great importance; it was labeled ''cognitive disorders'' and included mental retardation, attention deficit disorder, and specific learning disabilities. It is the specific learning disabilities that will be the focus of this presentation (Zuckerman & Chase, 1984).

Learning disabilities are not rare within the pediatric population. Culbertson and Ferry predicted that 3.5% to 5% of the school population have speech and language disorders, and 2% to 4% have learning disabilities (Culbertson & Ferry, 1982). It is important that these two problems be linked, since Mattis indicated that the frequency of specific diagnosis in learning disabilities include 39% with language disorder syndromes, 37% with articulation and grapho-motor disorders, 16% with visual perceptual disorders, and 10% unknown. Thus,

the area of language and articulation is extraordinarily important (Mattis, 1978). Cantrell and Forness corroborated this finding by noting that more than 50% of reading disabilities have underlying language disorders while a smaller percentage have visual perceptual problems (Cantrell & Forness, 1982).

The definition of specific learning disabilities as noted by Public Law 94-142 includes conditions such as perceptual handicaps, brain injury, minimal brain dysfunction, dyslexia, and developmental aphasia, and omits those youngsters whose learning problems are based upon sensory or motor handicaps, mental retardation, emotional disturbance, or environmental, cultural, or economic disadvantage. Since this definition is one upon which the school child's placement is based, we, as pediatricians, must consider this definition as indigenously important to our practice (Federal Law, 1980).

RESEARCH IN LEARNING DISABILITIES

Analyzing a group of inner-city children who were referred to a school health clinic for school failure problems, Kappelman and his group (1972) noted that 55.6% of the youngsters referred from the elementary schools came in with basically neurological etiologies as the primary causes. In breaking this down further, perceptual dysfunctions or specific learning disabilities accounted for 24.5%, with the male-to-female ratio being approximately two-to-one (Kappelman, Rosenstein, & Ganter, 1972). A subsequent study of a similar population of 100 consecutive youngsters appearing at a learning disabilities clinic found that perceptual handicaps or specific learning disabilities were the primary diagnoses for 33% of the children. What the authors found in addition, however, was that it was not appropriate to "label" the child with a single diagnosis, since there were multiple weaknesses that contributed to the learning handicap and could be noted as secondary and tertiary diagnoses. A good example of this was the fact that 81% of the youngsters presenting with a primary diagnosis of attention deficit disorder also had significant specific learning disabilities; therefore, chemotherapy only "slowed down the children to fail visibly" (Kappelman, Roberts, Rinaldi, & Cornblath, 1975). This has been corroborated by the long-range outcome work of Gabrielle Weiss, who has indicated that chemotherapy alone is insufficient to treat attention deficit disorder and that the educational and emotional aspects must gain our attention as well (Weiss, Minde, Werry, et al., 1972).

There are as many theories concerning categorization of learning disabilities as there are professionals working in the field. Two of the outstanding early leaders in the field were Johnson and Myklebust. These researchers divided learning disabilities into problems of sensation, problems of perception (the ability to identify immediately learned objects), imagery (the ability to recall accurately and appropriately past learned material), symbolization allowing categorization, and, finally, conceptualization which leads to problem solving. Defects in any of these five areas accounted for learning disabilities within their categories (Johnson & Myklebust, 1967).

SCREENING TESTS

Two groups of pediatricians have developed pediatric screening tests for neuromaturational problems that serve the pediatrician as predictors for potential future learning disabilities. One such instrument was developed by Sally Shaywitz (Shaywitz, Shaywitz, McGraw, & Grall, 1984) at Yale, while Melvin Levine at Boston (1983) has developed instruments known as the PEER, the PEEX, and the PEERAMID. These three tests for neuromaturational areas of concern deal with different age groups. Specifically, the PEER is a test for school readiness, the PEEX tests children 7–9 years of age, and the PEERAMID is for the young adolescent. Dr. Levine has identified areas of concern on the PEEX which, when abnormal, alert the pediatrician to potential learning disabilities. These are the minor neurologic indicators identified by Dr. Levine: temporal-sequential organization, visual-spatial orientation, auditory-language function, fine-motor function, gross-motor function, and memory (Levine, Meltzer, & Busch, 1983). Because of the vast diversity in the categorization of learning disabilities, the presenter has developed his own listing of possible problems identifying the weaknesses within the child's perceptual and processing ability that may have led to specific learning disabilities. Stated simply, the areas of concern are: auditory memory, comprehension, differentiation, association, processing, and expressive language. Additional areas of concern include: visual memory, comprehension, differentiation, association, and processing, with visual-motor coordination as the final area in that category. Somewhat higher level functioning includes abstract-concrete reasoning, short-term vs. long-term memory, sequencing, comprehension, integration, categorization, and the final, highest level of learning ability, problem solving. The auditory language was placed first because of its pre-eminent position in learning disabilities; short-term vs. long-term memory was given special placement because of the recent realization that this was an area leading to difficulty in mathematics (dyscalculia).

The pediatrician must recognize that the child who presents at the office with learning problems in preschool or school environments requires a systematized process for this child's clinical evaluation. The following procedures are essential for the pediatrician and his professional colleagues to use in order to effect a total "whole child" assessment relative to the learning problem. First, a medical assessment should be made by the pediatrician that includes medical history, physical exam, neurological exam, and vision and hearing tests. Often the pediatrician may make an assessment of the emotional status of the child but may request additional professional assistance. Generally, the school will provide the pediatrician with information about the child's academic achievement level. Again, outside help may be used in this area. Frequently, the pediatrician refers the child for an assessment of general cognitive functioning as measured by standardized tests and an assessment of information processing skills, including language. When all of this information is collated and analyzed, it may be possible for the pediatrician plus other professional colleagues to form an interdisciplinary assessment of the child's learning weaknesses and strengths. Among the helpful, but not consistent, physical findings are the so-called "soft neurological signs." These reflect motor awkwardness or neurological immaturity, and may include such physical findings as synkinesia, dysdiadochokinesia, right/left confusion, or difficulty with finger localization. Mild abnormal neurological signs may also be noted during the examination; these may include asymmetry of reflexes or muscle tone, mild tremors or ataxia, increased or asymmetrical deep tendon reflexes, an asymmetric gait or awkward posture or choreiform movements, or overall motor clumsiness. The pediatrician is aware that most neurological soft signs, if present, tend to diminish over time from an early age onward and may disappear by the time the child is 11 years old.

As noted above, during the pediatrician's approach to the diagnosis of learning disabilities, it becomes necessary for the pediatrician to become a team member with other professionals and family members whose observations and testing can add considerable information and evidence to an accurate final assessment of the child's learning ability and overall school and home adaptation. The team includes the parents as well as the classroom and/or special education teacher, principal, and school guidance counselor. In addition, the pediatrician frequently requests help from a communication specialist, audiologist, social worker, clinical psychologist, and educational specialist. Only on unusual occasions will the pediatrician need the consultation advice of the neurologist or child psychiatrist. It is essential for any pediatrician entering private practice to investigate the community and locate the "other professionals" necessary to obtain complete diagnostic assessments of youngsters with school learning disorders. Knowing where to go for psychological testing, language assessment, social work investigation, or educational testing, for example, can be extremely useful in facilitating the diagnostic assessment of these children.

CONCLUSION

The pediatrician needs to be aware that early identification of youngsters with learning disabilities is an essential part of pediatric practice. This is not a condition that will be "grown out of." It is a problem that requires the most sensitive and perceptive diagnosis and management by a team of professionals and parents at home, school, and within the pediatric office. Schiffman and Goldberg (1983) have indicated that children who are diagnosed as having learning disabilities as early as the first or second grade have approximately an 85% chance of remediation and maintenance at grade level; in contrast, children who are not diagnosed as learning disabled until the fourth grade have a less than 35% chance of remediation that allows them to be maintained at grade level (Schiffman & Goldberg, 1983). This is a frightening figure. It can be improved by pediatric awareness, sensitivity, and willingness to undertake the overall investigation as early as possible to assist the parents, school, and child in finding routes and pathways around a learning disability. Such an investigation allows for success rather than educational oblivion.

REFERENCES

Cantrell, D., & Forness, S. (1982). Learning disorders. *Journal of the American Academy of Child Psychiatry, 21*(4),417.

Culbertson, J.L., & Ferry, P. (1982). Learning disabilities. *Pediatric Clinics of North America, 29*(1),121.

Federal Law 94-142, December 29, 1980. Government Printing Office, Federal Register 65083.

Johnson, D., & Myklebust, H. (1967). *Learning disabilities*. New York: Grune & Stratton.

Kappelman, M., Roberts, P., Rinaldi, R., & Cornblath, M. (1975). The school health team and school health physician. *American Journal of Diseases of Children, 129*,191–195.

Kappelman, M., Rosenstein, A., & Ganter, R. (1972). Comparison of disadvantaged children with learning disabilities and their successful peer group. *American Journal of Diseases of Children, 124*,875–879.

Levine, M., Meltzer, L. J., & Busch, B. (1983). The pediatric early elementary examination: Studies of a neurodevelopmental examination for seven- to nine-year-old children. *Pediatrics, 71*(6),894.

Mattis, S. (1978). Dyslexia syndromes. A working hypothesis that works. In A. Benton & D. Pearl (Eds.), *Dyslexia: An appraisal of current knowledge*. New York: Oxford University Press.

Schiffman, G., & Goldberg, H. (1983). *Dyslexia. Problems of reading disabilities*. New York: Grune & Stratton.

Shaywitz, S., Shaywitz, B., McGraw, K., & Grall, S. (1984). Current status of the neuromaturational examination as an index of learning disability. *Journal of Pediatrics, 104*(6),819.

Weiss, G., Minde, K., Werry, J., et al. (1972). Studies of the hyperactive child, VIII: Five year follow up. *Archives of General Psychiatry, 21*,409–414.

Zuckerman, B. S., & Chase, C. (1984). Specific learning disability and dyslexia: A language-based model (pp. 249–280). *Advances in Pediatrics*. Chicago: Yearbook Medical Publishers.

Chapter 26

Neurological Basis of Learning Disorders

N. Paul Rosman

IT HAS BEEN ESTIMATED THAT 15% OF school-age children in the United States are learning disabled. When considering such children, terms that are commonly used include:

Learning: acquisition of information

Learning problem: difficulty in acquiring information with variably successful compensatory strategies

Learning failure: difficulty in acquiring information with failure to develop or to implement compensatory stretegies

Learning disability: diminished performance in (a) school subject(s), such as reading, writing, or arithmetic, with achievement two or more grade levels below that expected based on the person's intelligence.

CLINICAL PROCESS

History

A comprehensive history should be obtained from both parents and, when possible, from the child, with additional information drawn from health records (e.g., developmental milestones, numbers of episodes of otitis media) and school records (e.g., results of psychologic tests). Risk factors must be assessed, including ones in the prenatal period (e.g., intake of unprescribed drugs), the perinatal period (e.g., birth trauma), and the postnatal period (e.g., meningitis). Effects of chronic medical illnesses (e.g., asthma) and potential adverse effects of medications (e.g., phenobarbital) must be considered. A family history of similar learning problems should be sought.

General Physical Examination

Many signs observed from the general physical examination can suggest a probable basis for the child's failure to learn. Examples are:

1. Head: Small head size, for example, from underdevelopment of the brain or injury to the brain
2. Neck: Webbed, as in Turner syndrome
3. Face: Involuntary movements, indicating tics, chorea, or drug effect
4. Eye: Strabismus, causing or resulting from poor vision
5. Ear: Poor hearing, contributing to speech delay
6. Mouth: "Fish mouth" appearance, as in myotonic muscular dystrophy
7. Trunk: Dystonia, from perinatal hypoxia or hyperbilirubinemia
8. Limbs: Hemiatrophy, indicating abnormality of contralateral cerebrum
9. Spine: Overlying lesions, indicative of possible underlying defects
10. Skin: Brown, white, and red birthmarks, associated with seizures and learning problems

TREATABLE MEDICAL CONTRIBUTORS TO LEARNING DISABILITIES

There are numerous medical conditions that can contribute to learning disabilities and many are treatable. Examples of such disorders, their causes, and "cures," are outlined in Table 1.

Table 1. Treatable medical contributors to learning disabilities

Contributor	Cause	Cure
Asthma	Environmental trigger	Avoidance; desensitization
Anemia	Iron deficiency	Administer iron
Malnutrition	Psycho-social deprivation	Increase "supplies"
Medication	Lethargy from antihistamines	Change the drug
Drug	Alcohol intoxication	Abstinence
Toxin	Lead	Chelation ethylenediamine-tetraacetic acid (EDTA)
Sydenham chorea	Rheumatic fever	Administer penicillin; phenothiazine
Metabolic disorders: Hyperthyroidism	Toxic goiter	Subtotal thyroidectomy
Hypoglycemia or Hyperglycemia	Diabetes mellitus	Modify insulin schedule
Copper excess	Wilson disease	Chelation (penicillamine)

THE NEUROLOGY OF LEARNING DISABILITIES

Neurological assessment of the learning-disabled child is justified, based on the accumulated evidence indicating a neurological basis for many (most) learning disabilities and contributors to learning failure.

Learning Disabilities

Reading disability (*dyslexia*) has been correlated with developmental abnormalities of the cerebral cortex, mainly in the perisylvian region, especially on the left. *Delayed speech development* can be caused by early left cerebral lesions and is often associated with "pathological" left-handedness. *Verbal auditory agnosia,* whether congenital or acquired (from seizures), appears to be of temporal lobe origin, as is "epileptic aphasia." Speech and cognitive disturbances in childhood *autism* have been related to reduced size of the temporal lobes, especially the left, and to abnormalities of the forebrain, cerebellum, and inferior olive. *Mathematical disability* (*dyscalculia*) can be of right or left cerebral origin.

Impaired graphomotor skills (*dysgraphia*) can be caused by poor vision, poor coordination, or visuo-motor handicaps of perceptual type.

Recent studies by Geschwind and colleagues (Geschwind & Behan, 1982) indicate strong associations between *learning disabilities, left-handedness,* and *autoimmune disease.* If, upon further study, such associations seem firm, they should lead to important avenues of new research on the neurobiology of learning disorders.

Contributors to Learning Failure

Of the many contributors to learning failure, *poor vision* (refractive errors, strabismus, lesions of the anterior or posterior visual pathways) or *poor hearing* (conductive or neurosensory loss) are particularly important. *Unclear speech* (*dysarthria*) can be caused by anatomic defects, or bulbar and corticobulbar abnormalities. *Involuntary movements,* from medication, anxiety, chorea, or simple motor tics or Tourette disease, can contribute to clumsiness. *Attention deficit disorder* (ADD), without or with hyperactivity (ADDH), if not from a definable cause (medical, drug, toxic, dietary, neurologic, psychiatric, environmental, or other), appears to be explainable by a catecholamine deficiency in brain.

Neurological Examination

Basic to conducting a meaningful neurologic examination is an understanding of the functional and dysfunctional anatomy of the brain. An exhaustive neurological examination can be exhausting to the child and less helpful than a more directed examination. The latter should be focused on those areas most likely to lead to further understanding of the child's failure to learn. Thus, in the child with learning failure, testing of visuo-motor skills almost certainly will be more fruitful than looking for an asymmetry in ankle jerks. There are a number of pitfalls leading to a child's apparent "failing" of (part of) the neurologic examination, remembered by the letter "F." These causes of "*Factitious Failure*" include: *F*atigue, *F*amine, *F*ever, *F*ear, *F*amily, *F*idgetiness, *F*antasy, *F*its, and "*F*armaceuticals." Though so-

called "soft signs" of neurologic dysfunction are more frequent in children with learning disorders than in the general population, it should be noted that all such signs can be seen normally at earlier stages of development. The diagnosis of perceptual handicap of visuomotor type is frequently made correctly, but it is also often made incorrectly, for many conditions can mimic such handicaps. These include: poor hearing, poor attention, poor motivation, low intelligence, poor vision, and problems with motor control. "Organicity" should not be presumed or concluded based on psychologic test results or from the child's response or nonresponse to medication (such as those prescribed for symptoms of ADD).

Laboratory Tests

A number of laboratory tests may be appropriate and useful in assessing children with learning problems. Examples include testing of vision and hearing (sometimes including brain

Table 2. Treatable neurological contributors to learning disabilities

Category	Cause	Cure
Sensory deficit	Poor vision	Corrective lenses
	Poor hearing	Treat middle ear problems; amplification
Motor deficit	Spasticity	Physiotherapy; diazepam
	Chorea	Chlorpromazine
	Athetosis/ dystonia	Trihexyphenidyl
	Tremor	Propranolol
	Myotonia	Procainamide
	Clumsiness	Occupational and physical therapies; adaptive physical education
Speech deficit	Dysarthria (cleft lip/ palate)	Surgical repair
	Dysphasia	Speech therapy
Paroxysmal disorders	Seizures	Anticonvulsants
	Headaches	Acute or prophylactic medication
	Inattention/ overactivity	Dextroamphetamine; methylphenidate; pemoline; environmental management
	Tourette disease	Haloperidol
Emotional disorders	Primary or secondary	Diazepam for anxiety; amitriptyline for depression

stem auditory evoked potentials, *BAEPs*), comprehensive *psychologic testing* (intelligence, attention, memory, academic, perceptual, projective), and occasionally, additional tests, some of them quite specialized (e.g., of a child with a suspected progressive neurologic disease). Laboratory tests should not be ordered unless their potential usefulness seems clear. For example, an electroencephalogram (*EEG*) should probably never be obtained in a child with learning failure unless a seizure disorder is suspected clinically. The reason for this is that abnormalities on EEG, including seizure discharges, are sometimes found in children who do not have neurologic problems. When clinically indicated, however, an EEG should be done; additionally, topographic mapping of parameters derived from EEG and evoked potential (*EP*) data is now possible. This is known as brain electrical activity mapping (*BEAM*). Similarly, brain scanning by cranial computerized tomography (*CCT*) or magnetic resonance imaging (*MRI*) should not be obtained injudiciously, for minor abnormalities (e.g., asymmetry in ventricular size) bearing no relationship to a child's clinical problem may be found, serving only to heighten family anxiety.

Examples of the many neurological disorders that can contribute to learning disabilities, their causes and "cures," are outlined in Table 2.

SUGGESTED READINGS

Adams, R.M., Kocsis, J.J., & Estes, R.E. (1974). Soft neurological signs in learning-disabled children and controls. *American Journal of Diseases of Children, 128,*614–618.

Capute, A.J., & Palmer, F.B. (1980). A pediatric overview of the spectrum of developmental disabilities. *Journal of Developmental and Behavioral Pediatrics, 1,*66–69.

Culbertson, J.L., & Ferry, P.C. (1982). Learning disabilities. *Pediatric Clinics of North America, 29,*121–136.

Denhoff, E., Hainsworth, P.K., & Hainsworth, M.L. (1972). The child at risk for learning disorder: Can he be identified during the first year of life? *Clinical Pediatrics, 11,*164–170.

Drillien, C., & Drummond, M. (1983). Developmental screening and the child with special needs: A population study of 5000 children. *Clinics in Developmental Medicine* (Vol. 86). Philadelphia: J.B. Lippincott.

Duffy, F.H., Denckla, M.B., Bartels, P.H., & Sandini, G. (1980a). Dyslexia: regional differences in brain electrical activity by topographic mapping. *Annals of Neurology, 17,*412–420.

Duffy, F.H., Denckla, M.B., Bartels, P.H., Sandini, G., & Kiessling, L. S. (1980b). Dyslexia: automated diagnosis by computerized classification of brain electrical activity. *Annals of Neurology, 7,*421–428.

Ferry, P.C. (1981). On growing new neurons: Are early intervention programs effective? *Pediatrics, 67,*38–41.

Galaburda, A.M., Sherman, G.F., Rosen, G.D., Aboitz, F., & Geschwind, N. (1985). Developmental dyslexia: Four consecutive patients with cortical anomalies. *Annals of Neurology, 18,*222–233.

Geschwind, N., & Behan, P. (1982). Left-handedness: Association with immune disease, migraine, and developmental learning disorder. *Proceedings of the National Academy of Sciences, 79,*5097–5100.

Geschwind, N., & Galaburda, A.M. (1985). Cerebral lateralization: Biological mechanisms, associations and

pathology: A hypothesis and a program for research. *Archives of Neurology, 42,*428–459;521–552;634–654.

Golden, G.S. (1982). Neurobiological correlates of learning disabilities. *Annals of Neurology, 12,*409–418.

Gordon, N. (1975). Learning difficulties: The role of the doctor. *Developmental Medicine and Child Neurology, 17,*99–102.

Hagerman, R.J. (1984). Pediatric assessment of the learning-disabled child. *Journal of Developmental and Behavioral Pediatrics, 5,*274–284.

Hart, Z., Rennick, P.M., Klinge, V., & Schwartz, M. L. (1974). A pediatric neurologist's contribution to evaluations of school underachievers. *American Journal of Diseases of Children, 128,*319–323.

Herskowitz, J., & Rosman, N.P. (1982). Headaches (Chapter 11); Seizures (Chapter 12); Learning Disabilities and Disorders of Speech and Language (Chapter 17). In *Pediatrics, neurology and psychiatry—Common ground: Behavioral, cognitive, affective and physical disorders in childhood and adolescence.* New York: Macmillan.

Kandt, R.S. (1984). Neurologic examination of children with learning disorders. *Pediatric Clinics of North America, 31,*297–315.

Kemper, T.L. (1985). Anatomical basis of learning disabilities. *Otolaryngologic Clinics of North America, 18,*305–314.

Kinsbourne, M., & Caplan, P.J. (1979). *Children's Learning and Attention Problems.* Boston: Little, Brown.

Millichap, J.G. (1977). *Learning disabilities and related disorders: Facts and current issues.* Chicago: Yearbook Medical Publishers.

Resnick, T.J., Allen, D.A., & Rapin, I. (1984). Disorders of language development: Diagnosis and intervention. *Pediatrics in Review, 6,*85–92.

Rumsey, J.R., Dorwart, R., Vermess, M., Denckla, M. B., Kruesi, M. J. P., & Rapoport, J. L. (1986). Magnetic resonance imaging of brain anatomy in severe developmental dyslexia. *Archives of Neurology, 43,*1045–1046.

Rutter, M. (1980). School influences on children's behavior and development. *Pediatrics, 65,*208–220.

Schain, R.J. (1977). *Neurology of childhood learning disorders* (2nd ed.). Baltimore: Williams & Wilkins.

Shapiro, B.K., Palmer, F.B., Wachtel, R.C., & Capute, A.J. (1984). Issues in the early identification of specific learning disability. *Journal of Developmental and Behavioral Pediatrics, 5,*15–20.

Shaywitz, S.E., Grossman, H., & Shaywitz, B.A. (1984). Symposium on Learning Disorders. *Pediatric Clinics of North America, 31,*279–518.

Taylor, E.A. (1986). The overactive child. *Clinics in Developmental Medicine* (Vol. 47). Philadelphia: J.B. Lippincott.

Trehub, S.E. (1977). Infant antecedents: A search for the precursors of learning disabilities. In M.E. Blaw, I. Rapin, & M. Kinsbourne (Eds.), *Topics in child neurology* (pp. 175–188). Jamaica, NY: Spectrum Publications.

Younes, R.P., Rosner, B., & Webb, G. (1983). Neuroimmaturity of learning-disabled children: A controlled study. *Developmental Medicine and Child Neurology, 25,*574–579.

Chapter 27

New Tests of Vision Screening and Assessment in Infants and Young Children

Janette Atkinson

TESTING OF VISION IN EARLY CHILDHOOD may be undertaken for two rather different reasons. In *vision screening,* a large group of the population, in whom vision problems have not yet been identified or suspected, are tested to pick up the subgroup who either have a manifest vision problem, or who show precursors that place them at risk for developing such a problem. In *visual assessment,* tests are conducted on a relatively small number of children who have already been identified as being at risk. An assessment of the visual function of each child is needed either to guide diagnosis and treatment or to assess the implications of a visual disorder for the child's development and capabilities. Of course, assessment and screening should be considered as an integrated service in the sense that children who fail a screening test will require follow-up with a fuller visual assessment. However, screening and assessment lead to very different requirements for the tests to be used.

Because a screening test has to be applied to large numbers of children, it is not economically practical to use a test that requires extended testing time for each child. Furthermore, since the great majority of children will yield negative results, parents cannot be ex-

pected to make large investments of time and effort to participate; in particular, they will not generally be willing to travel far, so tests should ideally be portable. Acceptability to families is important, since, ethical issues aside, anything that diminishes participation in a screening program reduces its value. The screening test should yield clear-cut rather than 'doubtful' results in the vast majority of cases, and the number of 'false positives' should be small. False positives incur not only costs to the service of follow-up, but also unnecessary anxiety and inconvenience to the patient's family.

In the author's unit, a variety of behavioral and electrophysiological tests are used that can give information on acuity and binocular function in infancy. However, none of these have the simplicity, portability, or ease for general health care personnel that have been described above as criteria for a screening test. In contrast, the technique of isotropic photorefraction (Atkinson et al., 1981) allows refractive errors to be detected by orthoptic staff operating readily portable equipment after a modest period of training. We have therefore been using this instrument in a trial program of population refractive screening for infants of 6–9 months.

The research and studies reported in this chapter are the work of members of the Visual Development Unit in collaboration with the Child Development Centre, the Departments of Paediatrics, Ophthalmology and Community Health (Cambridge), and Dr. Sue Atkinson (Community Health) and the Ophthalmology Department at Bristol. The work was supported by the Medical Research Council of Great Britain.

This screening program, and its evaluation in terms of diagnostic and predictive utility, are discussed below.

Compared to screening, visual assessment is required for a substantially smaller number of children; there are good grounds for suspecting visual impairment in all of them. A much greater investment of effort in each case is therefore feasible and justified. Diagnosis, decisions on treatment, and advice on education or rehabilitation all require a global picture of the child's visual capabilities, and so a range of tests related to distinct visual functions is needed. Patients can come to a central assessment unit, thus, sophisticated nonportable equipment and specialist personnel are justified. While a screening test must end in a categorical decision (whether or not to refer the patient), the outcome of assessment is a much fuller quantitative and qualitative description. The issue of 'false positives' does not arise in the same form: the aim of assessment is to provide the best estimate available of the child's visual function, with any uncertainties that may be present explicitly stated.

In assessment, therefore, tests of monocular and binocular acuity, accommodation, refraction, oculomotor function, binocularity, and central visual function may all be appropriate, with the exact combination depending on the reasons why the child has been referred. Quite separately from our screening program, we have undertaken visual assessment on a range of infants and young children referred because of pediatric or ophthalmological problems; our procedures and goals in such assessments are outlined in a number of previous publications (see Atkinson, 1984a).

The preliminary results of the screening program and a summary of a cohort of recent assessments are described below.

INFANT REFRACTIVE
SCREENING PROGRAM

One goal of a screening program is to detect conditions that are manifest but that have not otherwise come to the attention of health services. Another goal may be to identify children who, although they may not have a problem that impairs vision at the time of screening, are at risk for developing such a problem. The screening will have its greatest value if treatment for the at-risk group is provided to prevent the later onset of a visual problem.

In the context of refractive screening, a group that may be at risk are infants having a moderate to high degree of hypermetropia and/or anisometropia. Such hypermetropia in infancy has been found to have a high correlation with later onset of strabismus and amblyopia (Ingram, Traynar, Walker, & Wilson, 1979). The existence of a correlation does not answer whether this link is causal, with the excessive accommodation needed to overcome hypermetropia leading to overconvergence, and thereby strabismus, or whether hypermetropia and strabismus are associated for some other reason. If the strabismus *is* of accommodative origin, then the detection of hypermetropia in refractive screening could allow prescription of a spectacle correction to reduce accommodation and thus prevent development of strabismus. Our refractive screening program therefore includes a randomized controlled trial of partial refractive correction of infant hypermetropia as a preventive measure for preschool strabismus and amblyopia.

The photorefractive screening program for 6–9-month-old infants, currently underway in Cambridge and Bristol, has a number of aims. These include:

1. Study of refractive changes in the population
2. Early identification of refractive errors and strabismus
3. Investigation of the predictive value of refractive screening for later visual disorders
4. Test of prevention of strabismus and amblyopia by spectacle correction in a randomized controlled trial
5. Evaluation of the acceptability of photorefraction in the context of community screening

The procedure for the screening and follow-up has been described in some detail by Atkinson, Braddick, Durden, Watson, and Atkinson

(1984), as have some of the early results. Thus, only a brief summary will be presented here.

Changes in Refraction in the Population

Data from the screening of 6–9 month-olds show that the average cycloplegic refraction at this age is between 1.0 and 1.5 diopter (D) hypermetropic, and that approximately 50% of this population shows 1.0 D or more of astigmatism (confirming earlier findings of Howland, Atkinson, Braddick, & French, 1978; Mohindra, Held, Gwiazda, & Brill, 1978). Analysis of the axis of astigmatism in a sample of these infants indicates that different populations may show markedly different ratios of the different axes (see Atkinson & Braddick, 1983).

We have conducted a pilot analysis of the first infants with significant degrees of hypermetropia (+4.0 D or more) but who have not worn spectacles. In this group, hypermetropia reduces by an average 0.75 D between 1 and 2 years of age. There is also a reduction in astigmatism over this period (as found earlier by Atkinson, Braddick, & French [1980]); however this reduction appears to occur at a slower rate in those children with against-the-rule or oblique astigmatisms than in with-the-rule astigmatisms. The reason for this difference is unknown, and it remains to be seen whether it will be substantiated by analysis of a larger group.

Early Detection of Refractive Errors and Strabismus

Figure 1 shows the refractive errors identified in Cambridge and Bristol in the initial period of the screening. The two populations look very similar: 5% have a significant degree of hypermetropia, while myopes and anisometropes are each 1%–2%. Partial analysis of a longer period of screening in Cambridge generally confirms the incidence of hypermetropia and of other refractive errors (see Figure 2). The orthoptic examination carried out alongside photorefraction found a small incidence of manifest strabismus in this age group, representing strabismus of early onset in around 1%

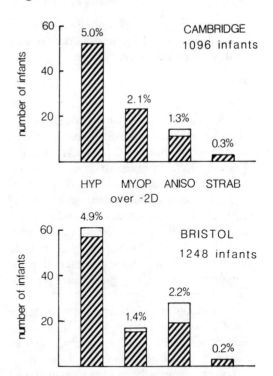

Figure 1.   Refractive errors found in photorefractive screening at 6–9 months of age: initial data from Cambridge and Bristol programs. HYP = hypermetropia + 4 D or greater in at least one axis. MYOP = myopia −2 D or greater in at least one axis. ANISO = 1.5 D or greater difference between corresponding axes in the two eyes. STRAB = manifest strabismus. Shaded areas = refractive errors confirmed by subsequent retinoscopy.

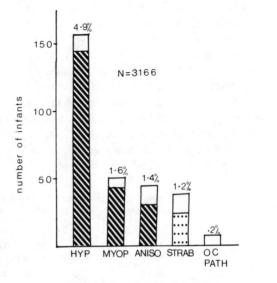

Figure 2.   Refractive errors found in photorefractive screening at 6–9 months of age in the Cambridge population. Categories are the same as in Figure 1.

of the population. We presume that in the majority of preschool children with strabismus the onset must be after 1 year of age.

Predictive Value of Refractive Screening

The regular follow-up examinations of children identified as having abnormal refractions at 6–9 months have been described in detail by Atkinson (Atkinson et al., 1984). All those followed-up have an examination of the fundus when first referred, and an orthoptic examination on every visit. We monitor acuity (using preferential looking on younger children) and accommodation (using noncycloplegic photorefraction). A child who at any stage is found to be strabismic or amblyopic is referred for the appropriate ophthalmological care immediately.

In addition to the children with refractive errors, one control infant with normal refraction is selected for every hypermetrope detected. This control group is also followed-up, in order to compare the incidence of later visual problems between infants who have refractive errors at 6–9 months and those who do not.

At the end point of our program, when the child is 3½ years of age, each child who has been followed-up is assessed to see whether vision is normal or abnormal. We use the Sheridan Gardiner single optotype test and a development using the same letters in a 'crowded' form (Atkinson, Pimm-Smith, Evans, Harding, & Braddick, 1986). From studies of visually normal children at this age, a single optotype acuity of 6/6 and 6/9 on our crowded test is regarded as acceptable performance. If any child fails to show these levels of acuity initially, their refraction is rechecked, and the child is retested with any new spectacle correction that may be required. Any child who fails

to show normal acuity on two such tests is considered amblyopic. Children are also tested for normal binocularity using the TNO stereo test.

The first hypermetropes detected in the Cambridge screening program, and their control cases, have now reached the age of 3½ years and have completed these tests. These results are shown in Table 1. Nearly all controls have normal vision at 3½ years, but this is not true for the hyperopic infants. Thus, from these early results, it does appear that refractive errors picked up in infant screening are indeed an effective predictor of later visual problems. The relation of these results to refractive correction is discussed below.

Randomized Control Trial of the Prevention of Strabismus and Amblyopia

In this trial, half the infants who had been identified in the screening as having a significantly hypermetropic refraction were offered a partial spectacle correction for their hyperopia. The correction given was not a full correction of the hypermetropia; rather, it brought their corrected refraction close to the norm for their age group. The other half of the infants were uncorrected.

Parents were carefully questioned at each follow-up examination about the time during which their children wore the spectacles, and a full record was kept. This has not often been done in studies of refractive correction of children, but in our view it is essential if the effectiveness of this treatment is to be evaluated. At the present time, the author estimates that approximately 50% of those given a prescription at 6–9 months wore the glasses most or all of the time, with the other 50% ranging from intermittent wearing to "never worn." We have found that very few infants under 1 year of age

Table 1. Visual outcome at 3½ years in children who were hyperopic at 6–9 month screening, and controls.

Sample tested	Total	Fail on		
		Single letter acuity test	"Crowded" acuity test	Binocular tests
Untreated hyperopes	36	20 (55%)	25 (69%)	9 (25%)
Controls	33	0	3 (9%)	1 (3%)

will persistently not tolerate spectacles, but that there is more frequent noncompliance if the spectacles are first prescribed at 1 to 2 years. In general, it was found that the parents' reluctance is the main factor leading to infants who do not wear their spectacles at all. Although this is an undesirable finding, it is understandable considering that these children show no obvious visual defect such as strabismus.

All children in the trial were tested at 3½ years to find out whether the early spectacle correction had improved their chances of normal vision at this age. Table 2 shows the results. There is a significant difference between hyperopes who have worn spectacles in infancy and those who have not, with the former having significantly better vision at 3½ years. Although there is much data still to be collected and analyzed from this program, the results to date showing the success of early intervention are encouraging.

INDIVIDUAL ASSESSMENT OF VISION

In contrast to screening, individual assessment is carried out with specific groups for whom detailed knowledge of visual function is required. One such group is infants and children with physical and mental disabilities for whom a high incidence level of visual disorders has been determined. Most of the previous studies (many of which are reviewed by Goble, 1985) have concentrated on specific isolated aspects

of vision, such as strabismus or acuity. Here we have taken a somewhat different approach, with an interdisciplinary team working together to look at a number of interrelated aspects of vision. The eventual aim is to help those involved in the care, treatment, and education of these children to understand the effect of the child's visual deficits on everyday life, so that every effort can be made to help the child to develop strategies to deal with his or her problems. The details of many of the tests that were used have already been published elsewhere (Atkinson, 1984a) and so will only be tabulated below.

Clinical Population

A total of 108 children were referred for assessment to the Visual Development Unit by pediatricians from the Child Development Centre and Addenbrooke's Hospital, Cambridge. The ages of these children ranged from 4 months to 12 years, but nearly all of them (100) were 4 years of age or younger. Many had the mental age of under 2 years. In 30% of the cases, a visual problem had already been diagnosed or was strongly suspected by the clinicians making the referral, while the remaining 70% were referred for a visual assessment as part of a more general battery of sensory and developmental tests. Children were referred with a wide variety of pediatric diagnoses; one-third were cases of cerebral palsy, one-third had general developmental delay, and the other third had a range of disorders.

Table 2. Relation between early refraction, spectacle correction, and outcome of vision test at 3½ years

			Number		Vision test at 3½ years	
					Pass	Fail[a]
Control group (normal refraction at 6–9 mo)	Not prescribed spectacles	Not consistently worn	33	36 Spectacles not worn	91%	9%
			24			
	Prescribed[b] spectacles	Consistently worn	12		31%	69%
Hyperopes (more than 4D at 6–9 mo)				13 Spectacles worn	69%	31%
			13			

[a]Pass/fail difference between controls and hyperopes without spectacles is significant on chi-squared, $p < .01$.
[b]Effect of spectacle correction on hyperopes is significant on chi-squared, $p < .05$.

Procedure

Table 3 shows the tests that were used in the procedure. Each examination starts with a discussion with the parents (or other relevant caregiver) about their observations of the child's behavior and what they think the child sees and perceives. Any relevant family history of eye problems is noted. We then watch the child playing and interacting with others in our small reception nursery. This is supplemented by informal testing of visually guided reaching and grasping for bright toys, visual attention to distance (e.g., awareness of parents entering or leaving the room, or response to peek-a-boo at 2 meters around the edge of a door) and informal field testing. For the latter test, a visually conspicuous but silent toy is brought in laterally from either side of the child and we observe when the child first notices its appearance. When perceptual and cognitive deficits are suspected, the child may be informally tested for the understanding of object permanence by hiding toys in different ways. Additionally, the child is tested for visual recognition of toys, objects, and people.

The other more formal tests are carried out in separate rooms away from the nursery, so that the child is not distracted by toys and other people. Frequent breaks are given between tests for playing so that the child does not become bored and the parents have time to relax and talk about their child's problem. The 'field testing' referred to in Table 3 has so far been carried out only when indicated by a history of

Table 3.   Individual assessment of vision

1. Discussion of child's history, including family history of eye problems
2. Observation of general visuo-motor behavior
3. Orthoptic examination
4. Isotropic photorefraction without cycloplegia
5. Acuity assessment (forced-choice preferential looking, STYCAR, Sheridan-Gardiner, "crowding")
6. Field testing
7. Optokinetic nystagmus (OKN)
8. Pattern VER
9. Binocular vision (monocular OKN; binocular VER)
10. Discussion of results

hemiplegia or by observations on informal testing. The testing is done by bringing Stycar Balls into the field of view from behind the child in a nondistracting environment, with the child's attention initially attracted forward by an observer who then notes when the first fixation towards the target is made. We have been primarily concerned with identifying children in whom there is consistent asymmetry between the points at which attention is attracted in the two lateral half-fields. As all these tests have already been described in a number of previous papers, they will not be described here (Atkinson, 1984a). However, two relatively new procedures will be briefly described below, and a summary table of results for the clinical group will be given.

Test of Changes in Focusing or in Visual Attention

We use isotropic photorefraction without cycloplegia (Atkinson et al., 1981), both to indicate possible refractive errors and to assess the child's ability to shift focus with changes in visual attention. A video photorefractor has been developed in our unit whereby photorefractive images are stored in a digital frame store; this enables the images to be immediately examined after each flash exposure. This immediacy is essential for looking at children wih multiple problems, since it allows the tester to make several rapid assessments of focusing with minimum effort on the child's part. From a series of photorefractive tests with targets (large, noisy, brightly illuminated toys) set at different distances from the eyes, it is possible to determine how reliably the child is able or willing to change focus and accommodate accurately on nearby targets. Of course, it is necessary to compare the results of this test with those of cycloplegic photorefraction in order to ascertain whether any lack of appropriate focusing is due to a significant myopia, or whether it is a consequence of motor difficulties or deficits in the control of visual attention. In nonmyopic children, one of three kinds of behavior were found when children were tested with target distances of 20 to 200 cm:

1. Normal focusing over the entire range
2. Fixed focus close to the position of cycloplegic refraction
3. Appropriate changes of focus for nearby targets (e.g., 20 to 75 cm) with little change of accommodation for targets beyond these distances. Behavior of type (ii) or (iii) is taken to indicate deficits of visual attention.

New VEP Test of Cortical Vision

Line or edge orientation is a very simple and basic aspect of spatial configuration. It is also one whose representation in an array of selective channels has been extensively explored in physiological (Hubel & Wiesel, 1977) and psychophysical (Braddick, Atkinson, & Campbell, 1978) studies. The development of this system in infancy is of interest both for its role in pattern perception and, from the point of view of developmental neurology, because it is specifically a cortical function; subcortical parts of the primate visual system do not contain orientation-selective neurons.

We have developed an evoked potential technique, applicable to children or adults, which is designed to test for the presence of orientation-selective cortical mechanisms. The problem is to isolate the response of such mechanisms from that of subcortical neural elements that lack orientation selectivity. Simply presenting a grating pattern that changed orientation would not achieve this, since there would be luminance and contrast changes at many points in the pattern. These local events could activate mechanisms that were com-

pletely unselective for edge orientation. However, changes in orientation can be embedded in a dynamic sequence of random displacements of the grating (Figure 3). Each displacement, on average, produces as much local contrast change as an orientation reversal. Any nonorientation-selective mechanisms may then be driven at the high frequency of the displacements, but these mechanisms do not "see" anything different at the transitions where an orientation reversal occurs, and so will not show any extra response at the lower frequency of the reversals. Any response at this frequency must arise from orientation-selective mechanisms that are cortical.

In recording from a normal 7-week infant (Figure 4), a clear and statistically reliable response to the reversals of orientation is present. Orientation selective mechanisms must therefore be present in the visual cortex by this age. In contrast, Figure 5 shows VEP records from a newborn infant. A pattern-appearance control condition (Figure 5, top) demonstrates that the newborn is sensitive to the spatial and temporal frequencies of the dynamic stimulus used and that VEP recording is possible, but the orientation-reversal display produces no VEP response (Figure 5, bottom).

The results illustrated in Figures 4 and 5 are typical of their age groups. In a group of twenty newborns selected as showing a statistically reliable pattern appearance response, we found none who showed any evidence of the orientation response found in older infants (Braddick, Wattam-Bell, & Atkinson, 1986). In the same study, we followed an additional group of thir-

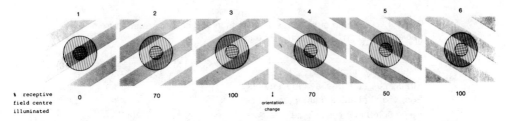

Figure 3. A sample from the stimulus used to elicit orientation-specific VEPs. Panels 1–6 show successive video frames superimposed on a hypothetical circularly symmetrical receptive field. With each new frame the grating undergoes a random displacement, and between frames 3 and 4 its orientation is reversed. The numbers below each panel show that, for the circular receptive field, the change in the percentage of the center area illuminated when the orientation is reversed cannot be distinguished from the changes due to the phase shifts with each new frame. A VEP synchronized with the reversals is therefore evidence for orientation selectivity.

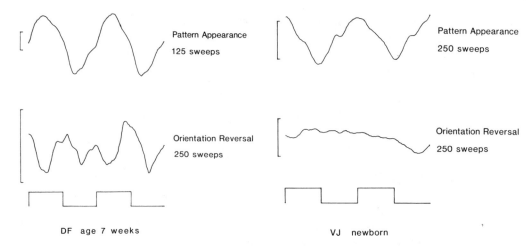

Figure 4. Visual evoked potential records from a 7-week-old infant. The middle record shows the response to the stimulus of Figure 3. For the top record, the grating underwent phase shifts as in panels 1–3 of Figure 3, but in frames 4–6 the field was blank (without a change of mean luminance). The bottom trace shows the stimulus alternation in the orientation shift condition.

Figure 5. Visual evoked potential records for a newborn. The top record shows a pattern appearance response, whereas the bottom trace shows a lack of orientation-reversal response.

thirteen infants longitudinally, testing VEPs at approximately 2-week intervals from 4–5 weeks of age. In this group, the first positive evidence of a VEP for the orientation-reversal stimulus was observed at a median age of 6 weeks.

Our method therefore gives no evidence of orientation specificity in the infant visual system before 6 weeks on average, and clear evidence thereafter. This is supportive evidence for the hypothesis that the onset of functional cortical responses does not take place at birth but some weeks later (Atkinson, 1984b). We have started using this test to look at the VER in visually unresponsive children as part of their visual assessments. The test may be particu-

larly appropriate for children with very limited responses, such as in children with severe cerebral palsy.

RESULTS

The results of these various tests have been summarized in Table 4. Many of the children failed more than one test, and only 19% showed no visual problems on any of the tests given.

Almost half the children showed abnormal eye movements or strabismus, and almost half had significant refractive errors. For some of these children, the strabismus may be associated with the refractive error. In at least some of these cases the disorder might be expected to be improved by treatment.

Only a small group of children have been

Table 4. Outcome of visual assessments in 108 children referred from pediatrics and child development center

Abnormal	Proportion abnormal
Visual acuity/amblyopia	45%
Strabismus/abnormal eye movements	46%
Poor visual attention/perceptual deficits	47%
Refraction under cycloplegia	44%
"Cortically blind"—no confirmed ocular pathology	11%
Confirmed ocular pathology	4%
(Visual fields:	9 deficits out of 12 children tested)
Children found to have one or more visual defects	81%

"field" tested. Of the 9 showing a field deficit, 7 were hemiplegics. In the future, more extensive field testing of children with cerebral palsy may reveal a higher incidence of such problems.

A high percentage of these children suffered from attentional and perceptual deficits (47%). These deficits were often nonspecific and could not be clearly defined from the tests that were used. New methods will need to be developed to split this large group into subgroups whose problems can be defined more specifically. The different classes of behavior in changing focus, found using noncycloplegic photorefraction, might provide a starting point for categorizing different types of deficit.

DISCUSSION AND CONCLUSIONS

In this paper, both our screening program and our methods of individual visual assessments for children suffering neurological impairments have briefly been described. It is apparent that there is a significant number of children in need of assessment and treatment both in the normal population and in the population of children with handicaps. While children with severe disability only represent a relatively small percentage of the population in the United Kingdom, we have found that most of these children have visual problems, some of which might be treated successfully if identified at an early stage. In our view, these children have not in the past received the attention they deserve, partly because adequate assessment of their visual function has not been available. Two new tests that we have devised in research and are now beginning to use for assessment are also described. It is the author's hope that by continuing to link research and clinical work in this way, we may eventually enable all children to receive good health care.

REFERENCES

Atkinson, J. (1984a). Assessment of vision in infants and young children. In S. Harel & N.J. Anastasiow (Eds.), *The at-risk infant: Psycho/socio/medical aspects* (pp. 341–352). Baltimore: Paul H. Brookes Publishing Co.

Atkinson, J. (1984b). Human visual development over the first six months of life: A review and a hypothesis. *Journal of Human Neurobiology, 3*, 61–74.

Atkinson, J. & Braddick, O.J. (1983). Vision Screening and Photorefraction—the relation of refractive errors to strabismus and amblyopia. *Behavioral Brain Research, 10*, 71–80.

Atkinson, J., Braddick, O.J., Ayling, L., Pimm-Smith, E., Howland, H.C., & Ingram, R.M. (1981). Isotropic photorefraction: A new method for refractive testing of infants. *Documenta Opthalmologica, 30*, 217–23.

Atkinson, J., Braddick, O.J., Durden, K., Watson, P.G., & Atkinson, S. (1984). Screening for refractive errors in 6–9 month old infants by photorefraction. *British Journal of Opthalmology, 68*, 105–12.

Atkinson, J. Braddick, O.J., & French, J. (1980). Infant astigmatism: Its disappearance with age. *Vision Research, 20*, 891–898.

Atkinson, J., Pimm-Smith, E., Evans, C., Harding, G., &

Braddick, O.J. (1986). Visual crowding in young children. *Documenta Opthalmologica, 45*, 201–213.

Braddick, O.J., Atkinson, J., & Campbell, F.W. (1978). Channels in vision: Basic aspects. In R. Held, H. Leibowitz, & H.L. Teuber (Eds.), *Handbook of sensory physiology, Vol. VIII: Perception*. Heidelberg: Springer-Verlag.

Braddick, O.J., Wattam-Bell. J., & Atkinson, J. (1986). Orientation-specific cortical responses develop in early infancy. *Nature, 320*, 617–619.

Goble, J.L. (1985). *Visual disorders in the handicapped child*. New York: Marcel Dekker.

Howland, H.C., Atkinson, J., Braddick, O., & French, J. (1978). Infant astigmatism measured by photorefraction. *Science, 202*, 331–333.

Hubel, D.H., & Wiesel, T.N. (1977). Functional architecture of macaque monkey visual cortex. *Proceedings of the Royal Society of London, Series B. 198*, 1–59.

Ingram, R.M., Traynar, M.J., Walker, C., & Wilson, J.M. (1979). Screening for refractive errors at age 1 year: A pilot study. *British Journal of Ophthalmology, 63*, 243–50.

Mohindra, I., Held, R., Gwiazda, J., & Brill, S. (1978). Astigmatism in infants. *Science, 202*, 329–331.

Chapter 28

Contributions of Auditory Nerve–Brain Stem Evoked Responses to the Diagnosis of Pediatric Neurological and Auditory Disorders

Haim Sohmer

E VOKED POTENTIALS ARE WIDELY USED TO-day in sensory and neurological diagnosis. As opposed to the spontaneous nature of the electroencephalogram (EEG), which also involves signal recording using skin electrodes, the evoked potential (EP) must be evoked through stimulation, usually by appropriate sensory stimuli. Since the skin electrodes are placed distant from the sites within the nervous system that generate the EP, the responses tend to be small in amplitude. The same electrodes also record the ongoing EEG, electrocardiogram (ECG), and electromyogram (EMG), the signals for which together constitute noise when one is interested only in the EP, leading to a poor signal (EP) to noise ratio. Several strategies are used to improve this signal to noise ratio. First, the researcher must choose sensory stimuli that synchronously activate a maximal number of the neural elements that contribute to the desired EP. The latency of these neural responses must also be constant in response to repetitive stimulation. Therefore, several types of stimuli may be used. For example, flash or alternating patterns of checkerboards are used to elicit the visual EP, short pulses of electrical stimuli to somatosensory nerve bundles situated close to the skin surface

(e.g., the median nerve at the wrist) are used to elicit the somatosensory EP, and click acoustic stimuli are used to elicit the auditory EP. The electrical activity recorded by the skin electrodes, usually on the scalp, head, or neck is then amplified differentially so that noise components that are in phase at both recording electrodes are cancelled. The electrical activity is then bandpass filtered so as to take advantage of possible differences in frequency spectrum between the signal and several of the noise components. For example, if the desired signal (EP) is a series of compound action potentials (as in the case of the short latency components of the auditory and somatosensory EP), most of the signal energy is around 1000 Hz, while most of the energy of the EEG (noise) is around 10 Hz. Therefore, a filter that passes frequencies greater then 100 Hz and below 3000 Hz will reduce the EEG components of the noise. Additional noise depression is achieved by means of signal averaging. By storing successive short increments of poststimulus recorded electrical activity in successive "cells" of a computor memory and adding to these identical increments of activity to repetitive stimuli, recorded electrical activity that is time locked to the stimuli (i.e., appears with identical latencies to repeated stimulation) is summed, while random electrical activity is cancelled (Chiappa, 1983; Sohmer & Zuckerman, 1979).

In applying these principles and strategies to the recording of the auditory nerve–brain stem evoked responses (ABR), repetitive click stimuli, 10–20 per second, at intensities of up to 75–80 dB above the threshold of the normal population (75–80 dB nHL), are applied by means of an earphone (see Figure 1). The short electrical pulses (50–100 μsec) that are transduced by the earphone into the clicks are often alternated in polarity so that possible electrical artifacts are cancelled in the averaged response. The electrical activity is recorded as the potential difference between a scalp vertex electrode and an earlobe (or mastoid) electrode. The activity is bandpass filtered between about 100 Hz and about 3000 Hz. The response averager is set to about 50 μsec per memory point or "cell" so that if the averager uses 256 such points, the response trace is made up of 12.8 msec of poststimulus time (duration of the "window"). The final response is usually the summated average of several hundred to a few thousand click stimuli.

The ABR trace (see Figure 2) is made up of a series of 6–7 vertex positive waves, the peak of the first wave at 1.3–1.5 msec after the stimulus, each wave coming about 1msec following the preceding wave. They are less than 1 μV in amplitude. Recordings of humans with

localized lesions (Starr & Hamilton, 1976) or during the course of neurosurgery (Hashimoto, Ishiyama, Yoshimoto, & Nemoto, 1981; Moller, Jannetta, Bennett, & Moller, 1981) and experiments with animals have clearly demonstrated that the first wave is the compound action potential of the auditory nerve, and it usually represents the firing of nerve fibers responding best to the higher frequency components of the click stimuli (Sohmer & Kinarti, 1984). The succeeding waves are generated by more rostral parts of the brain stem auditory pathway: waves II and III from the medulla and waves IV–VI from the pons-midbrain. Since waves I, III, and IV–V are the most replicable waves in normal subjects, they contribute most to diagnosis. The useful response parameters include the presence and absence of these waves, their latency (from stimulus time to wave peak), and their amplitude.

THE CONTRIBUTIONS OF ABR

The important contributions of ABR in auditory diagnosis stem from the fact that in normal subjects, responses can be recorded to very low intensity click stimuli and from the fact that the latency of each of the ABR components including the first wave increases by about 2.0 msec for a 60–70 dB decrease in click intensity. Furthermore, the electrophysiological (ABR) threshold is very close to the behavioral threshold (Sohmer, Feinmesser, Bauberger-Tell,

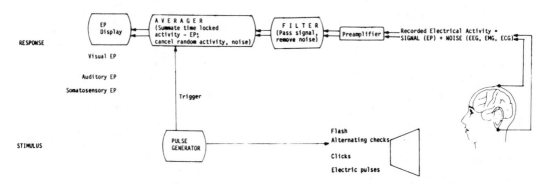

Figure 1. A diagram of the components of an evoked response system and their functions.

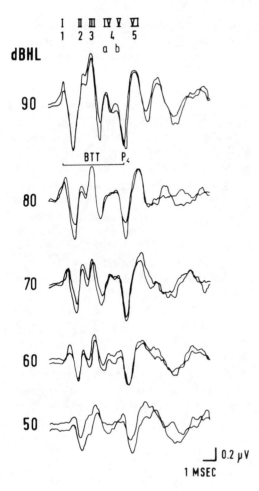

Figure 2. Auditory nerve–brain stem evoked responses (ABR) traces in a normal child in response to several click intensities. Note that as click intensity decreases, the latency of each wave increases and amplitude decreases. This continues until threshold (0–20dBHL), which is defined as the lowest click intensity which still elicits some ABR component (usually the IV/V complex). The interpeak latency BTT can be measured as the P₄-1 interval (shown) or as the V-I interval.

Lev, & David, 1972; Sohmer, Pratt, & Feinmesser, 1974), even in neonates. Therefore, the ABR can be used to determine hearing threshold in neonates and in other difficult-to-test patients.

An elevated ABR threshold is then an indication of the presence of a hearing loss; ABR can also be used to evaluate the cause of this hearing loss and to identify the site of lesion. For example, conductive hearing loss. a common type of loss in infants and children due to the presence of inflammatory or effusive fluid

in the middle ear cavity, leads to attenuation of incoming sound. Therefore, the conductive hearing loss is accompanied by prolonged ABR wave latencies, with the degree of prolongation more or less correlated with the degree of attenuation (Chisin, Gafni, & Sohmer, 1983; Mendelsohn, Salamy, Lenoir, & McKean, 1979). Such conductive losses can be alleviated by the introduction of a ventilating tube into the tympanic membrane. This leads to improved ABR thresholds and to a shortening in their latency (Chisin, Gapany-Gapanavicius, Gafni, & Sohmer, 1983). An additional type of hearing loss, due to a lesion of the receptor-hair cells of the inner ear, is called sensorineural hearing loss. When this type of loss is mild to moderate (up to 30–50 dB loss), it is usually not accompanied by prolonged latency of the auditory nerve response (wave I). However, in cases of more severe sensorineural hearing impairment with losses greater than 50 dB at higher frequencies (sloping, high frequency loss), the latency of the first wave is prolonged. The mechanism of the patterns of ABR responses seen in sensorineural hearing loss is relatively well understood (Sohmer & Kinarti, 1984; Sohmer, Kinarti, & Gafni, 1981). Thus, the different patterns of ABR abnormality are more or less specific for the different types of hearing loss seen.

Brain Stem Transmission Time (BTT)

When used in neurological diagnosis, more attention is paid to the brain stem components of the ABR. An ABR sign of neurological disorder can manifest as prolonged latency of the brain stem ABR components best described as prolongations of interpeak latencies. These are defined as the time interval between any two of the replicable waves (I, III, IV/V complex or P_4). One of the more commonly used interpeak latencies is called brain stem transmission time (BTT); this is defined as the time interval between wave I and either the IV/V complex or P_4 (see Figure 2). It is longer in neonates (I–V=5.3 msec; 1-P_4=5.9 msec) and approaches adult values at the age of 2–3 years (I–V=4.0 msec; 1-P_4=4.5 msec). This shortening of

BTT with age is probably due to the increase in myelinization in the brain stem during these ages. Therefore, normal values from groups of appropriate ages must be used in determining possible brain stem disorders in infants.

Even though it has been shown that BTT is often prolonged in several neurological disorders of infancy and childhood, the mechanism of this prolongation is generally not clear. For example, one could speculate that the prolonged BTT seen as sequelae of perinatal anoxic-ischemic insults may be due to a decrease in synaptic efficacy. This condition could also be due to uniformly delayed myelinization or, in demyelinating diseases, to uniform demyelination leading to slower axonal propogation. In addition, the local pressure due to a space-occupying lesion or a brain tumor could initially cause a slowing of axonal propogation seen as a prolonged BTT. With increased growth of the tumor, the pressure may cause the disappearance of components normally generated in or near that region and of components generated more rostrally in the pathway. The loss of brain stem ABR components may also accompany demyelinating diseases due to nonuniform demyelination of axons leading to a disruption in their ability to fire impulses synchronously (Matathias, Sohmer, & Biton, 1985). This may occur even though impulses are being propogated through the region of demyelination, as indicated by a normal pure tone audiogram.

This discussion of the various abnormal ABR patterns seen in neurological disorders has shown that even though the presence of abnormal brain stem components of the ABR can indicate the presence of a lesion in or near the auditory pathway, the particular pattern of ABR abnormality is generally not pathognomonic for any particular neurological disorder. Thus, the same type of disorder (e.g., brain stem tumor) can be accompanied by prolonged BTT or absent waves. Furthermore, the same type of ABR abnormality (e.g., prolonged BTT) can be seen in different disorders, such as brain stem tumors and demyelinating diseases.

Therefore, further research is required in order to determine the mechanism whereby particular insults or lesions give rise to abnormal ABR patterns.

REFERENCES

Chiappa, K.H. (1983). *Evoked potentials in clinical medicine*. New York: Raven Press.

Chisin, R., Gafni, M.. & Sohmer, H. (1983). Patterns of auditory nerve and brainstem evoked responses (ABR) in different types of peripheral hearing loss. *Archives of Oto-Rhino-Laryngology, 237*, 165–173.

Chisin, R., Gapany-Gapanavicius, B., Gafni, M., & Sohmer, H. (1983). Auditory nerve and brain stem evoked responses (ABR) before and after middle ear corrective surgery. *Archives of Oto-Rhino-Laryngology, 238*, 27–31.

Hashimoto, I., Ishiyama, Y., Yoshimoto, T., & Nemoto, S. (1981). Brain stem auditory evoked potentials recorded directly from human brain stem and thalamus. *Brain, 104*, 841–859.

Matathias, O., Sohmer, H., & Biton, V. (1985). Central auditory tests and auditory nerve brain stem evoked responses in multiple sclerosis. *Acta-Oto-Laryngologica, 99*, 369–376.

Mendelsohn, T., Salamy, A., Lenoir, M., & McKean, C. (1979). Brain stem evoked potential findings in children with otitis media. *Archives of Otolaryngology, 105*, 17–20.

Moller, A.R., Jannetta, P., Bennett, M., & Moller, M.B. (1981). Intracranially recorded responses from the human auditory nerve: New insights into the origin of brain stem evoked potentials (BSEPs). *Electroencephalography and Clinical Neurophysiology, 52*, 18–27.

Sohmer, H., Feinmesser, M., Bauberger-Tell, L., Lev, A., & David, S. (1972). Routine use of cochlear audiometry in infants with uncertain diagnosis. *Annals of Otology, Rhinology and Laryngology, 81*, 72–75.

Sohmer, H., & Kinarti, R. (1984). Survey of attempts to use auditory evoked potentials to obtain an audiogram. *British Journal of Audiology, 18*, 237–244.

Sohmer, H., Kinarti, R., & Gafni, M. (1981). The latency of auditory nerve-brain stem responses in sensorineural hearing loss. *Archives of Oto-Rhino-Laryngology, 230*, 189–199.

Sohmer, H., Pratt, H., & Feinmesser, M. (1974). Electrocochleography or evoked cortical responses: Which is preferable in diagnosis of hearing loss? *Revue de Laryngologie Otologie Rhinologie, 95*, 515–522.

Sohmer, H., & Zuckerman, B. (1979). Recording of auditory nerve and brain stem evoked responses with surface electrodes. In H.A. Beagley (Ed.), *Auditory investigation—The scientific and technological basis* (pp. 403–417). New York: Oxford University Press.

Starr, A., & Hamilton, A.E. (1976). Correlation between confirmed sites of neurologic lesions and abnormalities of far-field auditory brain stem responses. *Electroencephalography and Clinical Neurophysiology, 41*, 595–608.

Chapter 29

Syndrome Specific Remediation in Preschool Developmental Dysphasia

Doris A. Allen, Lois Mendelson, and Isabelle Rapin

DEVELOPMENTAL LANGUAGE DISABILITY (DLD), or dysphasia, is usually defined as a failure to acquire language normally despite normal hearing and nonverbal intelligence, lack of overt evidence of brain maldevelopment or acquired damage, and exposure to an adequate language environment. Children who fail to develop age-appropriate comprehension and/or production of language in early childhood are frequently diagnosed by professionals as being "language delayed." However, we consider these children to be dysphasic, not simply language delayed, because their receptive and/or expressive language differs substantially from that of normally developing children of any age. Furthermore, we have observed, in our clinical practices as well as in our ongoing research studies, patterns of deficit (dysphasic syndromes) that share some features with recognized acquired aphasias in older children and adults.

Despite the fact that there has been widespread recognition of a variety of acquired aphasic syndromes, developmental language disorder or developmental dysphasia has often been treated as though it were a single clinical entity. However, some investigators have suggested distinct language-deficit syndromes which, presumably, reflect dysfunctions of different neurological systems. The earliest attempts at subclassification of DLD closely followed the adult aphasiology model. Aram and Nation (1975, 1982), Ingram, (1972, 1975), and Myklebust (1954) identified six patterns of DLD through the use of standardized tests that assessed language expression, comprehension, and repetition at the levels of phonology, syntax, and semantics. Using a similar approach, Wolfus, Moskovitch, and Kinsbourne (1980) found two distinct patterns of expressive and mixed receptive-expressive deficits on measures of phonology, syntax, and semantics. Wilson and Risucci (1986) have identified seven cognitive-linguistic syndromes based on a clinical assessment of language deficits combined with performance scores on a wide battery of standardized neuropsychological tests.

The influence of developmental psycholinguistics can be seen in the work of Bloom and Lahey (1978) and Menyuk (1969); however, these authors do not postulate distinct DLD subtypes. In our own clinical studies of language disordered preschool children (Allen & Rapin, 1980; Rapin & Allen, 1982a, 1982b, 1986; Resnick, Allen, & Rapin, 1984), we have identified six DLD subtypes or dysphasic syndromes. These are based on a clinical assessment of comprehension, processing, and expression at the levels of phonology, syntax, semantics, and pragmatics.

This work was supported in part by The Peggy O'Malley Fund.

233

There are several reasons for attempting to subtype dysphasic children. One reason is the need to create homogeneous subgroups with tightly defined deficits in order to facilitate discovery of the pathogenesis of specific syndromes. By decreasing the variance among children, one maximizes the probability of making inferences about the brain dysfunction responsible for different syndromes. This is done by using such approaches as mapping electrical activity, blood flow, or glucose utilization during the performance of verbal tasks. A second reason for subtyping, and the one that concerns us here, is that it enables one to create specific intervention strategies based on the particular needs of children who fall into one or another of the clinical syndromes. In the present paper, we will describe the six syndromes that we have identified and discuss specific intervention strategies that we have developed based on our understanding of the core language deficits of each subtype. We have been applying these treatment strategies—often with dramatic results—in the Therapeutic Nursery at the Albert Einstein College of Medicine.

The Therapeutic Nursery

The Albert Einstein Therapeutic Nursery is designed to meet the needs of preschool children with moderate to severe language impairment and at least normal nonverbal cognition. While some mildly impaired children progress well with a combination of conventional individual speech-language therapy and a good nursery school program, more severely disordered children may require a more radical and far-reaching treatment approach. Such children, who often suffer from associated or concomitant behavioral and emotional difficulties, respond well to a nursery treatment modality that addresses not only their specific language deficits but also their broader social, cognitive, and behavioral difficulties. Their problems may include:

1. General lack of self-confidence
2. Lack of impulse control
3. Low frustration tolerance
4. Attention deficits

5. Social immaturity
6. Extreme avoidance of language-related tasks
7. Over-dependence on parents as receptive and expressive translators

Because of these difficulties, the children often resist formal language work. Thus, the initial task is to establish a therapeutic milieu within which the language problems can be addressed. Parents are engaged on a regular basis as active participants in the program in order to maximize the children's growth and development.

Autistic children (who, by definition, have communication disorders as well as social/emotional/behavioral deficits) are also accepted in our Therapeutic Nursery. This group of children exhibit specific abnormalities in socialization, relatedness, symbolic functioning, and extreme behavioral difficulties which distinguish them from the nonautistic dysphasic group. Before any specific language work can begin, it is necessary to address such autistic behaviors as social withdrawal or inappropriateness, lack of eye contact or mutual focus, perseveration, and inattention. Even for the verbal autistic children, language therapy must take into account their singular failure to acquire the social pragmatic rules of interpersonal communication such as turn-taking, choosing appropriate topics of conversation, and initiating and maintaining discourse. Some of the autistic children we have treated have eventually become verbal and literate (even those who were mute when they entered the program). Nonetheless, their language continues to be aberrant, and they continue to exhibit social and behavioral abnormalities that chronically interfere with their interpersonal communications.

The specific course of treatment for the behavioral and social difficulties of both autistic and nonautistic language impaired children is beyond the scope of the present paper. Instead, we will focus on the treatment of their language disorders. Virtually all language impaired children (whether or not they are autistic) share certain basic language deficits. Because the onset of expressive language is almost universally delayed in these children, it is not surprising that most of them continue to exhibit the following deficits throughout the preschool years: 1) impoverished vocabularies with intermittent word-retrieval difficulties; 2) difficulty with WH-question forms (*what, who, where, when, why,* and *how*), expressively as well as receptively; 3) difficulty with abstract language and with references to past and future events; and 4) difficulty in sustaining conversations, particularly with peers. While it is important to address these general issues of language impairment, we have found that we can design more powerful remediation strategies by identifying the specific dysphasic syndrome of each child, following our model as described below.

CLINICAL SUBTYPES
OF DEVELOPMENTAL DYSPHASIA

Our model for identifying subtypes of developmental language disorders is based on concepts from the fields of developmental psycholinguistics and aphasiology. We first identify the language level(s) in which deficits can be observed: phonologic, morphologic/syntactic, lexical/semantic, and pragmatic use as defined in the psycholinguistic literature. Secondly, we utilize the input/processing/output model from aphasiology, which broadly defines disorders as primarily expressive, receptive, or mixed expressive/receptive. Finally, we combine the models to look specifically at the language level(s) at which the expressive or receptive breakdowns appear to occur. For example, decoding deficits can occur at the phonologic, syntactic, semantic, or pragmatic levels, and the subsequent clinical picture differs accordingly. Thus, a child who cannot decode at the phonologic level is blocked from further receptive potential while a child whose decoding deficit occurs at the lexical/semantic level can have intact receptive and expressive phonology.

In the following sections, we briefly describe each of the six dysphasic syndromes identified through the combined psycholinguistic/aphasiology model:

1. Verbal dyspraxia
2. Phonological production deficit
3. Verbal auditory agnosia
4. Phonologic-syntactic deficit
5. Lexical-syntactic deficit
6. Semantic-pragmatic deficit

Following a description of the clinical picture, we present the key intervention strategies essential for treating the core language deficits in each syndrome.

Verbal Dyspraxia and Phonological Production Deficit Syndromes

Clinical Description We have identified two syndromes in which the impairment is almost totally in the expressive system, with comprehension relatively intact. One of these, which we call Verbal Dyspraxia, is a severe expressive disorder in which the child is extremely nonfluent. Utterances are usually limited to a few poorly-articulated single words and, in the most extreme cases, the child may be virtually mute. The second syndrome, which we call the Phonological Production Deficit syndrome, is a disorder in which the children are quite fluent but are nonetheless unintelligible. Their utterances are characterized by multiple sequencing errors, substitutions, and distortions, resulting in a stream of speech that merely approximates sentences. In both syndromes, the production of consonants (and particularly of consonant clusters) is more difficult than the production of vowels, and repetition of single consonant-vowel sequences poses less difficulty than more complex sequencing involving longer words and phrases.

There is widespread disagreement in the literature as to what actually comprises these expressive syndromes; even the terminology used is ambiguous at best. Such terms as "apraxia of speech," and "developmental misarticulation" may be used by professionals to refer to the same clinical phenomenon. Some clinicians characterize these syndromes as speech disorders, while others, including ourselves, view them as language disorders. We contend that both syndromes involve a failure to encode at the level of phonology. What is *not* clear to us, as yet, is whether Verbal Dyspraxia and the

Phonological Production Deficit Syndrome represent two extremes on a continuum of severity or two separate syndromes. There are arguments to be made for either position. In the discussion that follows, we treat the two simultaneously, since similar remediation strategies are appropriate for both groups.

Intervention Strategies Children in both expressive groups are usually aware of their lack of intelligibility and tend to resist direct speech and language work in individual sessions. The most severely verbally dyspraxic children often become so intensely anxious when asked to imitate with their mouths that, for them, formal language work, even in small groups, is virtually impossible. We first engage these children in games of sensory stimulation of the mouth, either face-to-face or using a mirror. We introduce pleasurable activities involving the mouth, such as blowing bubbles, sucking or blowing through a straw, and licking lollipops. We also imitate their sounds or mouth movements. We place the child's finger on our lips while we produce exaggerated language sounds. For some children, this procedure appears to facilitate imitation of our sounds, as if they read our lips with their fingers.

Gradually, the children's anxiety level decreases, and they are ready for language work in small groups. Activities include singing, production of nonverbal vocal sounds during play (such as animal and vehicle sounds), and simple chants in the context of such games as "Simon Says." Such nonvocal imitative games as rhythmic clapping, drum beating, and the like are also used, first alone and then accompanied by vocalizations. By working in groups, and by placing fluent and dysfluent children together, the children's self-consciousness and anxiety about verbal productions can be greatly reduced. Once this has been accomplished, the children are amenable to individual work in a more formal language therapy approach.

We begin formal language work with both expressive groups at the level of phonology rather than at the level of phrases or sentences. For the dyspraxic children, this is a necessary first step toward beginning to talk. For the fluent children, it is a way to "clean up" their inaccurate phonologic productions before proceeding to larger units. We begin where each child exhibits the greatest proficiency—usually with front and back vowels. We then add a single bilabial consonant to the front vowel (moo), reduplicate (moo-moo), and finally expand the sequence (moo-moo-moo, moo-moo-boo, moo-boo-moo). This sequencing is first done slowly and rhymically, increasing speed as the task becomes more familiar. Sequences are repeated frequently until the children can approximate the model with ease. Working with sounds and sound sequences ultimately helps the dysfluent children overcome their extreme difficulties in formulating language, while it helps the fluent children to formulate and then to control the rate of production. We begin at this simple level in order to give the children the confidence to attempt more complex language. With each success comes a greater willingness to try.

With appropriate group and individual therapy the fluent children usually acquire serviceable sentence production. The prognosis is not as good for the dysfluent children, although some do achieve greater fluency than one might expect given the severity of their deficits. All dyspraxic children—even those who progress dramatically—are difficult to treat, and many require speech and language therapy beyond the preschool years. Those who are unable to produce intelligible sound sequences of words and phrases, even after appropriate intervention, may need to be introduced to a visual-manual system (such as reading and writing) at an early age in order to make it possible for them to communicate with others. Many dyspraxic children come to us with rudimentary gestural systems that can be expanded to include, in the most severe cases, the use of formal sign language in conjunction with verbalization.

Verbal Auditory Agnosia

Clinical Description Verbal Auditory Agnosia (VAA), commonly called Word-Deafness, is a well-defined syndrome in both adults and children. The primary deficit lies in the inability to decode spoken language at the level of phonology. That is, despite normal peripheral hearing, the individual is unable to derive any meaning from the sounds he or she hears. The result is that all subsequent linguistic operations are blocked; these children comprehend virtually nothing and are essentially mute. Some children with VAA have histories of having acquired this disorder after reportedly normal early language development. The children described here appear to have been afflicted from birth or at least before the onset of expressive language. Children with *developmental* (as opposed to *acquired*) VAA often arrive for treatment in a most profound state of isolation because of their total incapacity to tap into any oral language system. Because they are so completely averbal, they often have not yet even grasped the fundamental concept that all things and persons have names. Some young VAA children invent a rich gesture language which they use to communicate with familiar persons. Others seem to turn away from interpersonal communication altogether. Fortunately, because the visual system is often intact in VAA children, language can be introduced through the visual as well as the auditory channel.

Intervention Strategies Since VAA children have no internalized language system in early childhood, and, since they have no access to the normal channels of language acquisition, remediation must begin at the most rudimentary level. Total Communication is the treatment of choice, utilizing such visual modalities as signs or gestures, communication boards, and written words accompanied by oral language. Whichever system, or combination of systems, is used, it is important to present visual language in conjunction with spoken language at all times.

We have developed a language program that uses written language as the primary modality. For some children, this program stimulates a dramatic onset of verbal language as well as greatly increased comprehension. This teaching strategy has certain advantages over those based on manual sign language. It provides the child with access to a more universal system of communication, and it can be used by children with manual clumsiness or by those who cannot grasp the concept of signing.

The first step in our program is to ascertain whether the child has any interest in the letters of the alphabet. Some of our mute preschool children actually have a precocious familiarity with letters and numbers. For those who do not, it is often possible to engender such an interest through playing with letters in matching and sorting games. In order to introduce the concept that all things have names, we present a familiar object to the child (e.g., apple, cup, car). We name the object and immediately draw a picture of that object and name the picture. Under the picture, we print the label, naming the letters as we print, and have the child repeat the letter names after us if he or she can. Next, the child is given a set of individual plastic letters and helped to match them to the printed letters, again repeating each letter name as it is placed. Finally, we repeat the name of the object, using the frame "that's a ____." We underscore the printed word and say "that says ____." The concept is to move through successive levels of abstraction from real object to picture to word. It is very exciting to witness a child who has never spoken a single word begin to associate sounds and meanings through configurations of letters and eventually to utter meaningful words for the first time.

Once the child understands that everything and every person has a name, there can be a tremendous spurt in language learning. We continue to build vocabulary (beginning only with immediately perceivable objects) and to help the child generalize his or her lexicon by attaching written labels to different kinds of chairs, cups, and other objects. Once the labeling function has been learned, we introduce the frame "I want ____" in order to help the child understand that he can use these labels to request. (Here again, we are utilizing the developmental stages of normal language acquisition.) Next, we introduce the easiest WH-question forms: "What's this?" and "Where's the ____?'' and add more abstract constructs such as feelings (angry, happy, sad), always in an appropriate context.

Through the program described above, our VAA children have often made impressive gains in expressive and receptive language, considering their level of functioning when they came to us. Nonetheless, this is a devastating disorder; in spite of their exposure to an intensive tailor-made program, and in spite of their parents' participation in the process, the ability of VAA children to acquire linguistic skills is often severely limited. Comprehension through the early school years frequently continues to be acquired almost solely through the visual channel. For example, it is not at all unusual for VAA children to learn to respond to questions in the form they have previously learned visually but, at the same time, be unable to respond to an oral paraphrase of that form. For example, they may learn "What's that?" and be unable to associate that question with the question "What do we call this?" There is no way of knowing exactly what the children perceive through the auditory channel or how they are able to accomodate what they hear with the written word. What *is* clear is that many VAA children are able to make these auditory-visual connections. Those who can do so have the potential of becoming speaking children.

Those VAA children who do acquire the ability to speak continue to have defective phonologic output. Vowels tend to be nasalized, and prosody is flat. Since their deficit is specific to decoding at the phonologic level, the children are unable to monitor their own speech, resulting in production which resembles that of hearing impaired children. It is our impression that many mute autistic children suffer from VAA as a part of their overall condition. These children fare worse than nonautistic VAA children. They tend to withhold language, perseverate on certain words or phrases, or use them with apparent lack of comprehension. For these children, the remediation process is even slower and more laborious. Many autistic VAA children remain essentially mute and uncomprehending of oral language throughout their lives.

Phonologic-Syntactic (Mixed Receptive-Expressive Deficit) Syndrome

Clinical Description The Phonologic-Syntactic Syndrome may be the most common of the developmental dysphasias in preschool children. Expressive language usually does not emerge until after the age of 3, is characteristically sparse, and exhibits multiple substitutions, omissions, distortions, and sequencing errors. Comprehension is also impaired, being limited to only the "here and now." As phrasal speech develops, the child frequently produces forms not heard in the speech of normally developing children. For example, a normal toddler would progress from "baby cry" to "baby is crying" to "the baby is crying." The child with phonologic-syntactic deficits might produce such utterances as "baby is cry." It is difficult for these children to learn to produce syntactically organized utterances. Function words such as articles, prepositions, and auxiliary verbs are regularly omitted, as are endings on both nouns and verbs, resulting in "telegraphic speech."

The children in this group who have *severe* impairment in either receptive or expressive language frequently cause diagnostic confusion. The children who have severe *receptive* deficits may resemble those with VAA. However, because receptive language in the Phonologic-Syntactic group appears to be disordered at the level of *words* rather than at the level of phonologic decoding, their ability to imitate single words and short phrases is superior to that of VAA children. Those with severe *expressive* deficits can be distinguished from the Dyspraxic children on the basis of their more severely impaired comprehension. Children in this group who do not also have autistic features are able to use appropriately whatever language they do acquire. Some produce jargon as a way of maintaining conversational turns or for imitating discourse which they can hear but can neither comprehend nor produce. Autistic children in this group may jargon without apparent communicative meaning or pragmatic intent.

Intervention Strategies Because children in the Phonologic-Syntactic deficit group have problems with both comprehension and production, clinicians must be certain, when planning remediation, that everything the children learn to say is imbued with meaning. That is, although the remediation of their phonologic output requires many of the same strategies described for the Verbal Dyspraxia group, one must be careful to provide, in addition, a consistent understandable context in which they are able to comprehend what we help them to produce.

We have developed paradigms for enhancing comprehension and production simultaneously. For example, in a group setting, we introduce a language framework for talking about a particular topic, such as who is present and who is absent on a given day. We present the children with the following sequence:

1. "Who is here today?" This concept can be presented in a simple and concrete manner by touching each child as we recite "Mary is here," "Johnny is here," and so forth.

2. "Who is *not* here today?" Since the children may have no grasp of this question form, we show a photograph of each absent child while saying, "David is *not* here."

3. Eventually, it is possible to go through the same routine without the visual prompt of the photograph, eliciting a spontaneous and appropriate (albeit memorized) phrase from the group. We repeat this sequence daily until we are certain that the children comprehend the question forms in this context.

4. We then introduce a follow-up question: "Where is David?" and the answer, "He is at home with his mommy." The children repeat this answer with adult support until the children are able to reproduce and comprehend both the question and the answer spontaneously.

5. Once the children can correctly identify who is not present and can volunteer the answer spontaneously, we begin to generalize this concept in other settings. For example, if a child's mother has gone to another room, and we are certain that the

child knows where she has gone, we ask "Mary, where is your mommy?" We provide her with the appropriate response, "Mommy is in the kitchen." Next, we expand the procedure to include questions about the whereabouts of someone who is not regularly in the nursery, such as, "Where is your sister?"

A different strategy is used to help the children express their own needs or wishes. When it is clear that they want something that they cannot talk about, we encourage mothers to provide them with sentence frames to imitate, such as "I want ____," "Don't do that," or "Mommy, come." This seemingly simple routine can produce dramatic results, not only in aiding the children's verbalizations, but also in reducing screaming and other acting-out behaviors. One child who could only scream when he wanted something was eventually able to produce the following sequence: "Mommy, come. Come with me. Come in the nursery. Open this door."

The strategies discussed above can only be used if a child is able (and willing) to imitate simple language models. Because the children's speech is often unintelligible, it is important to restrict models to very simple words and phrases. Aberrant pronunciation is not corrected until some communicative fluency is achieved. When the child is ready, however, the Speech-Language Pathologist works with the child's production of individual sounds as well as syllables. Because the vocabularies of these children are often quite impoverished, we must build a stock of needed words, using common objects as well as pictures of objects, persons, actions, and feelings. The use of gestures, communication boards, and, in some cases, written words to supplement oral language are also encouraged. The parents are encouraged to employ these strategies at home as well as in the Nursery.

Lexical-Syntactic Deficit Syndrome

Clinical Description   There are six characteristics of the Lexical-Syntactic syndrome:

1. Intelligibility is usually quite good.
2. The ability to label visually perceived ob-

jects is far superior to the ability to retrieve these words in a nonlabeling context.

3. Syntax is immature, but usually not aberrant.
4. Overlearned language is better than spontaneous language produced within the context of a discourse demand.
5. Comprehension of object names and simple sentences is intact.
6. Comprehension of abstract language may be quite poor.

The emergence of expressive language is typically late, and parents are likely to report that their children can comprehend much more than they can say. Labels for objects and people are acquired much more readily than action and function words, resulting in an impoverished expressive vocabulary. Even after a word has been learned, the child's ability to retrieve that word in an extended conversational context is inconsistent. This word-finding problem may result in expressive language that is dysfluent and characterized by multiple hesitation signals, false starts, and self-corrections. Other indicators of formulation deficits include: 1) frequent use of filler words such as *this, that,* and *thing* in place of nouns, and an impoverished stock of verbs in the lexicon; 2) semantic paraphasias such as *car* for all four-wheeled vehicles or *eating thing* for fork; and 3) confusion of sound-alike words, such as *stool* for *school* or *track* for *crack.* We assume that these difficulties represent word-retrieval rather than comprehension or recognition memory deficits, since the children are often able to point on demand to pictures or objects whose names they cannot spontaneously produce.

This syndrome is seen in both autistic and nonautistic children. The autistic group demonstrates additional specific language abnormalities:

1. They often echo words and whole sentences irrespective of meaning or social context.
2. They often produce long sentence-like utterances composed of nonword jargon in-terspersed with occasional identifiable words.
3. They suffer from impairment in prosody and communicative use of language.

Intervention Strategies Intervention for the Lexical-Syntactic syndrome capitalizes on the children's relatively good comprehension and ability to imitate adult speech. Children who jargon are encouraged to imitate real speech as a way to increase vocabulary and expand syntactic combinations. As they learn to produce recognizable words through repetition, the jargon tends to diminish. Syntactic relations are expanded through the use of syntactic frames into which words can be inserted. For example, in response to the question "What is John doing?" we move the child from "eating" to "he's eating" to "he's eating a cookie" to "he's eating a cookie in the kitchen." Children with this syndrome make much faster progress in learning syntactic relations than children with VAA or the Phonologic-Syntactic disorder.

We use several strategies to assist the children with their word-retrieval and formulation deficits, including phonologic and semantic cueing, feature analysis, and the use of questions to focus on the important information to be encoded. Complex WH-question forms pose considerable difficulty for these children, but Yes-No questions are relatively easy. Therefore, we use the Yes-No question forms to teach the WH- forms. For example, in teaching the concept of "where," we would ask a question such as "Where did you get your new shoes?" Initially, the child might offer a response which indicates that "where" is not being understood (such as "yesterday" or "because my old ones had holes"). We then simplify by asking: "Did you buy them in a toy store?", "Did you buy them in a shoe store?" Gradually we arrive at a formulation such as "Oh, I see. Your mommy bought them for you at the shoe store." Through repeated expansions and formulations, the children are provided with valuable strategies for searching their lexicons for appropriate responses.

Prognosis for dysphasic children with this

syndrome is variable. Many of them have difficulty in the school-age years learning letter names and grasping phoneme-grapheme correspondence. As in the other syndromes, prognosis for the autistic children is poorer than for their nonautistic peers. In the autistic group echolalia frequently persists even after the children have become quite fluent, and comprehension continues to be impaired. Nonetheless, the autistic as well as the dysphasic children with Lexical-Syntactic deficits regularly exhibit more expressive and receptive abilities than either the VAA or Phonologic-Syntactic cases.

Semantic-Pragmatic Deficit Syndrome

Clinical Description Children who suffer from semantic-pragmatic deficits present a puzzling picture for parents and professionals alike and are, therefore, more likely to be misdiagnosed than other dysphasic children. There are a number of reasons for this dilemma:

1. Some, though not all, children in this group begin to speak at the appropriate age or even precociously.
2. When expressive language does emerge, the children are usually fluent, often exhibiting hyperverbal or loquacious speech. Many of the children can remember nursery rhymes, songs, television commercials, and pieces of overheard conversation far beyond age-expectation.
3. Articulation and syntax in the early years are adequate.
4. Children in this group can often respond to simple commands and answer simple questions.

What, then, is disordered in the language of these children? On close examination, one is impressed with the real, but subtle deviance in their language production and comprehension. While their speech may be fluent, their communicative intent and semantic content tend to be limited, superficial, and often tangential. Their utterances are typically characterized by loosely chained associations rather than by the logical sequences of ideas. The words they speak are often approximately on target, but not quite, usually lacking in specificity despite being in the right semantic field. Jargon, neologisms, semantic paraphasias, and circumlocutions are common. Word retrieval difficulties are very much in evidence inasmuch as the names of objects and actions that can be labeled in isolation may not be recalled in conversational discourse.

Because children in this group have extremely well-developed auditory memories, they are able to repeat long and syntactically well-organized sequences as "delayed echoes" which may or may not be appropriate to the conversational topic. It is interesting that while their spontaneous nonechoed sentences are usually syntactically intact, they tend to be considerably reduced in length and syntactic complexity. Verbal production is frequently quite rapid, resulting in "cluttered" speech. In the Semantic-Pragmatic Deficit group, such basic rules as turn-taking, question asking and answering, giving and requesting information, and choice and maintenance of conversational topic may fail to be acquired even after extensive intervention. Comprehension of single words is frequently far superior to understanding those same words in conversation, and most WH-question forms are acquired late and with great difficulty, both expressively and receptively.

We have frequently seen the Semantic-Pragmatic Deficit Syndrome in high-functioning verbal autistic children as well as in nonautistic dysphasic children. Whether or not they are autistic, they may appear inappropriate and difficult to communicate with because of the special nature of their deficits. Their interpretations of other people's messages tend to be literal and concrete, missing the subtle semantic and/or pragmatic nuances. They may jargon or engage in long, rapid, rambling monologues with elusive content often based on remembered scripts.

Intervention Strategies The intervention strategies that we use to facilitate more socially appropriate and communicative use of language capitalize on the unusually strong auditory memories of these children. We listen carefully to their tangential scripts in order to determine what they are actually trying to communicate. Then we provide more socially appropriate scripts. For example, a child who repeats the same Band-Aid commercial each time he gets hurt might be taught to say "ouch, it hurts" instead. The children easily memorize and use these new phrases and are consequently rewarded by receiving social feedback from others. As we continue to shift them away from their long stereotypic speeches or rambling monologues, we provide them with a growing repertoire of more socially appropriate ways of interacting verbally.

Children in this group, like those in the Lexical-Syntactic Deficit group, require help with word retrieval, with acquiring greater semantic specificity, with strengthening their grasp of subordinate and superordinate categories, and with comprehension and production of more abstract language, including WH-question forms. Some remediation strategies for these deficits have been described above in the section on intervention for the Lexical-Syntactic Deficit syndrome. The more advanced children in the Semantic-Pragmatic group can also participate in higher level games such as "Twenty Questions" and in "same and different" feature analyses, as in "I am thinking about something that girls wear. It's *not* a skirt; it's a _____." These games can be made increasingly more complex in order to introduce more subtle semantic contrasts.

Since the children in this group have problems with interpersonal pragmatic uses of language, they are best treated within a social context. They must be taught to address others rather than speak to themselves, to look at others when they speak, to choose appropriate topics of conversation, and to maintain the topic in discourse. This remediation is most effectively implemented through well-structured games and activities involving peers.

SUMMARY AND DISCUSSION

In this chapter, six dysphasic syndromes have been identified in preschool children. We have indicated that subtyping the children allows us to design specific interventions to address the particular language needs of the children in each group. Finally, we have suggested that the developmental dysphasic syndromes result from brain dysfunction which selectively involves specific aspects of language. This last point deserves further elaboration.

Very little is known about the neurologic bases of the developmental dysphasias, but it is virtually certain that there is neither a single etiology nor a single pathogenesis of these syndromes. It is likely that some syndromes result from genetic or nongenetic aberrations in brain development, while early (prespeech) focal or multifocal acquired brain pathology may be responsible for others. The developmental syndromes we have identified share features with well-recognized *acquired* aphasias in older children and adults. For example, Verbal Auditory Agnosia is seen in patients with bilateral temporal lobe infarcts, the Phonologic-Syntactic syndrome has features seen in Broca's aphasia, and the Verbal Dyspraxia group resembles adults with aphemia. Similarly, the Semantic-Pragmatic Deficit syndrome has been observed in hydrocephalic children and shares some features with Wernicke's aphasia and with the syndrome of "isolation of the speech areas," and the Lexical-Syntactic Deficit syndrome presents similarly to transcortical aphasia in adults. Evidence for multiple syndromes rather than a single deficit disorder in developmental dysphasia derives from the fact that children who exhibit different clinical symptoms typically have distinct neuropsychological profiles (see Wilson & Risucci, 1986). These differences suggest the existence of dysfunction in distinct brain systems.

We have given considerable thought to the issue of how some of our preschool children (including some with autistic features) are able to make such impressive gains in the face of brain dysfunction. One hypothesis is that, in the course of providing sound therapeutic intervention at an early age, we may be able to enhance brain reorganization through the development of alternative pathways. For example, providing VAA children with a visual language system may, in the less severe cases, promote a bypass of areas of auditory dysfunction, enabling the children to acquire verbal language that would have been inaccessible through the auditory channel alone.

We must also consider why some children *fail* to improve significantly even after intensive remediation. These children may have a more extensive or bilateral brain involvement that prohibits reorganization. For example, children who are globally mentally deficient as well as language impaired have fewer resources available to them for recovering from developmental dysphasia than do children with normal nonverbal intelligence. Dysphasic children with *severe* comprehension deficits rarely progress as well as those with predominantly expressive disorders. Finally, those autistic children who exhibit *severe* social, attentional, and behavioral deficits have the most guarded prognosis.

In this chapter, we have suggested the kinds of remediation that are possible within the context of a parent-child therapeutic nursery. While such intensive treatment may not be necessary for mildly language impaired children, we believe it should be considered the treatment of choice for children with more severe deficits, particularly for those who exhibit associated social/behavioral problems. The physician, who is usually the first professional to see very young children with developmental disorders, is in the best position to make early referral for evaluations of hearing, speech/ language, and neuropsychological functioning— or for treatment in a therapeutic nursery. Such referrals are clearly essential for any child who fails to develop language on schedule.

REFERENCES

Allen, D., & Rapin, I. (1980). Language disorders in preschool children: Predictors of outcome. *Brain and Development, 2,*73–80.

Aram, D.M., & Nation, J.E. (1975). Patterns of language behavior in children with developmental language disorders. *Journal of Speech and Hearing Research, 18,*229–241.

Aram, D.M., & Nation, J.E. (1982). *Child language disorders.* St. Louis: C.V. Mosby.

Bloom, L., & Lahey, M. (1978). *Language development and language disorders.* New York: John Wiley & Sons.

Ingram, T.T.S. (1972). The classification of speech and language disorders in young children. In M. Rutter & J.A.M. Martin (Eds.), *The child with delayed speech,* (Clinics in Developmental Medicine), No. 43, pp. 13–32.

Ingram, T.T.S. (1975). Speech disorders in childhood. In E.H. Lenneberg & E. Lenneberg (Eds.), *Foundations of language development 2,* (pp. 195–261). New York: Academic Press.

Menyuk, P. (1969). *Sentences Children Use.* Cambridge, MA: M.I.T. Press.

Myklebust, H.R. (1954). *Auditory disorders in children: A manual for differential diagnosis.* New York: Grune & Stratton.

Rapin, I., & Allen, D.A. (1982a). Progress toward a nosology of developmental dysphasia. In Y. Fukuyama (Ed.), *Child Neurology* (pp. 25–35). Amsterdam: Excerpta Medica.

Rapin, I., & Allen, D.A. (1982b). Developmental language disorders: Nosologic considerations. In U. Kirk (Ed.), *Neuropsychology of language, reading, and spelling* (pp. 155–184). New York: Academic Press.

Rapin, I., & Allen, D.A. (1986). The physician's assessment and management of young children with developmental language disorders. *Padiatrische Fortbildungskurse fur die Praxis, 60,*1–12.

Resnick, T.J., Allen, D.A., & Rapin, I. (1984). Disorders of language development: Diagnosis and intervention. *Pediatrics in Review, 6,* 85–92.

Wilson, B.C., & Risucci, D.A. (1986). A model for clinical-quantitative classification. Generation I: Application to language-disordered preschool children. *Brain and Language, 27,*281–309.

Wolfus, B., Moskovitch, M., & Kinsbourne, M. (1980). Subgroups of developmental language impairment. *Brain and Language, 10,* 152–171.

Chapter 30

Pharmacological Intervention in Attention Deficit Disorder

Status of Current Research

Gerald S. Golden

THE USE OF PHARMACOLOGICAL AGENTS, especially psychostimulants, is common practice for the treatment of attention deficit disorder (ADD) in many countries. In some cities in the United States, up to 10% of all school-age boys have been treated with these drugs. It is not rare to have the school teacher recommend to the parents that they ask the physician to prescribe medication for the child.

The frequency with which a diagnosis of attention deficit disorder is made, and the degree of reliance on drugs for treatment, vary considerably on a country by country basis, however. These discrepencies will not be discussed, but are partially due to differing diagnostic criteria and conceptual frameworks. This is illustrated by the work of Sandberg, Rutter, and Taylor (1978) in the United Kingdom. Sandberg presents convincing evidence that many children diagnosed as having ADD in the U.S. would be labeled as having a conduct disorder in the U.K.

This review will be limited to an analysis of some of the recent work using methylphenidate and dextroamphetamine. An attempt will be made to answer the following questions:

1. Is there a specific effect of these drugs on children with ADD?
2. Which symptoms respond?
3. How can an optimum dose be determined?
4. What are the potential side effects of treatment with these drugs?

It is essential to note that the majority of these studies are short term, and say nothing about the therapeutic or adverse effects of the drugs administered on a long-term basis. What is perhaps the most critical problem, the long-term prognosis for children with attention deficit disorder, and whether or not this disorder can be modified with the use of drugs, will not be covered in this presentation.

PSYCHOSTIMULANT TREATMENT AND ADD

General pediatric textbooks state that stimulant drugs have an idiosyncratic action on children with ADD, producing a calming and focusing effect, while stimulating normal children and adults. It is further stated that depressant drugs also have an idiosyncratic effect, causing increased hyperactivity in children with ADD. The claim is sometimes also made that a therapeutic trial of psychostimulants can differentiate the child with organically based hyperactivity from the child in whom the symptoms are reactive to life stresses. The so-called organic group would respond positively, while the behavioral group would become even more disorganized and hyperactive.

These general concepts were challenged by Rapoport et al. (1978). Fourteen boys, ages 6–12 years, were treated with a single dose of dextroamphetamine, 0.5 mg per kg orally.

245

These children all had superior school performance, good motor skills, and good peer relationships, and they were without major behavior problems. In a placebo controlled double-blind crossover study, the drug significantly decreased reaction time and motor activity and increased cognitive performance. Five hours after the dose of medication was given, there was a behavioral rebound with excitability, euphoria, and talkativeness. It is of note that the children could identify the day the drug was administered with high accuracy, and stated that they "felt funny" or "did not feel like themselves."

The same group of investigators then carried out a similar experiment comparing normal boys, hyperactive boys, and normal college-age men (Rapoport et al., 1980). The boys all showed decreased motor activity. Both boys and men demonstrated increased vigilance and improvement on a learning test. The men reported that the drug made them euphoric while the boys felt tired or different. In general, except for the changes in perceived mood, the drug had similar actions in all of the groups.

In conclusion, the concept that psychostimulants have specific effects on children with ADD can be questioned. For this reason, it is obvious that all studies utilizing these drugs must have proper control groups. It is also clear that psychostimulants cannot be used in diagnostic testing for ADD.

Treatment Results

The next issue is that of determining which symptoms will respond to treatment with psychostimulants. These agents are not generally administered in a laboratory, but in a social environment. Almost all clinical observers would agree that the child on psychostimulant drugs is easier to manage in the classroom and is less of a burden on his or her teacher and peers.

Whalen, Henker, and Dotemoto (1980) examined the frequency of normal classroom interactions between teachers and students and those interactions that represented attempts to control behavior. The teachers were much more controlling towards hyperactive boys given placebo than towards either nonhyperactive boys or children being treated with methylphenidate.

Charles, Schain, Zelniker, and Guthrie (1979) studied 45 children ages 6 to 10 years with the use of parent and teacher rating scales and a vigilance task, the Children's Checking Test. Doses were started at a level of 0.2 mg per kg and increased by steps to a target dose of 0.8 mg per kg. Analysis of the behavior rating scales showed that all measures improved when the child was on medication and deteriorated when the drug was discontinued. This latter effect was most prominent on the teacher rating scales. Comparing the groups that were initially normal or abnormal on the Children's Checking Test, researchers found there was improvement in attention in the poor performance group but not in the normal group. It is of note that the parents' ratings were not as accurate as those of the teachers when comparing the results to the Children's Checking Test. Also of interest was the finding that although there was deterioration in the way a child's behavior was rated when the drugs were discontinued, there remained some residual improvement over the baseline level.

Many of the studies that look at target symptoms do so in the context of attempting to determine a dose-response relationship or optimum drug level. Sprague and Sleator (1977) used a short-term memory task and found that the peak enhancement of learning occurred at a dose of 0.3 mg per kg, and that there was a decrement in performance at higher doses. Social behavior, however, was best at a dose of 1.0 mg per kg. Brown and Sleator (1979) found quite similar results on the Matching Familiar Figures Test, a measure of impulsivity. The inverted U curve indicated that there may have been a dissociation of the dose response effect when looking at different measures, and that in clinical practice it is important to set treatment priorities.

Rapport, DuPaul, Stoner, Birmingham, and Masie (1985) obtained somewhat different results on the Matching Familiar Figures Test. Using a group of children who were all defined as "responders" on the basis of improvement in classroom status and in scores on the abbreviated Connors scale, they found fewer errors with a dose of 15 mgs. than when the children were given placebo (5 mgs. or 10 mgs.). There was a linear relationship, decreasing errors occurring with an increasing dose, using either the total dose or calculating the dose on a mg. per kg. basis. The researchers felt that their data differed from that of Brown and Sleator (1979) in that intermediate doses were used, the tests were administered so that no practice effect occurred with their subjects, and they restricted their subjects to those who were proven drug responders. Their overall conclusion was that one must look at the specific tasks and the characteristics of the child. This individualization is an important treatment principle.

The same workers assessed a group of subjects who responded to methylphenidate with improvement on a paired associate learning test (Rapport, Stoner, DuPaul, Birmingham, & Tucker, 1985). These children also showed significant positive effects on ratings by their teachers, as well as on time spent on-task, academic accuracy, and assignment completion. Improvement was best at higher doses. The investigators recommended that clinic-based testing should be used to determine the optimal medication effect for any given child.

PHARMACOKINETICS OF METHYLPHENIDATE

There has been little work on the pharmacokinetics of methylphenidate in hyperactive children. Shaywitz (Shaywitz et al., 1982) found that the drug had a peak blood level at approximately 2.5 hours and a half-life of about the same length. Doubling the dose also doubled the effectiveness of the drug. They demonstrated a linear relationship between blood level and improvement on the Connors Abbreviated Rating Scale. Future research could well be directed towards utilizing blood levels to determine an optimal range and to set an optimal dose for each child.

Although more striking therapeutic effects may be found at higher doses, Werry and Sprague (1974) have pointed out that side effects increase with dose level, and that at 1.0 mgs. per kg., 50% of children will have some side effects. Although these side effects are usually mild, they can be troublesome. The most common are weight loss, gastrointestinal distress, and adverse effects on behavior and personality.

Major life threatening effects of methylphenidate are extremely rare. There has been a good deal of controversy concerning the issue of growth suppression in children taking psychostimulant drugs, however. These data can be summarized as follows (Roche, Lipman, Overall, & Hung, 1979):

1. Untreated children with attention deficit disorder have weights and heights within the normal range.
2. There is temporary retardation of weight gain when these drugs are administered.
3. There is temporary slowing of growth in stature when these drugs are administered.
4. These effects are most prominent in the first few years of therapy.
5. The effects are dose related.
6. Growth suppression is most prominent in children who do not have drug holidays.
7. There does not appear to be any permanent effect on stature, but there are no long-term studies that have followed the growth of children who are maintained on therapy through pubescence.

The mechanism of this growth suppression is not clear, and does not appear to be entirely a function of appetite suppression. Schultz, Hayford, Wolraich, Hintz, and Thompson (1982) found normal growth hormone, somatomedin, and prolactin levels in children taking methylpenidate. There was an increased peak growth hormone response following administration of arginine, but this correlated only with acute administration of methylphenidate and was not present with chronic administration of the drug.

Kilgore et al. (1979) postulated that interference with cartilage metabolism was the major factor involved. Methylphenidate inhibits somatomedin-mediated sulphate uptake by cartilage. This effect is due to inhibition of xylosyltransferase and galactosyltransferase enzyme activities.

Cardiovascular responses to administration of methylphenidate have been reported by Ballard, Boileau, Sleater, Massey, and Sprague (1976). Both heart rate and blood pressure are increased, and this effect is dose related. It is important to note that there was no tolerance to this effect with periods of therapy up to 1 year in duration. No changes in the electrocardiogram, other than tachycardia, were present. The significance of these findings is not clear.

TREATMENT OF TICS AND TOURETTE SYNDROME

In recent years, there has been a great deal of interest in the role of psychostimulant drugs in the production of tics and Tourette syndrome. This area remains somewhat controversial. Denckla, Bemporad, and Mackay (1976) reported on 1,520 patients who had been given psychostimulant drugs for hyperactivity. Only 1.3% developed tics or had an increase in tics. Of the twenty patients adversely affected, fourteen developed a tic disorder for the first time. Six of the 45 patients with preexisting tics worsened.

Examining the issue from the opposite perspective, Erenberg, Cruse, and Rothner (1985) reported on 200 patients with Tourette syndrome. This group was of interest because many of these children also had attention deficit disorder and learning disabilities. Forty-eight of these patients had received stimulant drugs. Nine of the children had taken psychostimulants before tics first appeared, although only four were on medication at the time the tics actually developed. Thirty-nine additional patients had developed tics before stimulant drugs were introduced. When these drugs were given, tics

worsened in 11 patients, did not change in 26, and decreased in 2. Although the relationships are not completely clear, the parents of any child who is placed on psychostimulant drugs should be warned about the possible occurrence of tics. Furthermore, if tics begin, the situation should be reevaluated and the drug discontinued if at all possible.

CONCLUSION

In conclusion, the literature available at this time supports the following statements:

1. The effects of psychostimulant drugs on behavior and cognitive function do not appear to be completely specific to patients with ADD; similar effects are found with normal subjects.
2. Treatment reduces impulsivity and motor activity.
3. Treatment improves attention and vigilance.
4. The optimal dose is not clear and must be ascertained individually for each child.
5. Serious side effects are rare, but there have been no long-term follow-up studies of side effects, particularly in children who are treated through adolescence.

Psychostimulant drugs can clearly improve the classroom behavior of a child with attention deficit disorder. These drugs are powerful pharmacologic agents, however, and should be used only if the diagnosis is clear, the need for the drug can be justified, and the child has not responded adequately to nonpharmacologic treatment measures. Simple techniques of classroom management and behavior modification are often highly effective, and worthy of a trial.

REFERENCES

Ballard, J.E., Boileau, R.A., Sleater, E.K., Massey, B.H., & Sprague, R.L. (1976). Cardiovascular responses of hyperactive children to methylphenidate. *Journal of the American Medical Association, 236*, 2870–2874.

Brown, R.T., & Sleater, E.K. (1979). Methylphenidate in hyperkinetic children: Differences in dose effects on impulsive behavior. *Pediatrics, 64*, 408–411.

Charles, L., Schain, R.J., Zelniker, T., & Guthrie, D.

(1979). Effects of methylphenidate on hyperactive children's ability to sustain attention. *Pediatrics, 64*, 412–418.

Denckla, M.B., Bemporad, J.R., & Mackay, M.C. (1976). Tics following methylphenidate administration: A report of 20 cases. *Journal of the American Medical Association, 235*, 1349–1351.

Erenberg, G., Cruse, R.P., & Rothner, A.D. (1985). Gilles

de la Tourette's syndrome: Effects of stimulant drugs. *Neurology, 35*,1346–1348.

Kilgore, B.S., Dickinson, L.C., Burnett, C.R., Lea, J., Schedewie, H.K., & Elders, M.J. (1979). Alterations in cartilage metabolism by neurostimulant drugs. *Pediatrics, 94*,542–545.

Rapoport, J.L., Buschsbaum, M.S., Zahn, T.P., Weingartner, H., Ludlow, C., & Mikkelsen, E.J. (1978). Dextroamphetamine: Cognitive and behavioral effects in normal prepubertal boys. *Science, 199*,560–563.

Rapoport, J.L., Buschsbaum, M.S., Weingartner, H., Zahn, T.P., Ludlow, C., & Mikkelsen, E.J. (1980). Dextroamphetamine: Its cognitive and behavioral effects in normal and hyperactive boys and normal men. *Archives of General Psychiatry, 37*,933–943.

Rapport, M.D., DuPaul, G.J., Stoner, G., Birmingham, B.K., & Masie, G. (1985). Attention deficit disorder with hyperactivity: Differential effects of methylphenidate on impulsivity. *Pediatrics, 76*,938–943.

Rapport, M.D., Stoner, G., DuPaul, G.J., Birmingham, B.K., & Tucker, S. (1985). Methylphenidate in hyperactive children: Differential effects of dose on academic learning and social behavior. *Journal of Abnormal Child Psychology, 13*,227–243.

Roche, A.F., Lipman, R.S., Overall, J.E., & Hung, W.

(1979). The effects of stimulant medication on the growth of hyperkinetic children. *Pediatrics, 63*,847–850.

Sandberg, S.T., Rutter, M., & Taylor, E.L. (1978). Hyperkinetic disorder in psychiatric clinic attenders. *Developmental Medicine and Child Neurology, 20*,279–299.

Schultz, F.R., Hayford, J.T., Wolraich, M.L., Hintz, R.L., & Thompson, R.G. (1982). Methylphenidate treatment of hyperactive children: Effects on the hypothalamicpituitary-somatomedin axis. *Pediatrics, 70,* 987–992.

Shaywitz, S.E., Hunt, R.D., Jatlow, P., Cohen, D.J., Young, J.G., Pierce, R.N., Andersen, G.M., & Shaywitz, B.A. (1982). Psychopharmacology of attention deficit disorder: Pharmacokinetic neuroendocrine and behavioral measures following acute and chronic treatment with methylphenidate. *Pediatrics, 69*,688–694.

Sprague, R.L., & Sleator, E.K. (1977). Methylphenidate in hyperkinetic children. Differences in dose effects on learning and social behavior. *Science, 198*,1274–1276.

Werry, J.S., & Sprague, R.L. (1974). Methylphenidate in children: Effect of dosage. *Australia and New Zealand Journal of Psychiatry, 8*,9–19.

Whalen, C.K., Henker, B., & Dotemoto, S. (1980). Methylphenidate and hyperactivity: Effects on teacher behaviors. *Science, 208*,1280–1282.

Chapter 31

Attention Deficit Disorders, Hyperkinesis, and Learning Disabilities

Controversial Therapies

Marvin I. Gottlieb

CHILDREN DISABLED BY LEARNING IMPAIR-ments, attention deficit disorders, and/or hyperkinesis frequently become significantly and chronically handicapped in their educational, psychological, or social development. Developmental and behavioral problems of this type jeopardize a relatively large population of preschool and school-age children (estimates range as high as 15%–20%) and thereby constitute major pediatric health care issues. These disorders are the source of frequent referral complaints encountered by child neurologists and developmental pediatricians. Regardless of the particular area of specialty, these disorders are unquestionably challenging management problems. Prior to obtaining medical consultation services, parents often experiment with (or intend to explore) nontraditional therapies, that is, controversial interventions that have been popularized by the communications media and are touted by parent advocacy groups. Child neurologists and developmental pediatricians share a mutual concern and professional responsibility in clarifying and putting these various controversial therapies into a more scientific perspective for parents.

APPRECIATING PARENT VULNERABILITY

Parents of children with learning disabilities, attention deficit disorders, or hyperkinesis, as a group, have generally been described as being "overly anxious, apprehensive, and frustrated." There is indeed a basis for this generalization and a justification as well. These childhood problems characteristically disrupt family dynamics, often by creating an atmosphere of unremitting tension within the household. (The child in distress is a family in distress.) In attempting to secure the "traditional" services most often recommended for educational and behavioral disorders, the parents may encounter a myriad of procedural and bureaucratic frustrations. As Brown (1987) comments:

> Families are sometimes given the covert message from trusted sources that standard interventions are not likely to be beneficial and that they are invariably expensive, demanding and drawn out. Standard interventions include physical and occupational therapy, language training, orthopedic procedures and other chronic treatment efforts. (p. 432)

Traditional management strategies often necessitate coordinated combinations of various

251

therapies, including: special education, medications, and parent and child counseling. Parental disappointments and frustrations with these treatment modalities can be readily appreciated, inasmuch as medical, educational, and psychological interventions generally do not provide a "quick" resolution for problems such as learning disabilities, attention deficit disorders, or hyperkinesis. Furthermore, the traditional therapies cannot guarantee an ultimate "cure." More often than not, acceptable management approaches require monitoring and reevaluations, as well as periodic modifications of the originally designed treatment plan. The parent(s) may initially participate with enthusiasm in the recommended program, although they may frequently feel confused about the ultimate goals of the intervention and the nature of their particular involvement. However, anxieties are most often provoked by parental misconceptions about specific treatment approaches. Treatment approaches that engender parental anxiety include: *special education,* frequently perceived as a process that labels and stigmatizes, and that separates the child from the mainstream of acceptable educational and social environments; *medications,* which precipitate fears of drug dependency, and of producing a "zombie" and changing the child's personality; and *parent/child counseling,* interpreted as an admission of mental health problems, a "step toward divorce," and of parental weakness in coping with family problems.

The physician is often the first professional to be consulted regarding these issues, but he or she may be ineffective in resolving parental fears and anxieties. It is therefore understandable that many parents may enthusiastically embrace a controversial therapy, particularly one suggesting that there is "a quick cure that can do no harm." Nonstandard management approaches are especially appealing to vulnerable parents whose anxieties and apprehensions ultimately become a reality, such as: "the children at school call him dumb and MR"; "medications make him sleepy"; "since taking the pills, he's not the same child," or "we can't see any progress in his reading or writing"

(perhaps even after only a few weeks or months in a resource program). Parent vulnerability is the precursor for their experimentation with nonstandard therapies, often reflecting mutually weak support between the parents, poor professional-parent communication, and perceived evidence of professional management failures. Parents may "blindly" accept the nonstandard (controversial) therapy as a panacea for resolving their child's troublesome educational, psychosocial, and medical problems ("a quick cure"). The philosophy of "Let's give it a try because it can't hurt" may magnetically capture their enthusiasm and zeal for participation. The desire to try a novel approach is usually difficult to "lecture away." Efforts by the parents to relieve their child of the social pressures of "being different" may in effect represent their fears concerning the artificial educational and psychosocial environments which are sometimes constructed to assist the child with learning and behavioral problems.

APPRECIATING PHYSICIAN VULNERABILITY

The primary care physician, the consulting child neurologist, and/or the developmental pediatrician may be questioned by parents or referring professionals regarding the efficacy of a nonstandard therapy. On occasion, they are asked to provide medical reassurances that the questionable therapy is *really* "harmless." The physician may be requested (or expected) to initiate and monitor the controversial therapy, an approach that has either been selected by the parent or recommended by another professional. In essence, the parents are requesting that the medical consultant assume complete responsibility for management and outcome. The physician is consequently placed in the compromised position of being pressured to either participate in a program characterized by a weak scientific foundation and often recognized shortcomings, or risk disrupting a previously established patient-physician relationship.

The professional dilemma in either accepting or rejecting management responsibility has increased dramatically, as physicians have assumed more active roles in serving children with various developmental-behavioral disorders. In addition, there has been an unprecedented popularization of undocumented "medical breakthroughs" on television, in magazines, and in newspapers. These suggested advances have included questionable approaches that have been indirectly but convincingly touted as *the* therapy for learning problems, hyperactivity, and attention disorders. Occasionally, the physician who may be besieged with parent requests to help find a quick cure for these complex disorders succumbs to the empirical trial of a controversial therapy.

Effective advocacy, however, mandates that the physician have an understanding of both acceptable and controversial therapies, and that he or she assumes a defensive but knowledgeable attitude toward participation in therapies that are nonstandard (untested or documented as having no value). The primary care physician and medical consultants must be capable of assessing: 1) the designation of "standard" versus "nonstandard" therapy, 2) the scientific acceptability of *any* proposed management strategy, 3) factors that motivate parents to experiment with controversial therapies, 4) the effects (good or bad) of participation in nonstandard therapy programs, as well as traditional programs, and 5) the supports parents receive during the course of their child's therapy.

Parents and physicians are vulnerable partners in their efforts to assist children with learning disabilities, attention deficit disorders, and hyperactivity. The physician is expected to be the mediator when parents express interest in exploring controversial management approaches. The ability to counsel effectively mandates a sound knowledge base of the hypothetical constructs and scientific documentations of both standard and nonstandard therapies. An understanding and compassionate counseling atmosphere, when explaining facts to parents, is undoubtedly more effective than a pressured, demanding, rigid lecture on "why not to" elect a particular therapy.

GENERAL CHARACTERISTICS OF CONTROVERSIAL THERAPIES

The nonstandard (controversial) therapies characteristically share common shortcomings (Golden, 1984). These shortcomings include:

1. Their theoretical bases are not completely consistent with established scientific principles.
2. Treatment is liberally recommended for a broad range of developmental and behavioral disabilities.
3. Therapy is promoted as "not harmful."
4. Claims of efficacy are initially popularized in the communication media rather than in refereed journals.
5. Controlled studies do not replicate claims.
6. Lay groups enthusiastically and publicly promote the therapy (Table 1).

It should also be noted that controversial therapies generally promote a management approach in isolation. Standard therapies more often rely on adjunct supports and multidisciplinary interventions.

The novel nature of many of the controversial therapies often provides interesting copy for newspapers, magazines, and television. So-called data are commonly presented as various testimonials that claim dramatic improvements or cures. These generalizations are understandably more popular and convincing for the public than scientific reports published in inaccessible academic journals (the public is rarely familiarized with findings from the latter). Advocates of nonstandard therapies may publicly challenge their critics with provocative clichés, such as:

"If you don't agree . . . prove me wrong."
"Traditional medicine will not accept new and novel approaches."
"It can't hurt so why not try it."

Despite cautionary policy statements issued by various professional academies and societies, a plethora of controversial management approaches continue to flourish for children with educational and behavioral disorders.

Table 1. General characteristics of controversial versus acceptable therapies

Characteristic	Controversial therapies	Acceptable therapies
Theoretical construct	A "novel" approach with a weak underlying hypothesis	Constructed from an established neurological, biochemical, or educational basis
Therapy focus	Claims for "curing" a broad and diverse group of disabilities	Designed to treat a specific disorder
Side-effects (complications)	Reported to be a noninvasive, nonharmful, often a "natural" intervention	Recognized short-comings; patient alerted to the side-effects
Claims of efficacy	Usually popularized in the media. Rely on testimonials and case histories	Reported in peer-review journals; experimental design in keeping with the scientific method
Therapy design	Usually used as a single therapy approach. Failures blamed on inadequate compliance	Generally a combination of therapies (e.g., special education and counseling and/or medication)
Replication of data	Various studies fail to replicate claims	Results are similar in various studies
Lay group response	Promoted by lay groups as the panacea or quick cure. Frequently associated with lobbying activities	No strong lay advocacy group "pushing" the treatment modality
Professional response	Hesitant to recommend therapy. May lose patient by refusal to participate. May accept controversial approach if standard therapies do not produce positive results. May agree for limited time to participation in controversial therapy with periodic assessment of progress	Comfortable in recommending and monitoring therapy. Aware of shortcomings and the "no guarantee" clause

REVIEW OF SPECIFIC CONTROVERSIAL THERAPIES

Several professional journal articles have previously reviewed specific controversial therapies, particularly those recommended for learning disabilities, hyperactivity, and attention deficit disorders (Brown, 1987; Golden, 1984; Gottlieb, 1979; Silver, 1986). This chapter focuses primarily on two major categories of nonstandard therapies: 1) special dietary modifications, and 2) neurophysiological retraining.

Special Dietary Modifications

Food Additives Feingold (1975) hypothesized that certain food additives, and artificial food flavors and colors, could produce learning disabilities and hyperactivity in susceptible children (Feingold, 1975a; Feingold, 1975b). He postulated that the increased incidence of children with these particular developmental-behavioral disorders parallels the increased utilization of synthetic colors and flavors in the food supply. The "reaction" is attributed to a genetically-based nonimmunological sensitivity to various artificial food contaminants. Feingold further suggested that elimination of food additives would result in a dramatic improvement in both learning and behavior, and that the reintroduction of synthetic flavors, colors, and naturally occuring salicylates in the child's diet would result in a return of symptoms. The Feingold therapy has been energetically embraced and endorsed by the participating public, by some professionals, and in media presentations, possibly coinciding with a nationally changing lifestyle . . . a concern for "physiophilia" (Levine & Liden, 1976).

Numerous clinical studies have been conducted to test the claims of the Feingold hypothesis. In a double-blind, crossover design, (utilizing a baseline diet, a control diet, and the additive-free diet) results indicated that teachers were able to recognize changes in behavior when comparisons were made between control and test diets. However, parents were unable to detect differences between the two groups. Although the sample size was relatively small, the investigators concluded that the Feingold diet may reduce childhood hyperactivity, but they expressed caution in the interpretation of data because of the variables involved in their study (Connors, Coyette, Southwick, et al., 1976). Subsequent studies were less supportive of the Feingold hypothesis, concluding that additive-free diets were *not* effective in the management of hyperkinesis (Harley, Mathews, & Eichman, 1978; Harley, Ray, Tomasi, et al., 1978; Wender, 1977; Williams, Cram, Tavsig, et al., 1978). In 1982, the National Advisory Committee on Hyperkinesis and Food Additives convened a Consensus Development Conference at the National Institutes of Health to review existing data on this controversial issue (National Institutes of Health Consensus Development Conference, 1982).

Variables such as psychological factors may have contributed to the few reports associating improvement in behavior with utilization of the additive-free diet. However, nutritional, psychological and financial considerations (as well as time lost from participation in traditional therapies) are important factors for not recommending the Feingold therapy. Nevertheless, the controversy is unresolved for some professionals and for a larger number of parents. Physicians, however, must be prepared to respond meaningfully to those who promote the special diet, and to refer to the limitations of the hypothesis, based on better controlled clinical studies (Brenner, 1977; Spring & Sandoval, 1976; Wender, 1986).

Megavitamins   An orthomolecular management approach was originally proposed by Hoffer, Osmond, and Smythies (1954), who developed a treatment program for schizophrenia utilizing niacin, ascorbic acid, and pyridoxine hydrochloride. The concept of orthomolecular psychiatry was further supported and popularized by Pauling in a theoretical paper in 1968. Cott (1971) promoted the use of megavitamins, initially, for children with schizophrenia, and in subsequent reports, for children with learning disabilities. Cott's extension of the therapy involved escalating doses of various vitamins and medications in conjunction with a hypoglycemic diet. Study results were based primarily on patient testimonials, and on the reporting of successful outcomes in a variety of etiologically divergent disorders (schizophrenia, autism, brain injury, and learning disabilities). However, the research design lacked double-blind-crossover or placebo controls, that is, protocols usually employed in drug studies. The American Academy of Pediatrics Committee on Nutrition reviewed megavitamin therapy and concluded that this management strategy was *not* justified based on clinical studies (American Academy of Pediatrics, 1976). In a subsequent controlled study of 41 children with attention deficit disorder, it was concluded that megavitamin therapy was an ineffective intervention for that disorder (Haslam, Dalby, & Rademaker, 1984).

Megavitamin therapy should be discouraged because of its highly questionable effectiveness and its potential for adverse side effects, which can range from gastrointestinal complaints to hepatic toxicity (Haslam et al., 1984; Herbert, 1977; Herbert, 1978).

Mineral Therapy   Although generally supplied in adequate amounts in a balanced diet, deficiencies of calcium, copper, chromium, iron, magnesium, manganese, potassium, sodium, and zinc have all been postulated as causes of impaired learning and other neurodevelopmental disorders (Cott, 1971). Quantitative estimation of these trace elements is often determined by hair analysis (Phil & Parkes, 1977). Phil and Parkes concluded that learning-disabled children could be distinguished, with 98% accuracy, by a quantitative assessment of five minerals. Specifically, learning-disabled children exhibit increased amounts of cadmium, manganese, and chromium and decreased quantities of cobalt and lithium. For the most part, supportive data for the hypothesis is again based on patient testimonials rather than on data from scientifically designed research protocols. Golden (1984) noted that "the evidence supporting an abnormality in the body economy of minerals in children with learning disabilities is weak, and support for supplementary minerals in treatment is nonexistent" (p. 466). As with other interventions, the physician must be aware of the potential adverse side effects of prolonged administration of mineral supplements in excess of body needs.

Hypoglycemic Diets Hypoglycemia, regardless of etiology, has been hypothesized as adversely influencing neurological function, with resultant disorders of learning and behavior. Cott (1971) reported on an abnormally high incidence of hypoglycemia and dysinsulinism among learning-disabled children. Similarly, the ingestion of sugar per se has been postulated as an immediate cause of hyperactivity. However, data from controlled studies fail to support either hypothesis. In a study of 192 children referred for "reactive hypoglycemia," 129 experienced clinical episodes characterized by lightheadedness, sweating, "jitters," and/or weakness. Low blood sugar, and/or rapid rate of fall of blood sugar could not be documented in these patients (Johnson, Dorr, & Sivenson, 1980). The investigators concluded that many of the patients had emotional problems.

The therapy of dietary modifications to compensate for rebound hypoglycemia, as advocated by some centers, has been subject to criticism both in its hypothetical construct and as a documented effective therapy. Hypoglycemia can be caused by diverse etiologies and may require specific management with dietary, endocrine, and/or surgical interventions. A focus that concentrates solely on the possible effects of hypoglycemia on learning and behavior symptoms (ignoring causes), may deprive the patient of specific diagnostic and management services. It must be emphasized that the effects of prolonged utilization of special diets on growth and development have not been clearly defined. Indeed, it is possible that the special diet may potentially cause more problems than the difficulties for which it was prescribed.

Food Allergies Food allergy has been described as an important factor in learning disorders and behavioral problems; this theory implys that food elimination diets would improve these conditions (Crook, 1975). Various studies indicate that both the basic premise and the reported beneficial therapeutic effect of food-elimination diets are questionable. Psychological factors and observer bias appear to be significant variables in reports suggesting a "cause and effect" relationship between food allergy and learning/behavioral disorders (May, 1975). McLoughlin, Nall, Isaacs, et al. (1983) concluded that the impact of allergies and their therapies

> irrespective of ability and performance levels: affect general factors in learning (e.g., attention, alertness, energy, etc.) except in the case of an obvious one-to-one relationship, such as hearing disturbance due to eustachian tube dysfunction; and possibly exacerbate existing problems of the learning disabled or behavior-disordered children. (p. 510)

Neurophysiologic Retraining

Patterning The patterning theory suggests that neurological organization cannot be achieved until the stages of phylogenetic development have been completed (Doman, Spitz, Zucman, et al., 1966). The hypothesis proposes that children must achieve full development at each level without deviation from the normal sequence, and that variation from the sequential pattern, or incomplete development, interferes with cortical hemispheric dominance. The resultant deficit in neurological organization is believed to be ultimately reflected as deficits in neurodevelopmental areas, including: mental retardation, learning disabilities, and behavioral problems. A patterning therapy program has been designed (passive movements, sensory stimulation, rebreathing expired air, and various dietary restrictions) to correct the CNS disorganization. There is, however, no scientific foundation for either the basic concepts of the theory or the recommended therapy approach, that is, organization and reorganization of the central nervous system (Cohen, Birch, & Taft, 1970). Sparrow and Zigler (1978) noted that patterning has been employed for a heterogeneous group of disorders, including learning disabilities, hyperactivity, cerebral palsy, mental retardation, and a variety of neurodevelopmental disorders. In their evaluation of seriously retarded children, the patterning treatment proved to have no remedial value.

The American Academy of Pediatrics Committee on the Handicapped Child (1968) questioned the principles encompassed in the patterning theory. The Committee noted that:

1. Promotional methods challenge the adequacy of parents who refute the treatment.
2. The rigid program protocols neglect the needs of other family members.
3. There are anxiety-provoking pressures placed on parents to follow the program without deviation, thus rendering it useless.
4. The developmental profile employed by the Institute for the Achievement of Human Potential has not been validated or available for study.
5. Claims of "cures" have not been scientifically documented.
6. Patterning therapy is in conflict with acceptable child-rearing practices, thereby increasing parental anxiety and family tensions.

In addition, the therapy protocol requires numerous volunteer therapists to assist with the patterning exercises, thus involving rigid time schedules and strict adherence to program format. Therapeutic failures are attributed to the participant's inability to provide complete compliance with the program design. Patterning therapy has been criticized as an intervention that is time consuming and that offers false hopes. The policy statement of the American Academy of Pediatrics has critically reviewed and questioned this controversial therapy (American Academy of Pediatrics, 1982).

Optometric Training Abnormalities in visual perception, sensory-motor coordination skills, and eye movements have been suggested as specific causes of learning disabilities. It has also been suggested that these skills can be improved by neurological and visual training exercises. Theories implicating visual-neurological origins for specific learning disabilities and the use of optometric therapy for remediation have been questioned.

A critical issue "fueling" the controversy is the marked heterogenicity of impaired learning, and the utilization of a *single* therapy for all learning disabilities. Van Noorden (1976) noted that reading disability (dyslexia) is *not* caused by ocular problems. He suggested that evidence is lacking to support a hypothesis that reading disabilities are associated with problems in eye movement or eye balance. Learning is concluded to be a function of the brain and not of the eyes (Goldberg & Arnott, 1970). The type of ocular motility apparently does not determine the degree of comprehension, but "it is the ability to understand which determines the fluidity of the reading and that ocular motility simply denotes the degree of fluidity" (Goldberg & Arnott, 1970, p. 42). The optometric thesis generally recognizes that the special educator is the "primary care practitioner" for learning-disabled children. However, it stresses a rationale for treating the learning-disabled child by improving vision and "visual-functional and visual-perceptual factors related to learning" (Solan, 1981, p. 572). It is this latter optometric concept that has generated spirited controversy and periodic review (Keogh & Pelland, 1985; Levine, 1984).

The American Academy of Pediatrics issued a Joint Organizational Statement (1972) on "The Eye and Learning Disabilities", representing the viewpoints of the American Academy of Pediatrics, the American Academy of Ophthalmology and Otolaryngology, and the American Association of Ophthalmology. The statement emphasizes that learning disabilities and dyslexia are characterized by:

1. A need for multidisciplinary management ("eye care should not be instituted in isolation when a patient has a reading problem")
2. Lack of scientific data that supports cause

and effect relationship between all learning disabilities and peripheral eye defects
3. A weak base of scientific data that supports claims for improved academic abilities of learning-disabled children treated solely with visual training, and/or neurologic organizational training
4. No evidence that eyeglasses have value in the specific therapy of learning disorders, (excluding correctable ocular defects)
5. No *single* approach is applicable to treating children with impaired learning

The utilization of optometric training in isolation for learning disabilities should be viewed in the context of its potential adverse effects: diversion from traditional therapies, time investment, financial obligation, and engendering false hopes.

Sensory Integrative Therapy (Vestibular Stimulation) It has been postulated that there is an association between sensorimotor impairment and higher-level cognitive functioning (Finlayson & Reitan, 1976). It has also been suggested that perception and learning are dependent upon a functionally intact brain stem that can organize visual and auditory processes (Ayers, 1968). The normal development of visual perception is hypothesized to be dependent on intersensory integration from other sources, particularly vestibular and somatosensory sources. The postulate implies that if sensory integration is impaired (immediate postural reactions, poor eye muscle control, disturbed orientation and/or distractibility), the child will experience learning difficulties. An extension of the theory suggests that motor defects and underlying organic brain deficits can be treated by controlling sensorimotor behavior, thereby influencing neurosensory integration (Ayers, 1972). Activities that are suggested to be important in normalizing behaviors include: vestibular, postural, and tactile stimulation.

Within this neuro-organizational framework, Levinson (1980) proposed that children with cerebellar vestibular dysfunction will exhibit learning disabilities (dyslexia). He suggested that disturbances in the complex interaction of inner ear function, in coordination of eye-head movements, and in ocular fixation, tracking, and fixation are ultimately reflected as specific reading disorders (Frank & Levinson, 1976). The tests designed for evaluating this disorder, as well as the proposed therapy with anti-motion sickness medications (e.g., Dramamine), have been subject to scientific criticism.

Postrotary nystagmus (PRN; vestibular-ocular reflex following rotation), to differentiate children with vestibular processing dysfunction, appeared to support the Ayers hypothesis, specifically: "learning-disabled children with excessive PRN display greater or more extensive neurological involvement than learning-disabled children with normal or depressed PRN" (Ottenbacher, 1980, p. 44). Ottenbacher and Petersen (1983), from a review of the literature, concluded that there was quantitative evidence to support the value of vestibular stimulation. However, they noted that:

> despite the popularity of therapeutic intervention promoting the use of sensory stimulation and vestibular stimulation, in particular, only 14 studies that met the pre-established criteria for inclusion in the review were specifically developed to meet empirical standards commensurate with traditional inferential research in the behavioral and biomedical sciences. (p. 432)

The authors suggested the need for additional research in order to resolve questionable interpretations of their literature review.

Carte, Morrison, and Sublett, et al. (1984) attempted to replicate previous research on the effects of sensory integration therapy on learning-disabled children. They concluded that "sensory integration therapy had no statistically significant effect on hyponystagmus duration, perceptual processing dysfunction, or academic achievement" (p. 192). Carte et al. argued further that previous research did *not* utilize appropriate control group design. Polatajko (1985) assessed 40 children with learning disabilities and 49 normal children as matched controls, and concluded that: 1) there was no significant difference in vestibular function between the two groups, 2) there was no significant correlation between vestibular function and academic achievement, and 3) there was "no significant educational relevance in categorizing learning-disabled children according to vestibular dimensions." The hypotheses of Ayers and Levinson do not appear to be well documented (Brown, Haegerstrom-Portnoy, Yingling, et al., 1983; Carte, Morrison, Sublett, et al., 1984; Ottenbacher & Petersen, 1983). In the face of unresolved issues and contradictory data, recommendations for participation in these therapies must be cautiously reserved.

"ACCEPTABLE" THERAPIES: UNRESOLVED ISSUES

Although traditional management strategies (special education, pharmacotherapy, and psychological/psychiatric counseling) are based on more acceptable neuro-psychoeducational principles, several unresolved issues similarly persist. These are issues that are difficult to clarify because of research design limitations which prevent accurate assessment of intervention outcomes. Two major recognized research constraints are: 1) the absence of long-range follow-up studies, and 2) the characteristic heterogeneous nature of the disorders in question.

Frequent confusions in the choice of the most appropriate educational program for a child reflect the paucity of scientifically designed research studies. For example: *Which program is best for children with learning disabilities: mainstreaming or self-contained classrooms?* Self-contained special education classrooms have been criticized for promoting educational and social isolation of the child, that is, for "labeling" and "stigmatizing". In contrast, mainstreaming children with learning disorders may be inappropriate because of academically-induced child and family psychosocial stresses. In either educational environment, associated anxieties may seriously jeopardize the child's self-esteem and self-confidence. Advantages and disadvantages of each of these educational approaches have been variously debated (Ensher, 1976; Sarason & Doris, 1977; Winschel, 1976). Resource as-

sistance, which combines mainstreaming with intermittent utilization of a more constricted special education setting, often serves as an effective academic compromise.

The selection of an appropriate classroom placement, with a specific program design for the learning-disabled child, is frequently based on empirical decisions. *Which is academically more beneficial for the learning-disabled child: perceptual training or subject-oriented tutorial support?* Ideally, academic placement should be a scientifically constructed individualized educational program. This unresolved management issue has similarly provoked parental and professional concerns because visual and auditory perceptual training have not been unequivocally correlated with improved skills in reading or academic performance (Mann, 1972; Sullivan, 1972). Controlled studies are lacking, and a strong argument cannot be offered for differentially recommending either one of these specific educational therapies.

In general, clinical research protocols and study "end-points" for drug studies can be more accurately assessed. Nevertheless, pharmacotherapy for children with attention deficits, hyperactivity, and/or learning disorders is similarly characterized by significant unresolved issues. Major pharmacotherapy concerns are reflected by questions such as:

What is considered an appropriate drug response and how can it be measured?
Is the child's response truly a drug effect or a placebo effect?
Is an empirical trial of drugs with a favorable response a justifiable diagnostic test?
Should medications be used during weekends and during vacations?

The sole use of psychotropic medications to achieve a quick cure for psychoeducational problems has been severely and justifiably criticized. Total reliance on drugs to improve performance may in effect isolate the child from other necessary therapies that are critical in resolving underlying educational and psychosocial factors (Gottlieb, 1975; Muir, 1975). It is readily recognized that poorly defined criteria for the use of medications for learning disabilities, hyperkinesis, and attention deficits can create a management dilemma for the responsible physician (American Academy of Pediatrics, Committee on Drugs, 1970).

Counseling has traditionally been regarded as an established adjunctive therapy for children with attention deficits, hyperactivity, and learning disabilities. It is *not* a substitute for a well-constructed educational program or a soundly-based intervention with medication. Although generally recognized as an effective strategy for improving the child's self-esteem and for enhancing behavior control, it is often ineffective as an isolated therapeutic intervention. The long-term effects of psychostimulants and behavior therapy on academic and social development requires further research clarification. Positive short-term effects on academic performance have been reported as a result of behavioral interventions, but not as a result of drug therapy (O'Leary, 1980). The value of behavioral therapies over an extended period for the hyperactive child have not been defined. Psychologists and psychiatrists are similarly confronted with unresolved issues when selecting the most appropriate counseling approach. A combined therapeutic approach, rather than the single "simple cure" therapy design, appears to be most effective (Yang, Risch, & Lamm, 1973).

DISCUSSION

Several of the more popular controversial therapies recommended for attention deficit disorders, hyperkinesis, and learning disabilities have been reviewed. As a rule, these nonstandard management programs appear to reduce multifaceted, complex developmental-behavioral syndromes (e.g., dyslexia, attention deficits, hyperactivity) to a single biochemical or neurobiological variant (e.g., a vitamin deficiency, a mineral imbalance, a reaction to food coloring, a food allergy, or a specific neurological disorganization). Frequently, nonstandard remedies are enthusiastically endorsed as beneficial for a diverse spectrum of developmental and behavioral disorders, regardless of their very different etiological backgrounds. The "single" therapy is often employed as a specific remedy for a combination of psychoeducational, neuromotor, behavioral, and social problems. Brown (1979) commented that "The complex impairments are not only reduced to stark simplicity, but many cures are claimed for each impairment, i.e., each promoter with his own cure."

The powerful influence of the communication media in relating health information issues to the public has been universally acknowledged. At times, the public may be overwhelmed with commentaries on "new" and "exciting" breakthroughs. Magazine and newspaper articles, announcements on radio and television, as well as guest appearances by "experts" on television talk shows may serve as convincing endorsements for a particular therapy approach. The net effect of media popularization is the establishment of a pseudo-credibility for the nonstandard therapy. It is obvious that recognition by the communications media will have a much more profound influence on public perceptions and opinions than an article that is favorably reviewed but buried in a refereed scientific journal. The public may conclude that the time and concern devoted by the media to discussing a new remedy is in effect a proclamation of an exciting breakthrough in traditional medicine.

Physicians, however, are required to adopt a more conservative, analytical, and critical approach, evaluating therapeutic claims from data published in peer-review journals. A meaningful analysis of reported results and conclusions necessitates an appreciation of research design and method of subject control selection. Professionals are significantly less impressed (or should be) by testimonials of either promoter or patient. Most refereed journals discourage the one or two case history reports used to unequivocally support a hypothesis. Cautious professionals generally prefer to review several studies that test and retest initial reports of successful management approaches. Research protocols, data, and conclusions must be assessed within the context of acceptable scientific research designs (Table 2).

Therapies designated as controversial have undoubtedly been associated with occasional individual successful outcomes. The mechanisms for effecting the "cure," however, may not be attributed solely to modification of the presumed pathology (e.g., the influence of other variables, such as in the placebo effect, or in the interpretation of "remedy"). Professionals, despite claims of cures, are confronted with the dilemma of *not* endorsing or participating in a new and popular intervention, despite enthusiastic disclaimers of unpleasant side-effects. Parental concerns, apprehensions, and anxieties necessitate judicious counseling, thereby avoiding unpleasant confrontation when support is denied for a specific controversial therapy. However, in some situations, compromises can be formulated in which parents and professionals may agree to mutually monitor the child's responses over a limited time period. Nevertheless, the professional is obligated to first review with parents those factors contributing to the designation of "controversial" therapy, including a discussion of the scientific shortcomings of the novel management approach, the psychological and financial implications, and the diversion from more traditional approaches. Professionals will generally elect to disclaim responsibility for initiating or monitoring some of the nonstandard therapies. This decision requires sensitive counseling with the parent in order to clarify positions and to avoid feelings of abandonment.

Complex problems rarely have simple solutions. The search for a panacea, the quick cure, is a readily understandable quest for parents whose children may face profound psycho-educational and social complications of chronic handicapping disorders. Traditional management approaches characteristically cannot provide either short cuts or guarantees of improved function. However, therapies that offer false hopes serve to compound the tragedy of the child with a chronic handicapping disorder. Recommending and monitoring either acceptable or controversial therapies is undoubtedly a major management responsibility for primary care physicians, child neurologists, and developmental pediatricians. This relatively frequent therapy challenge is a significant issue of mutual concern for all professionals serving children with developmental-behavioral disorders. Professional confusion in recommending and conscientiously monitoring therapies may profoundly influence developmental outcomes, and may promote parental anxieties and frustrations.

Silver (1986) emphasized the need for meaningful medical intervention:

> "The pediatrician or family physician can play a critical role in coordinating the multidisciplinary evaluation and in being sure that the results are clearly explained to the patients. Also essential is anticipating guidance relating to what the child or adolescent will need and a willingness to be an advocate, helping their efforts with the school. Since these are long-term or even lifetime disabilities, the physician plays a critical role in monitoring the specific needs for each developmental stage." (p. 1051)

Perhaps the effectiveness of the challenge presented by Dr. Silver will ultimately be measured in the parents' reluctance to participate in scientifically undocumented, nonstandard therapies.

Table 2. Experimental design for assessing new therapies

1. Establish a rational hypothesis to justify the research study
2. Clearly define the conditions to be studied
3. Avoid sample bias by random selection of patients and matched controls
4. Interventions with control groups:
   a. Alternative therapy
   b. Inert placebo
   c. Untreated
5. Neutralizing sample bias:
   a. Therapist "blind" as to "who got what"
   b. Subject unaware of "what he/she got"
   c. Evaluator of outcome unaware of "who got what"
6. Measurement instruments or observations:
   a. Objective
   b. Replicable
   c. Protocols available
7. Analysis of data conforms to acceptable (standard) procedures
8. Data (research design, sample selection, etc.) published in peer-review journal

Adapted from Brown (1979).

REFERENCES

American Academy of Pediatrics, Committee on the Handicapped Child. (1968). The Doman-Delacato treatment of neurologically handicapped children. *Journal of Pediatrics, 72,*750–752.

American Academy of Pediatrics, Committee on Drugs. (1970). An evaluation of pharmacological approaches to learning impediments. *Pediatrics, 46,*142–144.

American Academy of Pediatrics, Joint Organizational Statement. (1972). The eye and learning disabilities. *Pediatrics, 49,*454–455.

American Academy of Pediatrics, Committee on Nutrition. (1976). Megavitamin therapy for childhood psychoses and learning disabilities. *Pediatrics, 58,*910–912.

American Academy of Pediatrics. (1982). The Doman-Delacato treatment of neurologically handicapped children. *Pediatrics, 70,*810.

Ayers, A.J. (1968). Sensory integrative processes and neuro-psychological learning disabilities. In J. Hellmuth (Ed.), *Learning disorders* (Vol. 3, pp. 43–58). Seattle: Special Child Publications.

Ayers, A.J. (1972). Improving academic scores through sensory integration. *Journal of Learning Disabilities, 5,*339–343.

Brenner, A. (1977). A study of the efficacy of the Feingold diet on hyperkinetic children. *Clinical Pediatrics, 16,*652–656.

Brown, G.W. (1979). Learning disabilities: Fads, fallacies and fictions. In M.I. Gottlieb & L.J. Bradford (Eds.), *Learning disabilities: An audio journal for continuing education* (Vol. 3:2). New York: Grune & Stratton.

Brown, G.W. (1987). Controversial therapy. In M.I. Gottlieb & J.E. Williams (Eds.), *Textbook of developmental pediatrics* (pp. 431–450). New York: Plenum.

Brown, B., Haegerstrom-Portnoy, G., Yingling, C.D., et al. (1983). Dyslexic children have normal vestibular responses to rotation. *Archives of Neurology, 40,*370–373.

Carte, E., Morrison, D., Sublett, J., et al. (1984). Sensory integration therapy: A trial of specific neurodevelopmental therapy for the remediation of learning disabilities. *Journal of Developmental and Behavioral Pediatrics, 5,*189–194.

Cohen, M.J., Birch, H.G., & Taft, L.T. (1970). Some considerations for evaluating the Doman-Delacato "patterning" method. *Pediatrics, 45,*302–314.

Conners, C.K., Coyette, C.M., Southwick, D.A., et al. (1976). Food additives and hyperkinesis: A controlled double-blind experiment. *Pediatrics, 58,*154–166.

Cott, A. (1971). Orthomolecular approach to the treatment of learning disabilities. *Schizophrenia, 3,*905–1005.

Crook, W.G. (1975). Food allergy—The great masquerader. *Pediatric Clinics of North America, 22,*227–228.

Doman, R.J., Spitz, E.B., Zucman, E., et al. (1966). Children with severe brain injuries: Neurologic organization in terms of mobility. *Journal of the American Medical Association, 174,*257–262.

Ensher, G.L. (1976). Mainstreaming: Yes. *Exceptional Parent, 6,*7–8.

Feingold, B.F. (1975a). *Why your child is hyperactive.* New York: Random House.

Feingold, B.F. (1975b). Hyperkinesis and learning disabilities linked to artificial food flavors and colors. *American Journal of Nursing, 75,*797–803.

Finlayson, M.A.J., & Reitan, R.M. (1976). Tactile-perceptual functioning in relation to intellectual, cognitive and learning skills in younger and older normal children. *Developmental Medicine and Child Neurology, 18,*442–446.

Frank, J., & Levinson, H. (1976). Seasickness mechanisms and medications in dysmetric dyslexia and dyspraxia. *Academic Therapy, 12,*133–152.

Goldberg, H.K., & Arnott, W. (1970). Ocular motility in learning disabilities. *Journal of Learning Disabilities, 3,*40–42.

Golden, G.S. (1984). Controversial therapies. *Pediatric Clinics of North America, 31,*459–469.

Gottlieb, M.I. (1975). Pills, pros and cons: Medications for school problems. *Acta Symbolica, 6,*35–65.

Gottlieb, M.I. (1979). The learning disabled child: Controversial issues revisited. In M.I. Gottlieb, P.W. Zinkus, & L.J. Bradford (Eds.), *Current issues in developmental pediatrics: The learning-disabled child* (pp. 219–259). New York: Grune & Stratton.

Harley, J.P., Mathews, C.H., & Eichman, P. (1978). Synthetic food colors and hyperactivity in children: A double-blind challenge experiment. *Pediatrics, 62,*975–983.

Harley, J.P., Ray, R.S., Tomasi, L., et al. (1978). Hyperkinesis and food additives: Testing the Feingold hypothesis. *Pediatrics, 61,*818–828.

Haslam, R.H.A., Dalby, J.T., & Rademaker, A.W. (1984). Effects of megavitamin therapy on children with attention deficit disorders. *Pediatrics, 74,*103–111.

Herbert, V. (1977). Megavitamin therapy. *Journal of the American Pharmaceutical Association, 17,*764–766.

Herbert, V. (1978). Facts and fictions about megavitamin therapy. *Resident Staff Physician, 24,*43–50.

Hoffer, A., Osmond, H., & Smythies, J. (1954). Schizophrenia: A new approach II: Results of a year's research. *Journal of Mental Science, 100,*29–54.

Johnson, D.D., Dorr, K.E., & Sivenson, W.M. (1980). Reactive hypoglycemia. *Journal of the American Medical Association, 243,*1151.

Keogh, B.K., & Pelland, M. (1985). Vision training revisited. *Journal of Learning Disabilities, 18,*228–236.

Levine, M.D., & Liden, G.B. (1976). Commentaries: Food for inefficient thought. *Pediatrics, 58,*145–148.

Levine, M.D. (1984). Commentaries: Reading disability: Do the eyes have it? *Pediatrics, 73,*869–870.

Levinson, H.N. (1980). *A solution to the riddle dyslexia.* New York: Springer-Verlag.

Mann, L. (1972). Perceptual training revisited. The training of nothing at all. In S. Chess & A. Thomas (Eds.), *Annual progress in child psychiatry and child development* (pp. 178–190). New York: Brunner/Mazel.

May, C.D. (1975). Food allergy: A commentary. *Pediatric Clinics of North America, 22,*217–220.

McLoughlin, J., Nall, M., Isaacs, B., et al. (1983). The relationship of allergies and allergy treatment to school performance and student behavior. *Annals of Allergy, 51,*506–510.

Muir, M. (1975). The consideration of emotional factors in the diagnosis and treatment of learning-disabled children. *Pediatric Psychology, 3,*6–9.

National Institutes of Health Consensus Development

Conference. (1982). Defined diets and childhood hyperactivity. *Clinical Pediatrics, 12,*627–630.

O'Leary, K.D. (1980). Pills or skills for hyperactive children. *Journal of Applied Behavioral Analysis, 13,*191–204.

Ottenbacher, K.J. (1980). Excessive postrotary nystagmus duration in learning-disabled children. *American Journal of Occupational Therapy, 34,*40–44.

Ottenbacher, K.J., & Petersen, P. (1983). The efficacy of vestibular stimulation as a form of specific sensory enrichment. *Clinical Pediatrics, 23,*428–433.

Pauling, L. (1968). Orthomolecular psychiatry. *Science, 160,* 265–271.

Phil, R.O., & Parkes, M. (1977). Hair element content in learning-disabled children. *Science, 198,*204–206.

Polatajko, H.J. (1985). A critical look at vestibular dysfunction in learning-disabled children. *Developmental Medicine and Child Neurology, 27,*283–292.

Sarason, S., & Doris, J. (1977). Dilemmas, opposition, opportunities. *Exceptional Parent, 1,*21–24.

Silver, L.B. (1986). Controversial approaches to treating learning disabilities and attention-deficit disorder. *American Journal of Diseases of Children, 140,*1045–1052.

Solan, H.A. (1981). A rationale for the optometric treatment and management of children with learning disabilities. *Journal of Learning Disabilities, 24,*568–572.

Sparrow, S., & Zigler, E. (1978). Evaluation of a patterning treatment for retarded children. *Pediatrics, 62,*137–150.

Spring, C., & Sandoval, J. (1976). Food additives and hyperkinesis: A critical evaluation of the evidence. *Journal of Learning Disabilities, 9,*28–37.

Sullivan, J. (1972). The effects of Kephart's perceptual motor-training on a reading clinic sample. *Journal of Learning Disabilities, 5,*545–551.

Van Noorden, G.K. (1976). Chronic vision problems of school-age children. *Journal of School Health, 46,*334–337.

Wender, E.H. (1977). Food additives and hyperkinesis. *American Journal of Diseases of Children, 131,*1204–1206.

Wender, E.H. (1986). The food additive-free diet in the treatment of behavior disorders: A review. *Journal of Developmental Behavioral Pediatrics, 7,*35–42.

Williams, J.I., Cram, D.M., Tavsig, F.T., et al: (1978). Relative effects of drugs and diet on hyperactive behaviors: An experimental study. *Pediatrics, 61,*811–817.

Winschel, J.F. (1976). Mainstreaming: No. *Exceptional Parent, 6,*9–10.

Yang, D.C., Risch, M.L., & Lamm, S.S. (1973). Rehabilitation of learning in a hospital class using psychoactive drugs. *Journal of Learning Disabilities, 6,*488–491.

Chapter 32

The Efficacy
of Early Intervention

John E. Williams

THE CONTROVERSY CONCERNING THE CON-
cept of altering developmental potential
through environmental manipulation dates
back to the Nature versus Nurture debate that
raged in the scientific community almost a century ago. More recently, in 1964, Project Head
Start was begun in the United States. It was
based on the belief that if the unstimulating
environment of underpriviledged preschool-
age children could be changed for several hours
a day to one that was stimulating and enriched,
the cognitive and educational potential of these
children would be enhanced. Since that time,
this concept has been carried over to include
biologically handicapped children. Over the
past 10 years, researchers have witnessed a
proliferation of early intervention programs
(EIPs) that provide therapies to children from
birth. Many of these programs are for children
who have been diagnosed as having developmental disabilities. However, some of the programs include children who are felt to be only
"at risk."

THE HEAD START PROGRAM

The Head Start program includes more than
100,000 children each year. Although several
studies that examine the long-term effects of
Head Start on IQ have been disappointing, it
has been shown that more durable IQ and
achievement score gains were achieved when
parents extended the remedial program to the
home through their own efforts. Gains were

also achieved when the preschool program was
followed by further special educational effort
once the child reached elementary school
(Ziegler, 1979). However, the rationale for
Head Start differs from that of early intervention for biologically handicapped children.

EARLY INTERVENTION
FOR CHILDREN WITH HANDICAPS

Across the United States, EIPs endeavor to
combine the provision of educational, health,
and social welfare services to children with a
wide range of biologic handicaps. Infants with
Down syndrome and other genetic abnormalities are served in EIPs along with infants
who have CNS injury of perinatal origin and
children with other developmental handicaps
of known and unknown etiologies. Conventional therapies, including, for example, physical therapy/occupational therapy (PT/OT),
language therapy, and special education, are
usually included in EIPs along with varying
degrees of parental involvement in therapy.
However, controversial therapies may also be
included under the rubric of early intervention,
for example, patterning and vestibular stimulation. There is also variability in the intensity of
how these therapies are applied; therapy frequency may vary from once a day to 40 hours
per week or more.

The factors outlined above raise several
basic questions about early intervention for biologically handicapped infants.

1. Can it work? Is there a malleable neurological substrate in the brain-injured infant?
2. Is there a generic intervention and a generic patient? If not, would all the different therapies and varying applications help an etiologically heterogeneous group of handicapped children?
3. Are researchers asking the right questions in the right ways? For example, do IQ scores adequately reflect the total adaptive, social, and emotional well-being of humans? If not, how can researchers more adequately describe the development of these attributes over time?

Neural Development and Plasticity

The question of whether or not the immature human brain can recover to some degree following an insult has been approached from several research avenues. Studies on lower vertebrates such as salamanders and fish have demonstrated the remarkable regenerative powers of their neural tissues (Berry & Spector, 1986; Szekely, 1979). Rats raised in "enriched" environments are measurably different in brain neurotransmitter concentrations and dendritic branching from those rats raised in less stimulating environments (Greenough, 1976). Animal studies have also demonstrated the CNS changes secondary to visual and auditory deprivation and restimulation (Innocenti & Frost, 1979; Webster & Webster, 1979). Another interesting insight into the possibility of plasticity of the CNS comes from the concept of embryonic overproduction of dendritic connections, and their subsequent partial elimination in postnatal life.

Exactly how neuronal regeneration research in lower vertebrates and animal studies involving sensory deprivation may relate to the neurodevelopment of brain-injured infants remains to be explained. For example, Huttenlocher demonstrated an increase in synaptic density in human frontal and visual cortical areas during infancy. After this period of proliferation, synaptic density decreased, reaching adult levels in later years (Huttenlocher, 1985). However, it would be presumptuous to assume that synaptic overproduction and elimination in the visual cortex connotes a "critical period" for brain plasticity in higher cortical function. Until the relationship between changes in the environment and neurotransmitter turnover and synaptogenesis can be elucidated, statements regarding changes in the CNS of brain-damaged infants relating to early intervention will remain hypothetical.

The Efficacy of EIPs

The question of whether or not EIPs have been responsible for changes in the developmental status of handicapped infants has been addressed by measuring various developmental attributes (e.g., IQ, motor skills, language development, behavior), and by conducting various types of analysis (statistical and deductive) involving judgments regarding the efficacy of the intervention type in question. When one considers the magnitude of difficulty involved in the design of studies of this nature, it is easy to see why the "definitive study" has yet to be published. Well-founded criticisms leveled at the methodology of most of these studies have appropriately prevented any single report from answering the questions of whether EIPs work, and if so, for whom.

Other efforts aimed at answering these questions have been directed at studying the results of groups of individual projects. In a review of 27 studies on the efficacy of early intervention, it was found that only two of the five prospective control/contrast group (random assignment) studies examined yielded results that statistically supported efficacy. The authors, however, concluded that this body of research provided "qualified" support for the effectiveness of early intervention for the biologically impaired infant (Simeonsson, Cooper, & Scheiner, 1982). Thus, when literature review is used as a method of hypothesis testing, the use of descriptive analysis of the reviewed data and narrative debate on the validity of the hypothesis will continue to yield equivocal answers.

EIPs and Quantitative Evaluation

In addition to the traditional narrative review approach to data interpretation, researchers have also made quantitative evaluations of the research on the efficacy of early intervention for biologically handicapped children. Ottenbacher and Petersen (1985) utilized such an approach to review 38 studies (1,544 subjects) using a total of 118 hypothesis tests of two group comparisons evaluating the effectiveness of EIPs. The individual studies were given numerical values based on how well they controlled for seven threats to their internal validity. For each hypothesis test, a size effect was calculated. They found that larger size effects were present in those studies that had poor internal validity. Conversely, those studies with "stronger" designs showed smaller effect sizes. This analysis revealed, however, that even in the most rigorously designed studies, the average performance of handicapped subjects in the treatment groups receiving early intervention was better than 67.7% of the subjects in the control or comparison groups. Ottenbacher and Petersen's conclusions were based on the quantitive aggregate of these studies. They found that: 1) measured treatment effects appear to be influenced by research design, and 2) effects were present.

The quantitative approach to literature review has not answered the question of what interventions should be used for which children. However, this approach has added a degree of objectivity to the interpretation of a body of research that includes large numbers of patients and treatments.

Perhaps the most important questions raised by the research methodologies applied to evaluating early intervention efficacy relate to the selection of outcome criteria. For example, IQ is frequently chosen as a dependent variable because it is easily measured and is a widely accepted construct. Reflex profiles and motor development inventories that have been previously standardized and that yield data that can be statistically manipulated are also frequently used. The use of such instruments in order to make judgments regarding the general value of EIPs implies that early intervention aspires to the unattainable goals of reversing mental retardation or of curing cerebral palsy. Thus, this area of behavioral research has unfortunately fallen into the trap of allowing methodological design to dictate the objectives by which the efficacy of early intervention is judged. Some researchers have argued that the proponents of early intervention do not themselves "know" exactly what benefits come from these therapies (Ferry, 1981, 1986; Russman, 1986). If this is in fact the case, then perhaps investigators should resist the temptation to rush from their armchairs to the testing laboratory in order to prove or disprove the efficacy of early intervention. Instead, they should begin the arduous and painstaking process of discovering which developmental-behavioral parameters should be examined and how they can be measured.

Early childhood development in the normal child is obviously multivariate in nature. Because behavior is the result of the complex interaction between endogenous (genetic, maturational) factors and exogenous (environmental) factors, the study of the altered development of organically impaired children can become entangled in a multitude of independent and dependent variables. Gallagher, Ramey, Haskins, and Finklestein (1976) have reviewed the literature describing how the longitudinal observation of children can be used to help solve this dilemma.

EIPs and Interdisciplinary Longitudinal Observation

Interdisciplinary longitudinal observation can not only elucidate the behavioral attributes that may be changing as a result of early intervention, but it can also help investigators develop new tools to measure these attributes. Thus, by enlarging the types of data collected, one is no longer limited to using standardized clinical measures such as IQ tests. Behaviors characteristic of children observed in typical settings could be utilized instead. Longitudinal observation should be used to collect this data on subjects in the wide variety of environmental contexts in which social, cognitive, affective, communicative, and motoric behaviors occur throughout the developmental period. The interdisciplinary longitudinal method of observing the behavioral changes in biologically handicapped children enrolled in EIPs is well suited to address many of the other issues that plague research on efficacy. Examples of these issues include:

1. Judging the cumulative impact of independent variables
2. Finding changes in the interrelationships between variables
3. Observing the variables that may demonstrate very small changes
4. Finding dimensions underlying behavioral changes
5. Discovering the delay or permanence of the impact of specific variables

CONCLUSION

The efficacy of early intervention may never be definitively judged until investigators are willing to follow a strategy that includes longitudinal observation. This approach permits the researcher to develop a sequential analysis of the behavior of biologically handicapped children that focuses on the interaction of many crucial variables over time. From this body of knowledge, new constructs can be integrated into existing models. Hypotheses can then be formulated based on this new conceptual framework and tested in carefully controlled experiments (Gallagher et al., 1976). By adhering to the observation/thinking/testing sequence as it relates to interdisciplinary longitudinal research design, researchers can begin to ask the right questions in order to fairly judge the efficacy of early intervention.

REFERENCES

Berry, M., & Spector, R. (1986). The nerve cell. *Developmental Medicine and Child Neurology*, Supp. 51, *28*,1.

Ferry, P.C. (1981). On growing new neurons: Are early intervention programs effective? *Pediatrics, 67*,38.

Ferry, P.C. (1986). Infant stimulation programs: A neurologic shell game? *Archives of Neurology, 43*,281.

Gallagher, J.J., Ramey, C.T., Haskins, R., & Finklestein, N.W. (1976). Use of longitudinal research in the study of child development. In T. Tjossen (Ed.), *Early intervention programs* (pp. 161–186). Washington, DC: National Institute of Child and Human Development.

Greenough, W.T. (1976). Enduring effects of differential experience and training. In M.R. Rosenzweig & E.L. Bennett (Eds.), *Neural mechanisms of learning and memory* (pp. 255–178). Cambridge, MA: MIT Press.

Huttenlocher, P.R. (1985). Synapse elimination and plasticity in developing human cerebral cortex. *American Journal of Mental Deficiency, 88*,5.

Innocenti, G.M., & Frost, D.D. (1979). Effects of visual experience on the maturation of the efferent system to the corpus callosum. *Nature, 280*, 231.

Ottenbacher, K., & Petersen, P. (1985). The efficacy of early intervention programs for children with organic handicaps. *Evaluation and Program Planning, 8*,135.

Russman, B.S. (1986). Are infant stimulation programs useful? *Archives of Neurology, 43*,282.

Simeonsson, R.J., Cooper, D.D., & Scheiner, A.P. (1982). A review and analysis of the effectiveness of early intervention programs. *Pediatrics, 69*,635.

Szekely, G. (1979). Order and plasticity in the nervous system. *Trends in Neurology, 2*,245.

Webster, D.B., & Webster, M. (1979). The effects of neonatal conductive hearing loss on brain stem auditory nuclei. *Annals of Otology, Rhinology and Laryngology, 88*,684.

Ziegler, E. (1979). Project Head Start: Success or failure? In E. Ziegler & J. Valentine (Eds.), *Project Head Start: A legacy of the war on poverty* (pp. 495–507). New York: The Free Press.

Chapter 33

Follow-Up Studies on Outcome of Hyperactive Children

Gabrielle Weiss

WHAT HAPPENS TO HYPERACTIVE CHILdren when they grow up? Theoretically, there are several possibilities:

1. They outgrow the symptoms of the hyperactive syndrome and become normal adults. This was the view of many pediatricians (Bakwin & Bakwin, 1966).
2. They continue to have symptoms of the syndrome to varying degrees but do not show evidence of psychopathology in other areas compared to normal children when grown up.
3. They are prone to develop serious disorders in adult life, such as antisocial or other personality disorders, alcoholism, or even psychotic states.
4. They show more general evidence of psychopathology (i.e., are more symptomatic) but do not develop distinct disorders in adult life.

Except for the first possibility, these four possibilities are not mutually exclusive and indeed, outcome may not be predictable. The question may not be answerable in any definitive fashion.

With respect to the existing literature on outcome, several controlled studies now exist. The purpose of this review is to summarize the main body of this literature in order to draw some pertinent conclusions.

TYPES OF FOLLOW-UP STUDIES

Retrospective Catch-Up Studies

The methodology of retrospective catch-up studies involves reviewing charts from several years back and selecting from them a child population diagnosed at that time as having the condition whose outcome is now being studied. As many as possible of the identified probands are then traced and evaluated. The main difficulty with this methodology is that of making retrospective diagnoses. In addition, most studies using this design have been unable to trace a large portion of the identified child population.

Retrospective Follow-Back Studies

Retrospective follow-back studies identify a deviant adult population, for example, alcoholics or patients attending an outpatient clinic, and then attempt to make retrospective diagnoses from their childhood histories. Many of these studies have been uncontrolled, and the problems are similar to those described for catch-up studies, namely, the difficulties of making diagnoses from histories that may go back 20 years or more.

Prospective Follow-Up Studies

Most prospective follow-up studies of hyperactive children begin to follow the children from the time the diagnosis is made. Some studies follow infants from birth (see McGee, Williams, & Silva, 1984; Nichols & Chen, 1981; Smith, 1977). In such studies, not only can the hyperactive syndrome be observed as it develops before referral, but the relative risks can be assessed as to their importance for the development of the syndrome.

Whatever methodology is chosen, outcome will vary considerably depending on the age of the probands at follow-up. The discrepancy of age range makes comparison among different studies difficult. In an attempt to deal with this, studies assessing outcome during adolescence will be described separately from those studying outcome in adulthood. For studies including both groups, the "mean age" of probands will be the determining factor; those studies in which the mean age of probands is 18 years or older will be considered under the section for adults.

FOLLOW-UP STUDIES ASSESSING HYPERACTIVE CHILDREN INTO ADOLESCENCE

Retrospective Catch-Up Studies

Mendelson, Johnson, and Stewart (1971) perused records in the Psychiatry Department of St. Louis Children's Hospital and selected 108 children who had been previously diagnosed as hyperactive. They were able to interview 83 of 140 children now age 12 to 16 years (mean age 13.4 years). Findings from this study indicated that 26% had long histories of antisocial behavior, 25% were in special classes, and the majority of the children still had problems of restlessness and distractibility, even according to the adolescents' self-reports (Stewart, Mendelson, & Johnson, 1973). About 40% had evidence of low self-esteem.

Blouin, Bornstein, and Trites (1978) compared drug and alcohol use in two groups of adolescents. One group had had a 5-year history of childhood "hyperactivity"; the other, a comparison group, were not "hyperactive" as children but had been evaluated as "not doing well at school." Results indicated that the "hyperactive" adolescents consumed more alcohol (although they were no more likely to be alcoholic), were frequently still hyperactive, and had significantly more conduct disorders.

A more middle-class group of adolescents, who had been diagnosed as having "minimal brain dysfunction with hyperactivity" 5 years earlier, was studied by Feldman, Denhoff and Denhoff (1979). Eighty-one previously diagnosed adolescents (mean age 15.5) were compared with their normal brothers. Over half of them were now "problem free," but 10% had antisocial problems and special education was required by one-third of the group.

Prospective Follow-Up Studies

Our own 5-year follow-up of 91 hyperactive adolescents (Weiss, Minde, Werry, et al., 1971) assessed the clinical picture for the age range 10 to 16 years (mean age 13.4 years). Scores on ratings of "hyperactivity" and "distractibility" had decreased but were still higher than those of normal controls. These problems were now rarely the presenting complaints; instead, the problems were "poor school performance" and "difficulties with peers." Clinically, the adolescents appeared immature for their ages, had no clear goals for themselves, showed poor self-image, and frequently became sad during interviews. They had failed more grades and had lower marks in all subjects on their report cards compared to matched normal controls (Minde, Weiss, & Mendelson, 1972). They showed no improvement on tests of intelligence and an actual decrement of performance on motor tasks. They continued to use more impulsive cognitive styles than controls (Cohen, Weiss, & Minde, 1972) on the Matching Familiar Figures Test. Most important was the finding, similar to Mendelson's (1971), that 25% had engaged in antisocial behavior. The biggest difference between the hyperactive and the control group was seen on the Psychopathy factor of the Peterson Quay Symptom Checklist.

An interesting study by Dykman and Ackerman (1980) assessed and compared three groups of 14-year olds who had been seen originally several years earlier. One of these groups ($N=31$) was a normal control group, and two groups ($N=62$) were learning disabled, with 23 also having the syndrome of hyperactivity. At follow-up at 14 years, there was little difference between the nonhyperactive learning-disabled group and the normal controls with respect to social deviancy and conduct problems. The hyperactive learning-disabled group, however, showed social deviancy and conduct problems in more than half their members. Dykman and Ackerman's study (1980) indicated that the presence of the hyperactive syndrome in the learning-disabled cohort predicted more social deviancy in adolescence. Learning disability itself did not predict conduct disorders in adolescence.

The fourth study to be described assessed older adolescents 14 to 21 years (mean age 17.3 years). This study was carried out by Satterfield, Hoppe, and Schell (1982), who followed up 110 hyperactive adolescents and 88 normal controls. In this population, approximately half of the hyperactive probands (whose actual court records were studied) had committed serious felonies. More hyperactive subjects than controls were also in delinquent training schools. The percentage of hyperactive adolescents arrested at least once for a felony was 58% for the lower class, 36% for the middle class, and 52% for the upper class, as compared to 11%, 9%, and 2% respectively, in the normal controls. All the offenses were considered serious, since running away, possession of less than one ounce of marijuana, getting drunk, or petty thefts were excluded.

A very recent study of adolescents was carried out by Lambert and colleagues (N. Lambert, personal communication, January, 1985) who found that 43% of the children diagnosed as hyperactive in childhood were still considered to be hyperactive in early adolescence. Twenty percent of the total were considered to be problem-free with respect to learning disabilities and behavior problems. The rates of delinquency and conduct problems were significantly higher for adolescents still being treated for hyperactivity and for those no longer being treated, than for normal controls.

This study also found that lower IQ, lower school achievement, lower performance on "perspective-taking" tests, lower levels of formal reasoning, and more field dependency predicted continued evidence of learning and behavior problems in early adolescence. There was no difference between hyperactives and controls with respect to nonaggressive or delinquent disorders, but the hyperactive adolescents showed more mood depression than normal controls. On measures of substance use and abuse at age 17, the only difference was more cigarette smoking among the hyperactive group.

From these studies of adolescents who were diagnosed as having the hyperactive syndrome as children, we draw the following conclusions:

1. About half or more of most proband groups continue to have symptoms of the syndrome, although frequently these are no longer the chief complaints.

2. Continued poor school performance is common; similarly, poor self-esteem and actual depression (one study) are common.

3. Significantly more conduct or antisocial behaviors were displayed by the adolescent probands across all studies. However, there were considerable differences among studies in the percentages who were antisocial as well as in the severity of the antisocial behavior. Satterfield's study showed about 50% as having committed felonies, whereas no differences in antisocial behaviors between former hyperactives and normals at age 17 were found by Lambert (N. Lambert, personal communication, January, 1985). It is very hard to explain these differences, which may be sociocultural, but they are most likely due to different initial intake criteria. Possibly the study most out of line with the others, that of Satterfield and colleagues (1982), followed hyperactive children who initially had more serious conduct disorders.

FOLLOW-UP STUDIES ASSESSING HYPERACTIVE CHILDREN INTO ADULT LIFE

Retrospective Catch-Up Studies

The first published study to assess hyperactive children well into their adult lives, tracing 14 to

18 subjects seen 25 years earlier in the Johns Hopkins Child Psychiatry Outpatient Clinic, was carried out by Menkes, Rowe, and Menkes (1967). While this study is frequently cited, its findings are strikingly different from subsequent studies that evaluated larger numbers of subjects and employed control groups. In this study at follow-up, four subjects were psychotic, two were retarded and economically dependent on their families, and four of the eight who were currently independent had spent time in an institution. Three subjects complained of hyperactivity.

Another 20 to 25 year retrospective study was carried out in 1976 by Borland and Heckman. By perusing old charts, they designated 37 boys as having had the hyperactive syndrome and were able to trace and interview 20 of the boys in adulthood as well as 19 of their brothers. These investigators found that about half of the probands still had some symptoms of the hyperactive syndrome, although the majority were steadily employed and self-supporting. The hyperactive subjects had not attained as high a socioeconomic status as their brothers, although the gap was narrowing slowly over time. Four of the twenty probands had some antisocial behavior.

Feldman and co-workers (1979) described a retrospective study of 81 children followed into adulthood. The mean age at follow-up was 21 years; 32 older siblings of the probands were interviewed as a comparison group. The subjects were middle class and had received various forms of therapy including special education and stimulant therapy. Results obtained were fairly similar to those of the study previously described. The majority of probands (91%) were working or at school. Half of the group was problem free. However, a significantly higher percentage of hyperactives had lower self-esteem, and 10% were considered to have serious emotional or behavioral problems. Treatment with stimulants was not associated with increased nonmedical drug or alcohol use, though a significantly higher percentage of hyperactives had used marijuana.

In another study, Loney and co-workers (Loney, Whaley-Klahn, Kisier, & Conboy,

1981), with the use of multivariate statistics, were seeking predictors of antisocial outcome in young adulthood. To date, 22 proband brother pairs, age 21 years, had been compared on measures of self-reported aggressive and antisocial acts. The Schedule for Affective Disorders and Schizophrenia-Lifetime Version (SADS-L) was used to assess antisocial personality disorders, alcoholism, and drug abuse. Results indicated that significantly more probands than brothers met 9 of 11 antisocial criteria on the SADS-L before the age of 15 years. Significantly more probands met three of the ten adult criteria for antisocial personality (lack of a permanent address, significant employment, and impaired interpersonal relationships). When one required criterion for the diagnosis of antisocial personality disorder was omitted (namely, lack of an intimate relationship with another person), 45% of probands versus 18% of the brothers met the criteria for antisocial personality disorder. The two groups did not differ significantly on the 19 individual items for alcoholism, although it was noted that both groups scored worse than controls from a collaborative depression study. Significantly more probands than brothers reported carrying hand guns or knives, and 54% of probands versus 15% of brothers had been in a fight resulting in bodily harm and the services of a physician. While probands did not commit more crimes against property or traffic offenses, their antisocial behaviors were more serious than those of their brothers. Forty-one percent of the former versus 5% of their brothers had spent time in jail.

Follow-Back Studies

For the sake of brevity, follow-back studies will be reviewed only briefly. Wood, Reimherr, Wender, and Johnson (1976) selected from among various outpatient groups 15 adults whose main presenting complaints were impulsivity, restlessness, poor attention span, and emotional lability. The parents of these probands were then asked to rate their children's behaviors between ages 6 to 10. Scores on the Conners Abbreviated Rating Scale placed two-thirds of the group in the upper 95th percentile. This finding suggested that adult patients were manifesting continued problems of the hyperactive syndrome. The limitations of this interesting study are due to its lack of a control group (e.g., outpatients with different symptoms) and to the uncertain validity of parents scoring the childhood problems of their now grown-up children.

Shelley and Riesler (1972) studied 16 young men in the United States Air Force who were referred for anxiety and self-depreciation as well as for their difficulty in performing certain tasks, such as marching, judo, and other gross and fine motor activities. After neurological examination, most were found to be clumsy, and 50% had finger apraxia or dysdiadochokinesis. The parents of these men reported that as children they had been restless, distractible, and had difficulties in school. They had improved during adolescence, but when they entered the Air Force, the tasks they were expected to perform proved too difficult for them. The limitations of this study are similar to those of Wood's study (Wood et al., 1976).

A Swedish study (Goodwin, Schulsinger, & Hermansen, 1975) assessed adoptees of whom 14 were diagnosed as alcoholic. The alcoholic adoptees had experienced significantly more childhood problems than the nonalcoholic adoptees with respect to school performance and hyperactivity. Additionally, they experienced conduct problems such as impulsivity, disobedience, shyness, insecurity, and sensitivity. There was no difference between the two groups of adoptees with respect to birth complications, childhood neurotic illness, depressive episodes, suicidal thoughts, unusual attitudes, or sexual deviation. Like the above two studies, this investigation relied on the memory of childhood events many years later, but unlike the above two studies, a normal control group was available. The findings suggest that some alcoholics have a childhood history of hyperactivity.

A fourth study evaluated 100 psychiatric inpatients in a Veterans Administration hospital and compared them with 28 normal matched controls (Gomez, Janowsky, Zeitin, et al.,

1981). The patients (age 20 to 65 years) were divided into four groups: psychotics, affective disorders, alcholics, and character disorders. Only organic brain syndromes were excluded. The authors used selected items from the 61 behavioral items of the Utah Personality Inventory, which they felt would most sensitively screen out the childhood hyperactive syndrome. Each item (rated on a 5-point scale) related to attention deficit, hyperactivity, and impulsivity. Results of this study showed 32% of the patient group versus only 4% of the controls reported a childhood history of hyperactivity. Furthermore, 20% of the patients versus none of the controls reported both a childhood and an adult hyperactive syndrome. The incidence of childhood hyperactivity did not differ significantly among the four patient groups, although character-disorder patients reported the highest percentage of the childhood syndrome. This study suggests that the hyperactive syndrome may predispose children to a number of different adult disorders. The lack of a significant correlation between character disorders and hyperactivity in childhood may have resulted from too few adults diagnosed as having antisocial personality disorder (the number of patients with this disorder is not given).

Prospective Studies

The following is a summary of the 10- to 12-year Controlled Prospective Follow-up Study conducted at the Montreal Children's Hospital.

This study reports on a series of outcome variables for 76 hyperactive subjects age 17 to 24 years (mean age 19.5 years) and 45 control subjects age 17 to 24 years (mean age 19.0 years). The two groups were matched with respect to age, sex, socioeconomic class, and IQ (Wechsler Adult Intelligence Scale [WAIS]). The 104 hyperactive subjects included in the study had been initially assessed in the Department of Psychiatry of the Montreal Children's Hospital 10 to 12 years previously (1962 through 1965). At that time, the children were 6 to 12 years of age. Children admitted into the study met the following criteria:

1. Restlessness and poor concentration were their main complaints; these complaints had been present since their earliest years.
2. The complaints were a major source of problems both at home and at school.
3. All children had IQs above 85 (WISC Full Scale).
4. None of the children were psychotic, borderline psychotic, epileptic, or had cerebral palsy.
5. All children were living at home with at least one parent.

The control group was first selected at the time of the 5-year follow-up study of the hyperactive children. Thirty-five children were matched with the hyperactive children on age, sex, IQ (Wechsler Intelligence Scale for Children [WISC]), and socioeconomic class. Criteria for inclusion in the control group required that the children had no significant academic or behavior difficulties in the home or at school. This control group was expanded to 45 subjects at the time of the 10-year follow-up study, using the same matching variables and criteria for inclusion.

The results of our 10- to 12-year follow-up study will be summarized under the following categories:

1. Biographical data
2. Psychiatric assessment
3. Physiological measures
4. Psychological tests

Biographical Data (Weiss, Hechtman, Perlman, et al., 1979) Fewer hyperactive subjects than controls were still living with their parents (76% vs. 95%), and hyperactives made significantly more geographic moves during the 5 years before follow-up assessment. They had significantly more car accidents (mean 1.3 vs. 0.07), although the number of subjects in each group who had car accidents was not significantly different.

Their school histories indicated that they had completed less education and more were still in high school at follow up evaluation. Their average marks were lower, and more hyperactives discontinued participation in high school

for this reason. They failed more grades in elementary and high school, but no particular subject or subjects were associated with their failure.

There was a trend for the hyperactive subjects to have more court referrals during the 5 years preceding follow-up (45% vs. 32%) but there was no difference between the groups as to the number of subjects who had court referrals during the year before follow-up.

A significantly greater percentage (74% vs. 54%) of hyperactive subjects had tried some form of nonmedical drug (mostly marijuana or hashish) in the 5 years preceding follow-up, but there was no difference between the groups with respect to nonmedical drug use in the year preceding follow-up. Interestingly enough, significantly more controls had used hallucinogens in the prior 5 years. There was no significant difference between the groups with respect to extent of drug or alcohol use (3-point scale: mild, moderate, or abuse) in the 5 years preceding follow-up.

Psychiatric Assessment The psychiatric evaluations indicated that more hyperactive subjects were diagnosed as having personality trait disorders. Two hyperactive subjects were diagnosed as borderline psychotic (this was not significant), but no subject in either group was diagnosed as psychotic. Significantly more hyperactive subjects felt restless than did controls, and significantly more were observed by the psychiatrist to be restless during their assessment, although getting up from their chairs was rare. Hyperactive subjects rated their childhoods as unhappy more often than did controls (Weiss et al., 1979).

Physiological Measures There was no difference between the groups with respect to height, weight, blood pressure, or pulse rate. Serial comparison of electroencephalograms (EEGs) of both groups at the 10-year follow-up revealed no significant differences. Comparison of EEGs of hyperactive subjects at initial evaluation, 5-year follow-up, and 10-year follow-up indicated that normalization of the EEG tended to occur during adolescence (Hechtman, Weiss, & Metrakos, 1978).

Psychological Tests Subjects rated themselves on the California Psychological Inventory (Gough, 1975) which was designed to tap cultural ideals of self-esteem and social interaction, and on the Symptom Checklist (SCL-90) (Derogatis, Lipman, & Covi, 1973), designed to tap classical psychopathology and test of self-esteem (Davidson & Lang, 1960; Hoy, Weiss, Minde, & Cohen, 1978). On both the California Psychological Inventory and on tests of self-esteem, hyperactives rated themselves as feeling significantly more inferior than controls. However, on the SCL-90, the ratings of the two groups did not differ, indicating that hyperactives see themselves as functioning less optimally, but not more pathologically, than do controls.

On social skills tests, hyperactives performed worse only on oral tasks, and performed equally to controls on written tasks. The social skills tests used were the Situational Social Skills Inventory in written and oral form and the Means-End Problem Solving (MEPS) test.

Cognitive style tests were also administered. Matching Familiar Figures test (MFF), Embedded Figures Test (EFT), and the Stroop Test indicated that the problems hyperactives had during childhood and adolescence persisted into adult life (Hopkins, Perlman, Hechtman, & Weiss, 1979).

This outcome study suggests that while a few hyperactive children did become grossly disturbed or chronic offenders of the law, none were diagnosed as psychotic or schizophrenic. However, the majority of young adults continued to have various symptoms of the hyperactive child syndrome. Impulsivity. lower educational achievement, poor social skills, low self-esteem, and restlessness remained problems.

SUMMARY OF THE 15-YEAR FOLLOW-UP STUDY AT THE MONTREAL CHILDREN'S HOSPITAL

The 15-year controlled follow up of this group of children has recently been completed (Hechtman & Weiss, 1986; Weiss & Hechtman. 1985). Sixty-three hyperactive adults and 41 matched controls were evaluated by means of a psychiatric interview, SADS-L (carried out blind). self rating scales, SCL-90, and the California Personality Inventory. A detailed history of nonmedical drug use and abuse, alcohol use and abuse, type and frequency of antisocial or aggressive acts, and employment records were obtained. The two groups no longer matched on WAIS IQ; at 15-year follow-up, the hyperactives scored significantly lower on the WAIS. This had not been true initially, nor at the 5- and 10-year follow-up evaluations. The results of this study will only be briefly summarized, as they form the content of several papers yet to be published, as well as a text published by the authors in 1986 (Weiss & Hechtman, 1986).

With respect to psychiatric status, the main findings of the 10- to 12-year follow-up were confirmed as follows:

1. More than half of the hyperactive subjects (66%) still had at least one disabling symptom of the original syndrome, compared to 10% of the controls.

2. Using the Diagnostic and Statistical Manual-(3rd. ed., 1980) criteria for diagnosis (which was not used in the 10-year follow-up study), 23% of the hyperactive adults had antisocial personality disorders. This classification did not rate a disorder on Axis I or II as mild or severe. If it had, most of the four adults diagnosed as antisocial would have been considered "mild." Using the modified SADS-L criteria, the numbers were similar: 23% (same subjects) when the same modification as that made by Loney and co workers (1981) was made, namely, omitting the criterion of having "no significant relationship."

3. On several measures, the hyperactive adults scored significantly worse than the controls. This was true for the California Personality Inventory (on which every factor distinguished the two groups), for the SCL -90, and for the Global Assessment Scale of the SADS-L. In addition, hyperactive adults were given more diag-

noses than controls and had more presenting complaints—including symptoms unrelated to the syndrome—than did controls. No one psychiatric disorder distinguished the two groups, with the exception of "Antisocial Personality Disorder" which was more frequent in the hyperactive adults. On the history, there was a trend toward more court referrals and more physically aggressive acts among hyperactive adults than among controls. The probands also had less years of education.

4. The formerly hyperactive children had made more suicide attempts than controls, and one subject died from suicide. (Two other subjects died from accidents which may have been suicide.) Although the number of deaths does not reach statistical significance in this study, verbal and printed reports by other investigators also cite one or more deaths in the hyperactive group but not in the control group. Some collaborative evaluation would help in assessing the significance of this finding. The employment records of the hyperactive adults confirm Borland and Heckman's (1976) findings that most subjects are employed and are economically independent. However, the work experiences of hyperactive subjects are inferior to controls with respect to employers' ratings of performance, duration of jobs, and work status as measured on the Hollingshead scale.

5. Data were collected from detailed interviews as well as court records. A trend was seen for more hyperactives to have had court appearances, and a greater number of court appearances than controls. There was no difference between the hyperactives and the controls on the degree of current use of alcohol, nor was alcoholism more frequent during the adulthood years of hyperactive children.

Rachel Gittelman-Klein has recently reported findings from her long-term, controlled follow-up study of 101 children diagnosed 7–11 years ago as having the hyperactive syndrome. All but two subjects were traced, and the age at follow-up was 16–23 years (mean age 18.3 years). One hundred controls were also assessed. The controls turned out to have significantly higher IQs and were slightly older, but these differences are unlikely to have influenced the findings.

An interesting finding from this study is that the full syndrome Attention Deficit Disorder with Hyperactivity (ADD-H) occurred in 31% of the probands and in 3% of the controls. Conduct disorders or antisocial disorders occurred in 27% of hyperactive probands and in 8% of the controls. Substance use disorder occurred in 19% of probands and in 7% of controls. Forty-five percent of the hyperactive subjects had histories of antisocial problems at some time during their lives. The investigators noted that those probands who had continuing symptoms of the syndrome at the time of the outcome evaluation were also much more likely to have an antisocial or a substance-use disorder. In fact, when those with persisting ADD-H were disregarded, no significant differences were found between probands and controls with respect to antisocial or substance-use disorders. In almost all cases, antisocial and substance-use disorders coexisted in the same individuals with the antisocial disorder preceding the substance-use disorder.

GENERAL CONCLUSIONS

The following conclusions can be drawn from the various studies that have been described assessing the outcome of the hyperactive syndrome in adulthood:

1. Most studies show that about half of the probands have "outgrown" the syndrome. However, one-third to two-thirds of the subjects continue to show symptoms of the syndrome. In the two studies that assessed work record, the majority of probands were working and were self-supporting, although their employment records on the whole were not as good as those of the controls. Evidence of this

poorer work record was demonstrated by their having a lower "work status" than controls (two studies), by their poorer ratings on employers' questionnaires (one study), and by their more frequent job changes (one study).

2. Most studies indicate that hyperactives have lower self-esteem, and rate themselves and are rated worse by others on various indicators of pathology. However, in no study was either alcoholism or schizophrenia more prevalent in adults who had been hyperactive as children. The follow-back retrospective studies suggest that hyperactivity in childhood may possibly predispose individuals to various adult disorders, including alcoholism and schizophrenia, but this finding is not borne out by the prospective studies.

3. In all studies, it is evident that for a significant minority, hyperactivity in childhood leads to adult antisocial personality disorders or antisocial behaviors. However, studies differ greatly on the percentage of subjects who are antisocial (ranging from 10% to 55%) and on the severity of the antisocial behavior. The difference among studies in this respect may be sociocultural (e.g., the likelihood of carrying guns or knives may vary from place to place), or it may be due to initial differences in the presence and degree of severity of conduct problems in the proband group.

The two studies most atypical are those of Menkes and co-workers (1967) and Feldman and colleagues (1979). The former study, with its very poor outcome, lacked a control group and included subjects who were initially retarded and who came from extremely chaotic homes. The Feldman study (1979) has an unusually favorable outcome; this may be due to the high economic class of subjects, the amount of treatment they received, and the possibility that some of the subjects initially had minimal brain damage without hyperactivity. Dykman and Ackerman (1980) have shown that hyperactivity in conjunction with learning disabilities predicts social deviancy in adolescence, whereas learning disabilities without hyperactivity have a good prognosis with respect to prosocial behavior.

In summary, despite the different methodologies of the studies reviewed in this paper, the majority of studies indicate fairly similar outcomes for probands when compared with matched normal controls. This suggests a fair degree of predictive validity for the hyperactive syndrome. The different outcomes among some of the studies are best explained by differences between the groups of hyperactive children at initial intake. Examples of such differences include: low versus high socioeconomic class, presence or absence of severe conduct disorders coexisting with the hyperactive syndrome, and inclusion or exclusion of the retarded. In fact, the extent of variability of the methodologies among the different studies is such that the amount of general agreement concerning adolescent and adult outcome of hyperactive children is surprising.

REFERENCES

Bakwin, H., & Bakwin, R. (1966). *Clinical management of behavior disorders in children.* Philadelphia: W.B. Saunders.

Blouin, A., Bornstein, R., & Trites, R. (1978). Teenage alcohol use among hyperactive children. *Journal of Pediatric Psychology, 3,*188–194.

Borland, H., & Heckman, H. (1976). Hyperactive boys and their brothers: A 25 year follow up study. *Archives of General Psychiatry, 33,*669–676.

Cohen, M., Weiss, G., & Minde, K. (1972). Cognitive styles in adolescents previously diagnosed as hyperactive. *Journal of Child Psychology and Psychiatry, and Allied Disciplines, 13,*203–209.

Davidson, H., & Lang, G. (1960). Children's perceptions of their teachers' feelings towards them related to self-perception, school achievement and behavior. *Journal of Experimental Education, 29,*107–116.

Derogatis, L., Lipman, R., & Covi, L. (1973). SCL-90: An outpatient psychiatric scale: Preliminary report. *Psychopharmacology Bulletin, 9,*13–28.

Dykman, R., & Ackerman, P. (1980). Long-term followup studies of hyperactive children. *Advances in Behavioral Pediatrics* (Vol. 1). New York: Kai Press.

Feldman, S., Denhoff, E., & Denhoff, F. (1979). Minimal brain dysfunction: A developmental approach. In E. Denhoff & L. Stern (Eds.), *The attention disorders and* related syndromes: Outcome in adolescence and young adult life (pp. 133–148). New York: Masson Publishing Co.

Gittelman-Klein, R., Manuzza, S.D., Skenker, R., & Bonagum, N. (1985). Hyperactive boys almost grown up. Archives of General Psychiatry, 42, 937–947.

Gomez, R., Janowsky, D., Zeitin, M., et al. (1981). Adult psychiatric diagnosis and symptoms compatible with the hyperactive child syndrome: A retrospective study. Journal of Clinical Psychiatry, 42, 389–394.

Goodwin, D., Schulsinger, F., & Hermansen, L. (1975). Alcoholism and the hyperactive syndrome. Journal of Nervous and Mental Diseases, 160, 349–353.

Gough, H. (1975). California Psychological Inventory (rev. ed.). Palo Alto: Consulting Psychologist Press.

Hechtman, L., & Weiss, G. (1986). Controlled prospective 15 year follow up of hyperactives as adults: Nonmedical drug and alcohol use and antisocial behavior. Canadian Journal of Psychiatry, 31, 557–567.

Hechtman, L., Weiss, G., & Metrakos, K. (1978). Hyperactives as young adults: Current and longitudinal electroencephalographic evaluation and its relation to outcome. Canadian Medical Association Journal, 118, 1247–1250.

Hopkins, J., Perlman, T., Hechtman, L., & Weiss, G. (1979). Cognitive types in adults originally diagnosed as hyperactives. Journal of Child Psychology and Psychiatry, 20, 209–216.

Hoy, E., Weiss, G., Minde, K., & Cohen, L. (1978). The hyperactive child at adolescence: Emotional, social and cognitive functioning. Journal of Abnormal Child Psychology, 6, 311–324.

Loney, J., Whaley-Klahn, M., Kisier, T., & Conboy, A. (1981, November). Paper presented at meeting of the Society for Life History Research, Monterey.

McGee, R., Williams, S., & Silva, P. (1984). Background characteristics of aggressive, hyperactive and aggressive-hyperactive boys. Journal of the American Academy of Child and Adolescent Psychiatry, 23, 270–279.

Mendelson, W., Johnson, N., & Stewart, M. (1971). Hyperactive children as teenagers: A follow up study. Journal of Nervous and Mental Disease, 153, 272–279.

Menkes, M., Rowe, J., & Menkes, J. (1967). A 25 year followup study on the hyperkinetic child with minimal brain dysfunction. Pediatrics, 38, 383–399.

Minde, K., Weiss, G., & Mendelson, H. (1972). A five-year follow-up of 91 hyperactive school children. Journal of the American Academy of Child and Adolescent Psychiatry, 11, 595–610.

Nichols, P., & Tu-chan Chen (1981). Minimal brain dysfunction: A prospective study. Hillsdale, NJ: Lawrence Erlbaum Associates.

Satterfield, J., Hoppe, C., & Schell, A.M. (1982). A prospective study of delinquency in 110 adolescent boys with attention deficit disorder and 88 normal adolescent boys. American Journal of Psychiatry, 139, 797–798.

Shelley, E., & Riester, A. (1972). Syndrome of MBD in young adults. Diseases of the Nervous System, 33, 335–338.

Smith, R. (1977). Kauai's children come of age. Honolulu: University of Hawaii Press.

Stewart, M., Mendelson, W., & Johnson, N. (1973). Hyperactive children as adolescents: How they describe themselves. Child Psychiatry and Human Development, 4, 3–11.

Weiss, G., & Hechtman, L. (1985). The psychiatric status of hyperactives: A controlled prospective 15-year follow-up of 63 hyperactive children. Journal of the American Academy of Child and Adolescent Psychiatry, 24, 211–220.

Weiss, G., & Hechtman, L. (1986). Hyperactive children grown up: Empirical findings and theoretical considerations. New York: Guilford Press.

Weiss, G., Hechtman, L., Perlman, T., et al. (1979). Hyperactives as young adults: A controlled prospective ten-year follow-up of 75 children. Archives of General Psychiatry, 36, 675–681.

Weiss, G., Minde, K., Werry, J., et al. (1971). A five year follow-up study of 91 hyperactive school children. Archives of General Psychiatry, 24, 409–414.

Wood, D., Reimherr, F., Wender, P., & Johnson, G. (1976). Diagnosis and treatment of MBD in adults. Archives of General Psychiatry, 33, 1453–1460.

Chapter 34

Neurological Theories of Dyslexia

Marcel Kinsbourne

IT HAS LONG BEEN KNOWN THAT SOME CHIL-
dren find it unusually difficult to learn to
read even though they apparently have normal
intelligence (reviewed by Kinsbourne, 1985).
The speculation (nearly a century old), that
these children have disorders of cerebral organization, has only in recent decades been taken
seriously by more than a few theorists
(Kinsbourne, 1983). An increasingly intensive
research effort is now being invested in the
study of left cerebral hemisphere representation of language processes presumably essential to reading acquisition (Satz, 1976). Are
these processes underdeveloped within the left
hemisphere of dyslexics, or are they anoma-
lously represented topographically (for instance bilaterally (Orton, 1937), or represented
in the "wrong" (i.e., subdominant) right
hemisphere?

CONTINUITY AND
DISCONTINUITY APPROACHES

Theoretical approaches to dyslexia vary with
the vantage point of the theorist. The neurologist, who by referral typically sees only the
most severe cases, is impressed by an apparent
discontinuity between the normal range of
reading skills and a deficit of dyslexic propor-
tions, and is therefore attracted by a neuropsychological and even neuropathological
point of view. He or she suspects an underlying
lesion, perhaps one analogous to that which, in
a previously normally reading adult, would

generate one of the varieties of acquired alexia.
The educator, more familiar with the wide
range of reading aptitude in the general school
population, and with interactive and multiply
determined outcomes, thinks in terms of con-
tinuity of degree of reading aptitude perhaps
even normally distributed in the population.
The dyslexic would be at the lower end of a
normal distribution of aptitude for reading acquisition in an essentially normal brain. His
adaptive problem would probably result from
genetic diversity, though it could be aggravated by inappropriate teaching, undermotiva-
tion, or a lack of interest in literacy in the family. These opposing views might nevertheless
find common ground at the neurological level.
Genetic diversity presumably exerts its effects
at the neural level of organization. Nothing is
known about the brain basis of individual differences in any facet of intelligence. A range of
possibilities could therefore be entertained,
from disordered selective activation of pertinent modules through anomalous interhemispheric conductivity to dysgenesis of
the relevant neuronal population.

Galaburda, Sherman, Rosen, Aboitiz, and
Geschwind (1985) reported four consecutive
postmortem examinations of brains of dyslexics. They found variously distributed dysgenesis of neurons, implicating, though by no
means limited to, the language area of the left
hemisphere. They speculate that the neuronal
dysgenesis is the cause of the reading problem.
But the functional implications of these neu-

ronal anomalies are not yet known. Further, the question of whether these anomalies are specific to dyslexia remains to be established by the application at autopsy of the painstaking and time consuming techniques involved, to a sufficient number of normal readers. A surprising but interesting outcome of such work might even be that neuronal dysgenesis explains some of the "normal" individual differences in a variety of intellectual domains. In any case, unilateral impairment is an insufficient explanation, because it does not explain why the other hemisphere does not compensate, as early lesion data lead us to expect (Aram & Ekelman, 1986). Pending confirmation of the relevance of neurohistological variations, I will focus on the other tradition of neurological theorizing: the view that the representation of language-related processes is *topographically* abnormal in the dyslexic's brain (Orton, 1937).

TOPOGRAPHICAL THEORIES: SPECIALIZATION OR ACTIVATION?

Topographical theories have focused on reading/language representation at the cerebral level. But a further relevant distinction has generally escaped notice. It is necessary but perhaps not sufficient for the neuronal machinery to be in place for proper function to result. Particularly in effortful processing, which reading acquisition must be considered to be (even if fluent reading is not), it is probably necessary for the appropriate cerebral area to be selectively activated by projections ascending from the brain stem, granting it ascendancy over other areas that potentially compete for control of behavior (Kinsbourne, 1980). It could be the topography of selective activation that is disordered in dyslexia. This might result in a cognitive deficit even if the necessary cerebral processors are in place, intact, and able to function. I shall therefore consider, as I review relevant experimental evidence, whether any of it resolves the conflict between abnormality of cerebral structure and abnormally distributed ascending activation.

If the topography of functional specialization is abnormal in learning disabilities, this would become apparent from the sequelae of

focal brain damage. For example, if dyslexics have bilateralized or right lateralized language areas, then lateralized lesion effects on language would reveal this. However, children rarely present for study with clear-cut focal unilateral acquired brain damage, and once they reach adulthood, dyslexics are typically lost to follow-up. So this relatively direct source of information is simply not available. An alternative methodology would be to use event-related measures of the distribution of electrophysiological or metabolic activation during language processing by dyslexics.

EVENT-RELATED MEASUREMENTS

Duffy, Denckla, Bartels, and Sandini (1980) have performed brain electrical activity mapping on reading disabled children. They found activation differences in some left hemisphere areas as compared to controls. A more recent study from this group (Duffy, Denckla, McAnulty, & Holmes, 1987) raises intriguing issues. The investigators subtyped dyslexics according to Denckla (1977) into: 1) anomic-repetition disorder, with associated naming difficulty characterized by incorrect word choice or circumlocution, difficulty in sequential verbal memory, but no comprehension problem; 2) dysphonemic-sequencing disorder, with fewer naming difficulties but worse sequential function and some syntactic comprehension deficit; and 3) global-mixed language disorder, with a broader language impairment. All three subtypes differed electrophysiologically from controls over the left sided classical language area. Subtypes of dyslexia could be discriminated by deviant function frontally and occipitally (anomics), centrally and parietally (dysphonemics), and over wider areas of cortex (globals). Two findings stand out. One is that virtually all dyslexic-control differences were bilateral. If one adheres to the conventional view that cerebral malfunction in dyslexics is left hemisphere based, one might attribute right sided differences to compensatory activity. Duffy and colleagues (1987) computed correlations between degree of deviance over a given cerebral territory and test scores. Areas functioning defectively should yield negative correlations between the neurophysiological and the performance variable, whereas compensating areas should yield positive correlations. Significant correlations of both types were found, but the signs did not assort by hemisphere. Types 1 and 2 yield almost totally positive correlations, type 3 yields negative correlations. We must provisionally conclude that type 3 involves a broad bilateral uncompensated malfunction. Types 1 and 2 show compensation bilaterally, whereas the areas of malfunction remain obscure. In any case, the assumption of a unilateral processing abnormality is not supported.

Cerebral metabolism measurements could be even more revealing of an abnormal brain, or at least abnormal brain use, in reading disabled children. Fluent readers reading silently exhibit activation of the occipital cortex (bilaterally) only (Peterson, Fox, Posner, Mintun, & Raichle, in press). This finding is itself of interest, in that there was no evidence of involvement of the classical language area (or even of one hemisphere more than the other). The familiar assumption that in reading, information flows from occipital to superior temporal cortex (Geschwind, 1970) may not hold, at least when reading is fluent. The nonfluent reader may show additional areas of activation. For instance, like the fluent reader reading aloud (Peterson et al., in press), the nonfluent reader may exhibit activation of several cortical and subcortical areas involved in control of the speech act (note that poor readers tend to whisper or move their lips when reading). Other findings related to task difficulty might also appear. Thus, a sufficient psychophysiological data base is not yet available. We therefore have to rely on less direct evidence. This is derived from three sources: 1) neuropsychological testing, 2) laterality testing, and 3) association with sinistrality.

NEUROPSYCHOLOGICAL TESTING

The neuropsychological testing basis of reading disability rests on the premise that the hypothesized hemisphere deficit is not confined to mental operations unique to reading and

writing. It also taps additional processes for which the same hemisphere is specialized, or ones which have application outside, as well as within, the reading domain. This view is antithetical to the older concept of pure developmental dyslexia (Critchley, 1970), which was itself modeled on the equally outdated concept of "pure alexia" arising from acquired brain damage. The contemporary assumption is that a skill deficit (e.g., in reading) is the surface manifestation of a process deficiency.

Processing ability can be tested within or outside the reading domain. Diagnostic educational tests that differentiate between types of difficulty in reading and writing could give hints as to the nature of the underlying disorder of function and could even permit an analogy with a known syndrome of left (or even right) hemisphere deficit. Neuropsychological tests outside the reading domain could muster evidence for deficient maturation of one hemisphere. They could even show how deficiency in a general form of processing for which that hemisphere is specialized can account both for the profile of neuropsychological test deficit and the particular difficulties the child experiences in learning to read and write.

Within reading, analyses of the prevalence of different error types have led to a distinction between difficulty in the analytic (phonics) aspect of reading acquisition and difficulty in whole word identification (Boder, 1971). The latter "dyseidetic" subtype has, on shaky grounds, been attributed to right hemisphere dysfunction. More recently, in relation to a vogue for developing a taxonomy of acquired reading disorders, some parallels are being drawn between subtypes of acquired alexia and patterns of difficulty experienced by children with selective reading disability (Temple & Marshall, 1983).

When fluent readers abruptly begin to make mistakes in reading on account of acute focal brain damage, the preexisting skill gives a basis for conjectures about what mental operation has suddenly become impaired. In contrast, when a child experiences difficulty in learning to read, the situation is complicated by a diversity of efforts to teach before the child comes to clinical notice. The error pattern is as likely to reflect the child's attempts to apply devices he or she has been taught to directly reflect the defective function. "Dysphonetic" reading, in which extraneous sounds are read instead of the correct ones, may reflect a whole word approach with some rather wild guesses by a child whose word attack skills are defective, are not being used, or have not been taught. "Dyseidetic" errors may conversely reflect too slavish an adherence to a phonics decoding approach, the child not having learned, or been unable to apply, the ability to go beyond the initial word attack so as to acquire fluency as the decoded words become familiar. Conversely, if a child cannot master the whole word route to reading, he or she might overuse word attack on irregularly spelled words; the child's errors will be dysphonetic. If the child has a phonemic handicap, he or she might overapply the whole word approach to words not in his or her sight vocabulary, and make dyseidetic errors (Kinsbourne, 1984). It is hard to determine exactly how a child has been taught, but in the absence of this information, evidence from error patterns is inconclusive for purposes of neuropsychological analysis.

Neuropsychological test deficits that probe disabilities outside reading and writing found in selectively disabled readers fall into the following categories: 1) language, 2) sequencing, 3) visuo-spatial, and 4) eye movement. The preponderance of opinion favors an account of the dyslexias as language-related dominant hemisphere disorders (Vellutino, 1979), and there is only a little evidence relating any dyslexia subtype to right hemisphere disability (Bakker, 1979). If anything, right hemisphere-based visuo-spatial skills tend to be superior in these children (Gordon, 1983; Symmes, 1972). Small samples of well analyzed cases do seem to show different types of reading problems (Kinsbourne, 1986a), but the larger scale studies that attempt to determine whether subtypes really exist, and identify them by cluster analysis (reviewed by Satz & Morris, 1981), all lack an essential ingredient. Clusters inevitably emerge (because it is inherent in the mathematics that they must), but it is not proven that the particular area of cognitive deficit that characterizes a cluster will identify a processing difficulty that is sufficiently severe to account for a very severe problem in learning to read. This is because although there are statistically significant differences between groups, there is usually substantial overlap between experimental and control samples. When arbitrary cut-off points are used to define abnormality on a test, these are often apt to overdiagnose, given criteria as generous as one standard deviation below the mean (Mattis, French, & Rapin, 1975). Many children with a test profile similar to that which characterizes a dyslexia subtype seem to learn to read without difficulty. This validity problem could be mitigated by demonstrating that within a subtype there is a highly significant correlation between the degree of deficit on the allegedly critical tests and the degree of reading backwardness (or of measured difficulty in teaching the child to read). This usually is not done (but see Tallal, 1980). Another promising approach is to follow the subtyped children longitudinally and to demonstrate consistency in the taxonomy (Morris, Blashfield, & Satz, 1986).

LATERALITY

Laterality paradigms of dichotic listening and hemi-field viewing have been widely used to assign roles in different forms of processing to the two hemispheres. They are taken to reflect the balance of activation between the hemispheres while the task is being done (Kinsbourne & Hiscock, 1983b). Thus, during a verbal task the engaged left hemisphere will usually be more activated, yielding a right ear and right field advantage in the dichotic and hemi-field tasks respectively. The method of dual-task verbal-manual interference (Kinsbourne & Hiscock, 1983a) more directly indicates speech lateralization. Concurrent speech will interfere more with manual activity if both are controlled by the same hemisphere (usually the left).

Both structural and activational insufficiency of the left hemisphere would be expected to manifest in the form of a shift of lateral asymmetries in verbal perception and performance toward the left. The mechanisms possibly involved include: 1) a bilateralized or right sided language area, and 2) ascending activation that projects bilaterally or to the wrong (right) side. In either type of case, there would be no asymmetry or left sided advantage either for verbal hemi-field or for dichotic stimuli.

Although in the more severe developmental language delays the usual language-related right sided ear advantages are often reported to be absent (Rosenblum & Dorman, 1978), this is not the typical finding in selective reading disability, where asymmetries in the normal direction are usually found (e.g., Caplan & Kinsbourne, 1981). This argument still holds, even though one study reports their absence in the "language" subtype of dyslexia (Pirozzolo, 1979) and another study suggests opposite asymmetries for two dyslexic subtypes (Malatesha & Dougan, 1982). So there is no reason to doubt that, structurally, the usual left sided lateralization of language is present in those dyslexic children who are right handed. That still leaves the question, how do dyslexics *use* their left lateralized language faculty?

When the left hemisphere is activated for purposes of language function, its rightward directed orienting facility is also activated: attention is biased rightward (Kinsbourne, 1970). As a consequence, normal adults find it harder to monitor speech signals on the left ear channel than on the right ear channel, when the two are in competition (Treisman & Geffen, 1968). This is true of normal children, who show a bias toward the right ear message, even when instructed to listen selectively to the concurrent message to the left ear (Hiscock & Kinsbourne, 1977). However, when, for purposes of a verbal task, dyslexic children adopt a verbal mental set, they fail to show the usual bias toward the right ear during selective listening for verbal material (Obrzut, Hynd, Obrzut, & Pirozzolo, 1981). They are better able to listen selectively to the left ear, screening out right sided input, than are normal readers, who include many right ear intrusions in their responses. It appears that the selective activation of the left hemisphere for purposes of verbal

processing is less intense and more easily overridden by other influences. This could be a clue as to why their language skills are weak or their cognitive styles are relatively nonverbal (Caplan & Kinsbourne, 1982). Is this weakness in selective hemisphere activation bilateral or restricted to the left? Smith and Griffiths (1987) presented dyslexics with dichotic environmental sounds for identification. They found the expected left ear advantage for this "right hemisphere" task. But whereas the control children could at will identify many stimuli from the right by listening selectively, the dyslexics could not do this at all. This suggests a hemisphere imbalance, with right hemisphere orienting tendency much the stronger. The dyslexics can easily override the "preprogrammed" rightward bias for a verbal task, but could not override the leftward bias for an environmental discrimination. This outcome is consistent with the hypothesis that ascending activation is right biased in dyslexics.

The most direct information on the lateralization of reading processes derives from the use of the verbal-manual interference paradigm (Kinsbourne & Hiscock, 1983a). This relies on the now well established fact that interference between two concurrent activities ("dual-task performance") is greater when both are programmed by the same hemisphere than when they are programmed in separate hemispheres. If a right handed child finger-taps while performing a verbal task, the secondary (verbal) activity will decrease tapping rate of both hands, but more of the right hand (Hiscock & Kinsbourne, 1978). If the secondary task is not verbal, interference is equal on the two sides (Hiscock, Antoniuk, Prisciak, & von Hessert, 1985) or greater on the left (McFarland & Ashton, 1978). So if poor readers are less lateralized for language processes, as has so often been suggested, they should fail to show the expected laterality effect in verbal-manual interference (even though they are right handed). If the failure to establish laterality affects the brain basis of reading only, the child will exhibit the usual laterality when the secondary task requires speaking, but not when it involves reading. In fact, poor readers show as much right lateralized interference in speech while tapping, and even more on reading while tapping (Hiscock et al., 1985). Even in poor readers, speech and reading laterality seem to be left-hemispheric. The excess of selective right hand interference observed in the poor readers was probably a consequence of the greater difficulty they experienced in performing the reading task.

Further studies of severely dyslexic children along the above lines are still needed. But to this point in time, evidence for diminished lateralization of reading-related cerebral activity in poor readers is lacking. In contrast, evidence for decreased left lateral activation is mounting.

COGNITIVE STYLE

If hemisphere specialization is not deviant in dyslexics, perhaps hemisphere use *is* deviant in dyslexics. Event-related measures (behavioral, electrophysiological, or metabolic) of how dyslexics use their brains could reveal an unusual pattern of hemispheric usage when the subject is reading or performing language tasks. One might attempt to explain the disability accordingly. Or the deviant hemisphere use might be secondary to the disability, representing the child's attempt to cope or compensate. It has often been implied that reading disabled individuals tend to use nonverbal (allegedly right hemisphere) strategies, when a left hemisphere approach would have been more effective. Ambiguity exists about cause and effect in these claims. Are these individuals reading disabled because they use the wrong hemisphere, or do they use the wrong hemisphere because they are reading disabled? The latter possibility implies that style follows substance: people chose the tactic in which they are best versed. But a recent study (Knolle, Gordon, & Gwany, 1987), finds no positive correlation between the hemispherically related pattern of skills on neuropsychological tests and cognitive style classified as right or left on two popular (though unvalidated) questionnaires. The possibility that people who use the wrong hemisphere

could have done better had they used the correct hemisphere is more intriguing, as it suggests latent aptitude waiting to be uncovered.

Poor readers certainly adopt a less verbal style than good readers (as do more younger than older readers, and more male than female readers) according to Caplan and Kinsbourne (1982). But here again, cause and effect remain to be disentangled. Also to be disentangled is a further question. When subjects use inappropriate strategies, is that why they fail, or do they use them in a desperate last resort when they fail to solve the problem in the usual way? For instance, there is much evidence that females tend more often than males to deploy verbal strategies when attempting to solve spatial problems that they find difficult. Yet, when cognitive style is assessed by observing the direction of reflective eye movements for questions permitting either verbal or spatial solution (Bakan, 1969; Day, 1964, 1967), no reliable sex differences in hemispheric preference emerge.

Bakker (1979, 1983), taking the view that each hemisphere contributes in its own unique way to fluent reading, distinguished between P-type dyslexics, who confine their attention to the visual aspect of words (ignoring their auditory-verbal aspect), using the right hemisphere, and L-type dyslexics who exhibit the reverse processing and hemispheric bias. Bakker explains the reading disability accordingly, as undue reliance on one hemisphere only. Zenhausern (in press) has further explained these two types of biased cerebral utilization. He classified dyslexics into left-lookers and right-lookers. The direction of gaze observed while subjects reflect on the answer to a question indicates which hemisphere is in control of behavior (Bakan, 1969), or the distribution of activation across the hemispheres (Kinsbourne, 1972). Zenhausern observed left gaze shifts, indicating right hemisphere use, in dyslexics who performed in a P-type manner, and right shifts in the alternate, L-type performers. Although it could be, in accord with Bakker's theory, that extreme hemisphere-related cognitive styles are responsible for the reading disability, an alternative explanation is more conservative, and perhaps more plausible. Zenhausern's observations may indicate a typology of styles of coping with an existing (and otherwise to be explained) reading disability. Given his inability to learn to read normally, the child whose cognitive bias is right hemispheric attempts to compensate by overextending the use of word-shape-meaning associations, bypassing the formation of intermediate phonological representations (which, even if not needed by the fluent reader, might be useful to the learner). The dyslexic whose bias is toward use of the left hemisphere might labor at grapheme-phoneme correspondence. With attention invested in this processing, the dyslexic has few resources left over to note meanings or infer them from context. In that sense the dyslexic may merit Zenhausern's classification as phonetic dyslexic.

Although much propaganda in the field of education is focused on the possibility of accomodating instruction to the hypothesized right hemispheric learner (Kinsbourne, in press) this would hardly be justifiable (even if feasible) if the nonverbal bias found in some reading disabled children were merely secondary to their reading problem.

SINISTRALITY

The long-standing suspicion that reading disability more commonly occurs in left handers and sinistral families has recently been confirmed (Kinsbourne, 1986b). In a questionnaire study based on the families of a large sample from a residential school for the learning disabled, we found the prevalence of dyslexia and other disorders of cognitive development to be highest in left handers with other left handed family members (familial sinistral). next highest among sporadic left handers, less among "familial right handers, and least among right handers from exclusively dextral families. This pattern conforms to a genetic model for the relationship between sinistrality and whatever immaturity of brain-based cognitive development underlies reading disorders. A role for pathological lefthandedness, due to early left-sided brain damage in the gen-

otypic dextral (Satz, 1972), is not ruled out, because there is reason to believe that sinistrality is a risk factor for early brain damage, which could then generate lefthandedness of the pathological type (Bradshaw-McAnulty, Hicks, & Kinsbourne, 1984). However, the prediction from pathological lefthandedness that dyslexia would be most prevalent in the extreme lefthander (presumably the person most impaired in left hemisphere development) was not borne out. Mixed handedness was more of a risk factor for dyslexia (a phenomenon earlier observed by Harris [1957] and Orton [1937] among many).

Further evidence for a genetic influence derives from the finding that sinistrality is also a risk factor for diseases of the immune system (Geschwind & Behan, 1982), which we confirmed in the questionnaire study. Geschwind & Galaburda (1985) have elaborated this view into sweeping theories that implicates testosterone effects in the genesis of sinistrality, and reading disability and immune disorder, and explains the male preponderance in the prevalence of the former (if not the latter). They speculate that testosterone has a retarding effect on left hemisphere maturation in the uterus, and that sinistrality, reading disability, and autoimmune diseases are all consequences of left hemisphere insufficiency. The data they cited for this theory have been shown to be inadequate (Satz & Soper, 1986). Nevertheless, this theory has the merit of being testable, based on the prediction that male gender, extreme left handedness, dyslexia, and immune diseases should all coincide by more than chance. Obvious problems arise: if there was enough testosterone in some females to render them dyslexic, why are not all males, who presumably generate more testosterone, dyslexic? If males generate more testosterone than females, why are not male sinistrals more extremely left handed than female sinistrals? Indeed, if intrauterine testosterone is sufficient to render some females left handed, why are all males not left handed? And, in our data, why did the excess of immune disorder and of cognitive delay related to sinistrality distribute independently, negating the idea that they are attributable to a common factor? That a single agent accounts for so many variables is an elegant but insufficient explanation.

Left hemisphere maldevelopment is not the only way in which nonrighthandedness associated with reading disability may be explained. Brain stem maldevelopment could cause ascending activation to be more diffuse (or right biased), so that right hand preference fails to develop, and selective activation of the left hemisphere is incomplete.

PERFORMANCE DEFICITS CORRELATED WITH READING ABILITY IN DYSLEXICS

Neuropsychological analysis attempts to identify an underlying mental operation impairment accounting for the clinical presenting symptom (e.g., dyslexia). Such deficits as difficulties in processing oral speech (Vellutino, 1979), rapid formant transitions (Tallal, 1980), serial ordering (Corkin, 1974), auditory or visual temporal order (Bakker, 1973; Hammond, 1982) pattern of a temporal sequence (Rudel, Denckla, & Spalten, 1974) or eye movements (Pavlidis, 1981), could still, with some stretching of the imagination, be attributed to a process plausibly critical for the acquisition of reading skill. But we have recently found reading retarded children to be inferior in performance on a set of tasks that do not even remotely relate to what one has to do to learn to read. These results call into question the assumed selectivity of reading disability, and suggest that the underlying cognitive impairment may be broad indeed.

Neff, Kinsbourne, and Languis (n.d.) compared teenage dyslexics with younger normal children on tasks including transfer of maze learning, tactile and visual matching, and selectivity of finger movement. In each case, the experimental group behaved like much younger normal children. Not only was the learning disableds' overall performance inferior to that of age-matched controls, and comparable to that of children 3–7 years of age, but, like these, or even younger normal children, they had more difficulty when the task included an across the midline component than when it was limited to one side of the body. The findings suggest that reading disability is in many cases not selective, but may be due to a wide ranging immaturity of selective processes, implicating behavior at the sensorimotor as well as the cognitive level. If this is so, one should be thinking more in terms of specialization (e.g., selective inhibition within) of the whole cerebral cortex than of any problem confined to one cerebral area or "module." Sinistrality might induce vulnerability to such cerebral organization, which also would represent the immature base state from which normal selectivity gradually emerges during development.

Within the normal range of school achievement, low achievers lag behind high achievers on several indices of cognitive and sensorimotor maturation; those differences remain even when Wechsler IQ is held constant (Dudek, Strobel, & Thomas, 1987). Thus, the conventional Wechsler matching is no guarantee that any remaining experimental control group difference is selective. The dyslexic, defined as underachieving in reading while of "normal" (Wechsler measured) intelligence, could still be lagging in development on a wide neurocognitive front (just as, but to a more severe extent than, the low achiever in the regular school population). If so, the study of the brain basis of dyslexia would gain in potential significance. Rather than only explaining a rather rare disorder, the brain-variants in question might be relevant to a wide continuum of neurological findings, ranging from within-normality to selective learning disability of the utmost severity.

CONCLUSION

There is circumstantial evidence from several sources for a brain-based deficiency of left hemisphere cognitive processes in children with reading disabilities. Although in some cases this may be due to structural abnormality, it seems likely that the problem is more often one of initiating and maintaining the selective cerebral activation necessary to perform verbal tasks and to learn verbal material of a difficult nature. The deficit may also implicate other, less conspicuous, mental operations and even accomplishments at the perceptual-motor level of organization. The attempt to remediate by the biological route should therefore focus on physical maneuvers and neurotransmitter agonists that enhance selective cerebral activation, particularly of the left hemisphere.

REFERENCES

Aram, D.M., & Ekelman, B.L. (1986). Cognitive profiles of children with early onset of unilateral lesions. *Developmental Neuropsychology, 2,*155–172.

Bakan, P. (1969). Hypnotizability, laterality of eye-movements, and functional brain asymmetry. *Perceptual and Motor Skills, 28,*927–932.

Bakker, D.J. (1973). Hemispheric specialization and states in the learning-to-read process. *Bulletin of the Orton Society, 23,*15–27.

Bakker, D.J. (1979). Hemispheric differences and reading strategies: Two dyslexias? *Bulletin of the Orton Society, 29,*84–100.

Bakker, D.J. (1983). Hemispheric specialization and specific reading retardation. In M.N. Rutter (Ed.), *Developmental Neuropsychiatry.* New York: Guilford Press.

Boder, E. (1971). Developmental dyslexia: Prevailing diagnostic concepts and a new diagnostic approach. In H.R. Myklebust (Ed.), *Progress in Learning Disability II.* New York: Grune & Stratton.

Bradshaw-McAnulty, G., Hicks, R.E., & Kinsbourne, M. (1984). Pathological lefthandedness and familial sinistrality in relation to degree of mental retardation. *Brain and Cognition, 3,*349–356.

Caplan, B., & Kinsbourne, M. (1981). Cerebral lateralization, preferred cognitive mode, and reading ability in normal children. *Brain and Language, 14,*349–370.

Caplan, B., & Kinsbourne, M. (1982). Cognitive style and dichotic asymmetries of disabled readers. *Cortex, 18,*357–366.

Corkin, S. (1974). Serial ordering deficits in inferior readers. *Neuropsychologia, 12,*317–354.

Critchley, M. (1970). *The dyslexic child* (2nd ed.). London: Heinemann.

Day, M.E. (1964). An eye-movement phenomenon relating to attention, thought, and anxiety. *Perceptual and Motor Skills, 19,*443–446.

Day, M.E. (1967). An eye-movement indicator of individual differences in the physiological organization of attentional processes. *Journal of Psychology, 42,*51–62.

Denckla, M.B. (1977). Minimal brain dysfunction and dyslexia: Beyond diagnosis by exclusion. In M.E. Blau, I. Rapin, & M. Kinsbourne (Eds.), *Topics in Child Neurology.* New York: Spectrum.

Dudek, S.Z., Strobel, M., & Thomas, A.D. (1987). Chronic learning problems and maturation. *Perceptual and Motor Skills, 64,*407–429.

Duffy, F.H., Denckla, M.B., Bartels, P.H., & Sandini, G. (1980). Dyslexia: Regional differences in brain electrical activity by topographic mapping. *Annals of Neurology, 7,*412–420.

Duffy, F.H., Denckla, M.B., McAnulty, G.B., & Holmes, J.M. (1987). Neuropsychological studies in dyslexia. In F. Plum (Ed.), *Language, communication, and the brain.* New York: Raven Press.

Galaburda, A.M., Sherman, G.F., Rosen, G.D., Aboitiz, F., & Geschwind, N. (1985). Developmental dyslexia: Four consecutive cases with cortical anomalies. *Annals of Neurology, 18,*222–233.

Geschwind, N. (1970). The organization of language and the brain. *Science, 170,*940–944.

Geschwind, N., & Behan, P. (1982). Left-handedness: Association with immune disease, migraine, and developmental learning disorder. *Proceedings of the National Academy of Sciences of the United States of America, 79,*5097–5100.

Geschwind, N., & Galaburda, A.M. (1985). Cerebral lateralization. Biological mechanisms, associations and pathology, II. *Archives of Neurology, 42,*521–552.

Gordon, H.W. (1983). Learning disabled are cognitively right. In M. Kinsbourne (Ed.), *Topics in learning disabilities* (Vol. 3, pp. 29–39). Gaithersburg, MD: Aspen Systems.

Hammond, G.R. (1982). Hemispheric differences in temporal resolution. *Brain and Cognition, 1,*95–118.

Harris, A.J. (1957). Lateral dominance, directional confusion, and reading disability. *Journal of Psychology, 44,*283–294.

Hiscock, M., Antoniuk, D., Prisciak, K., & von Hessert, D. (1985). Generalized and lateralized interference between concurrent tasks performed by children: Effects of age, sex, and skill. *Developmental Neurology, 1,*29–48.

Hiscock, M., & Kinsbourne, M. (1977). Selective listening asymmetry in preschool children. *Developmental Psychology, 3,*217–224.

Hiscock, M., & Kinsbourne, M. (1978). Ontogeny of cerebral dominance: Evidence from time-sharing asymmetry in children. *Developmental Psychology, 14,*321–329.

Kinsbourne, M. (1970). The cerebral basis of lateral asymmetries in attention. In A.F. Sanders (Ed.), *Attention and Performance III.* Amsterdam: North Holland.

Kinsbourne, M. (1972). Eye and head turning indicates cerebral lateralization. *Science, 176,*539–541.

Kinsbourne, M. (1980). A model for the ontogeny of cerebral organization in non-righthanders. In J. Herron (Ed.), *Neuropsychology of left handedness.* New York: Academic Press.

Kinsbourne, M. (1983). Brain basis of learning disabilities. In D.K. Reid & W.P. Hreska (Eds.), *Topics in learning and learning disabilities, 3.* Gaithersburg, MD: Aspen Systems.

Kinsbourne, M. (1984). The Boder Test of Reading-Spelling Patterns: A diagnostic screening test for subtypes of reading disability. *Developmental Medicine and Child Neurology, 26,* 263–264.

Kinsbourne, M. (1985). Learning disabilities. In P.J. Vinken, G.W. Bruyn, & H.L. Klawans (Eds.), *Handbook of clinical neurology II*. Amsterdam: Elsevier/North Holland.

Kinsbourne, M. (1986a). Models of dyslexia and its subtypes. In G. Th. Pavlidis & D.F. Fisher (Eds.), *Dyslexia: Neuropsychology and treatment*. London: John Wiley & Sons.

Kinsbourne, M. (1986b, October). *Sinistrality and risk for immune diseases and learning disorders*. Paper presented to the Child Neurology Society, Boston.

Kinsbourne, M. (in press). Right brain, left brain: Practical implications from infancy to adulthood. In M.I. Gottlieb (Ed.), *Developmental behavioral pediatrics: Selected topics*. New York: Plenum.

Kinsbourne, M., & Hiscock, M. (1983a). Asymmetries of dual-task performance. In J. Hellige (Ed.), *Cerebral hemisphere asymmetry: Method, theory and application*. New York: Academic Press.

Kinsbourne, M., & Hiscock, M. (1983b). The normal and deviant development of functional lateralization of the brain. In P. Mussen, M. Haith, & J. Campos (Eds.), *Handbook of child psychology* (4th ed., Vol. 2). New York: John Wiley & Sons.

Knolle, L., Gordon, H.W., & Gwany, D. (1987). Relationship between performance and preference measures of cognitive laterality. *Perceptual and Motor Skills, 61*, 215–223.

Malatesha, R.N., & Dougan, D.K. (1982). Clinical subtypes of developmental dyslexia: Resolution of an unresolute problem. In R.N. Malatesha & G. Aaron (Eds.), *Reading disorders: Varieties and treatment*. New York: Academic Press.

Mattis, S., French, J.H., & Rapin, I. (1975). Dyslexia in children and young adults: Three independent neuropsychological syndromes. *Developmental Medicine and Child Neurology, 17*, 150–163.

McFarland, K., & Ashton, R. (1978). The lateralized effect of concurrent cognitive and motor performance. *Perception and Psychophysics, 23*, 344–349.

Morris, R., Blashfield, R., & Satz, P. (1986). Developmental classification of reading-disabled children. *Journal of Clinical and Experimental Neuropsychology, 8*, 371–392.

Neff, L.S., Kinsbourne, M., & Languis, M. (n.d.). *Do dyslexics have deficient interhemispheric communication?* Manuscript in preparation.

Obrzut, J.E., Hynd, G.W., Obrzut, A., & Pirozzolo, F.J. (1981). Effect of directed attention on cerebral asymmetries in normal and learning disabled children. *Developmental Psychology, 17*, 118–125.

Orton, S.T. (1937). *Reading, writing, and speech problems in children*. New York: Norton.

Pavlidis, G. Th. (1981). Do eye movements hold the key to dyslexia? *Neuropsychologia, 19*, 57–64.

Peterson, S.E., Fox, P.T., Posner, M.I., Mintun, M., & Raichle, M.E. (in press). Positron emission tomographic studies of the cortical anatomy of single word processing. *Nature*.

Pirozzolo, F.J. (1979). *The neuropsychology of developmental reading disorders*. New York: Praeger.

Rosenblum, D.R., & Dorman, M.F. (1978). Hemispheric specialization for speech perception in language deficient kindergarten children. *Brain and Language, 6*, 378–389.

Rudel, R.G., Denckla, M.B., & Spalten, E. (1974). The functional asymmetry of braille letter learning in normal sighted children. *Neurology, 24*, 733–738.

Satz, P. (1972). Pathological left-handedness: An explanatory model. *Cortex, 8*, 121–135.

Satz, P. (1976). Cerebral dominance and reading disability: An old problem revisited. In R.M. Knights & D.J. Bakker (Eds.), *The neuropsychology of learning disorders*. Baltimore: University Park Press.

Satz, P., & Morris, R. (1981). Learning disability subtypes: A review. In F.J. Pirozzolo & N.C. Wittrock (Eds.), *Neuropsychological and cognitive processes in reading*. New York: Academic Press.

Satz, P., & Soper, H.V. (1986). Left-handedness, dyslexia, and autoimmune disorder: A critique. *Journal of Clinical and Experimental Neuropsychology, 8*, 453–458.

Smith, K., & Griffiths, P. (1987). Defective lateralized attention for non-verbal sounds in developmental dyslexia. *Neuropsychologia, 25*, 259–268.

Symmes, J.S. (1972). Deficit models, spatial visualization and reading disability. *Bulletin of the Orton Society, 22*, 54–68.

Tallal, P. (1980). Auditory temporal perception, phonics and reading disabilities in children. *Brain and Language, 9*, 182–198.

Temple, C.M., & Marshall, J.C. (1983). A case study of developmental phonological dyslexia. *British Journal of Psychology, 74*, 517–533.

Treisman, A., & Geffen, G. (1968). Selective attention and cerebral dominance in perceiving and responding to speech messages. *Quarterly Journal of Experimental Psychology, 20*, 139–150.

Vellutino, F.R. (1979). *Dyslexia, theory and research*. Cambridge: MIT Press.

Zenhausern, R. (in press). Instructional strategies and the causes of reading disability. *International Journal of Neuroscience*.

Index

Phonologic-syntactic syndrome
  Broca's aphasia and, 242
  clinical description, 238
  intervention strategies, 238–239
Photorefractive screening program, infant,
    220–223
Physicians
  role in controversial therapies, 260–261
  vulnerability of, appreciation for, 252–253
Phytanic acid oxidase activity deficiency, 71,
    76–77
Pipecolic acid, abnormal catabolism, in Zellweger
    syndrome, 69
Plasma cell lysosomal acid maltase activity, 30
Plasmalogens, abnormal biosynthesis, in Zell-
    weger syndrome, 70
Platelet aggregation, in Fabry's disease, 25–26
Polymicrogyrias, 169–171
POMC (proopiomelanocortin), 119
Pompe's disease, case study, 57–58
Porencephalies, 171–172
Postrotary nystagmus, 258
Potter syndrome, with total renal dysplasia, 167
P0 protein, 101
P1 protein, 101
P2 protein, 101
Prader-Willi syndrome, 6–7
Prednisone, 124
Pregnancy, extra-abdominal, 201
Premature infant
  psychological aspects of parents and infant,
    147–149
  very low birth weight, biological aspects of
    intraventricular hemorrhage and brain
    growth, 145–147
Prenatal disorders
  central nervous system
    neuronal migration disturbances, 165–167
    pathogenetic analysis, disturbances of neu-
      ronal-glial production, 161–165
    perfusion failures and hypoxias, 168–172
  neuropathology, 153–156
  postnatal survival and, 153
  see also specific disorders
Preschool children, Albert Einstein Therapeutic
    Nursery and, 234–235
Presumptive peroxisomal disorders, 77
Primidone, for neonatal seizures, 133–134
Proopiomelanocortin (POMC), 119
Pseudo-NALD, 76
Pseudo-Zellweger syndrome, 76
Psychological aspects, of neurodevelopmental out-
    come, 147–151
Psychostimulants
  for attention deficit disorder, 248
  long-term effects, 260
  in production of tics and Tourett syndrome, 248

Pyridoxine dependency, 131
Pyruvate metabolism, defects, in encepha-
    lomyopathies, 45

Quinolinate, 114
Quisqualate, 114

Radial glial cell, 157–160
Radial microbrain, 163
Rapid Golgi-gold substitution method, 157
Reading disability, 214
Recombinant vaccinia vaccine, 96
Reeler mouse, 167
Refraction
  changes in the population, 221
  errors, early detection of, 221–222
Refractive screening, predictive value of, 222
Refsum disease, 76–77
  see also infantile Refsum disease
Respiratory chain defects, in encephalomyopa-
    thies, 45
Restriction fragment length polymorphisms
    (RFLP)
  affected individuals, 3
  description, 1–2
  diagnosis of neurological disease, 83
  informative individual for, 3
  use for gene mapping, 2–4
Retroviruses, 89
Rett's syndrome, 141
RFLP, see Restriction fragment length
    polymorphisms
Rhizomelic chondrodysplasia calcificans punctata
    (RCDP), 73, 75
Ricinus communis agglutinin-I (RCA-I), 65
Rimmed vacuoles, 58
Risk assessment, cumulative, 203–206

Salla's disease
  endothelial cell involvement, 39
  epidermal cell involvement, 37
Sandhoff's disease
  endothelial cell involvement, 39
  epidermal cell involvement, 37
  gene cloning in, 8
Sarcoplasmic body myopathy, 59
School-age performance, outcome prediction and,
    206
Seizures
  ACTH and, 122–123
  corticotrophin releasing factor and, 123
  in fragile X syndrome, 13
  myoclonic, 129
  neonatal, see Neonatal seizures